Plants: Diet and Health

Plants: Diet and Health

The Report of a
British Nutrition
Foundation Task Force

Edited by Dr Gail Goldberg

Blackwell
Science

Published by Blackwell Science
for the British Nutrition Foundation

Editorial offices:
Blackwell Science Ltd, 9600 Garsington Road, Oxford OX4 2DQ, UK
  Tel: +44 (0) 1865 776868
Blackwell Publishing Professional, 2121 State Avenue, Ames, Iowa 50014-8300, USA
  Tel: +1 515 292 0140
Blackwell Science Asia Pty, 550 Swanston Street, Carlton, Victoria 3053, Australia
  Tel: +61 (0)3 8359 1011

First published 2003
Transferred to digital print, 2007

Library of Congress Cataloging-in-Publication Data
Diet and health : the report of a British Nutrition Foundation Task
Force/edited by Gail Goldberg.-- 1st ed.
    p. cm.
  ISBN 0-632-05962-1 (Paperback : alk. paper)
  1. Vegetables in human nutrition. 2. Plants, Edible. I. Goldberg, Gail.
II. British Nutrition Foundation.

  TX557.D54 2003
  613.2'62--dc21

                                                          2003012031

ISBN 978-0-632-05962-1

A catalogue record for this title is available from the British Library

Typeset in Times and produced
by Gray Publishing, Tunbridge Wells, Kent

The publisher's policy is to use permanent paper from mills that operate a sustainable forestry policy, and
which has been manufactured from pulp processed using acid-free and elementary chlorine-free practices.
Furthermore, the publisher ensures that the text paper and cover board used have met acceptable
environmental accreditation standards.

For further information on Blackwell Publishing, visit our website:
www.blackwellpublishing.com

Contents

This report is the collective work of all the members of the Task Force.
Authors of the first draft of each chapter are given below.

Foreword

The important place that fruit, vegetables, grains and other plant foods have in the human diet has been recognised for a considerable time and there has been clear evidence that diets rich in these foods offer health benefits. This appears particularly true in relation to the risk of premature development of chronic diseases such as cardiovascular disease and cancer. Despite substantial investment of time, effort and resources, the factor or factors responsible for this reduction in risk and the mechanism(s) of action have remained elusive. Initially attention focused on the so-called antioxidant nutrients such as vitamins E and C and β-carotene, but more recently a large array of plant substances, sometimes referred to as phytochemicals or plant bioactive substances, have become the focus of attention. Examination of the available information about these has been the primary topic considered by the Task Force. The Task Force was charged with considering the bioactive substances in foods that are not usually considered to be nutrients and to place these in the context of what is already known about antioxidant nutrients. Whilst the overall context is the promotion of good health through appropriate diet, protection against chronic disease, particularly cancer and cardiovascular disease, has also been addressed. This Report records the findings of the group of eminent scientists listed on pages xiii–xv.

The Task Force has been completely independent. The members are experts in their fields and between them cover a range of topics from the chemistry of plant bioactive substances to public health nutrition. The Report is aimed at a wide variety of professionals who may not be familiar with all the details and so has been written in a way that recognises that some of the complex underpinning chemistry and biochemistry will not be of interest to all readers. Rather than categorising the subject by chemical grouping, a food group approach has been adopted in order to bridge between the introductory chapters on intakes of plant foods, epidemiology and mechanisms and the final chapters which discuss the public health implications and the conclusions and recommendations of the Task Force. As has become practice with recent BNF Task Force Reports, a Question and Answer Section has been included which aims to cover the main aspects discussed within the Report in a way that we hope will be helpful to journalists and other non-specialist readers who need a concise and jargon-free explanation.

I am very grateful to the members of the Task Force who have all contributed a considerable amount of their time and expertise to this Report. The support provided by the Secretariat has also been outstanding and I would like to thank them most sincerely.

Professor Malcolm J. Jackson

Dedication

This book is dedicated to the memory of Professor Tony Diplock, a member of the Task Force who sadly died in February 2000. I had the pleasure and honour of being Tony's postdoc researcher for three-and-a-half years in the early 1980s, based at Guy's Hospital Medical School. On a personal level, he was a generous man who took every opportunity to support and encourage me in my work. On a professional level, he made an immense contribution to the field of anti-oxidant biochemistry, particularly in relation to vitamin E and selenium, both in Britain and internationally. He was also responsible for encouraging the then Ministry of Agriculture, Fisheries and Foods to fund a ground-breaking programme of research on antioxidant nutrients, for which he was still Programme Adviser at the time of his death. He is missed by friends and colleagues, but his contribution to science lives on.

Dr Judy Buttriss
Science Director, BNF

Terms of Reference

The Task Force was invited by the Council of the British Nutrition Foundation to:

(1) Review the present state of knowledge of bioactive substances in foods (that are not usually considered to be nutrients) and to place this in the context of what is already known about antioxidant nutrients; the promotion of good health through appropriate diet; and protection against chronic disease, particularly cancer and cardiovascular disease.

(2) Prepare a report and, should it see fit, draw conclusions, make recommendations and identify areas for future research.

British Nutrition Foundation Plants: Diet and Health Task Force Membership

Chair:

Professor Malcolm Jackson, Dean of the Faculty of Medicine, University of Liverpool, Liverpool, L69 3GA

Members:

Dr Louise Bourne
Lecturer
Department of Food Science
and Technology
Hugh Sinclair Unit of Human
Nutrition
University of Reading
PO Box 226
Whiteknights
Reading RG6 6AP
(until June 2000)

Dr Judith Buttriss
Science Director
British Nutrition Foundation
High Holborn House
52–54 High Holborn
London WC1V 6RQ

Dr Aedin Cassidy
Head of Molecular Nutrition
Unilever Research
Colworth House
Sharnbrook
Bedford MK44 1LQ

Professor Alan Crozier
Professor of Plant Biochemistry
and Human Nutrition
Plant Products and Human
Nutrition Group
Graham Kerr Building
Division of Biochemistry and
Molecular Biology
Institute of Biomedical and
Life Sciences
University of Glasgow
Glasgow G12 8QQ

Dr Garry Duthie
Principal Research Scientist
Antioxidants and DNA
Damage Group
Rowett Research Institute
Greenburn Road
Bucksburn
Aberdeen AB21 9SB

Professor Ian Johnson
Head of Intestinal Growth and
Function Programme
Institute of Food Research
Norwich Research Park
Colney
Norwich NR4 7UA

Dr David Lindsay
Food Science and Technology
Department
CEBAS (CSIC)
Apartado de Correos 4195
30080 Murcia, Spain

Dr Barrie Margetts
Reader
Institute of Human Nutrition
Level B, South Academic Block
Southampton General Hospital
Southampton SO16 6YD

Professor Brian Ratcliffe
Professor of Nutrition and
Associate Head of School
School of Life Sciences
The Robert Gordon University
St Andrew's Street
Aberdeen AB25 1HG

Mr Mike Saltmarsh
Director, Inglehurst Foods
53 Blackberry Lane
Four Marks
Alton
Hampshire GU34 5DF

Professor Klaus Wahle
Research Leader
Lipid and Cell Biology Unit
The Rowett Research Institute
Greenburn Road
Bucksburn
Aberdeen AB21 9SB
   (Until 2003, now at the
   Robert Gordon University)

Professor Ron Walker
School of Biological Sciences
University of Surrey
Guildford
Surrey GU2 7XH

Professor Martin Wiseman
Visiting Professor in Human
   Nutrition
University of Southampton
Institute of Human Nutrition
Level B, South Academic Block
Southampton General Hospital
Southampton SO16 6YD

Observers:

Dr Sheela Reddy
Senior Scientific Manager
Department of Health
Room 426A
Wellington House
133–155 Waterloo Road
London SE1 6LH

Mr Steven Wearne
Food Standards Agency
Aviation House
125 Kingsway
London WC2B 6NH (until April
   2000)

Contributors:

Dr Colette Kelly
Nutrition Scientist
British Nutrition Foundation
High Holborn House
52–54 High Holborn
London WC1V 6RQ

Ms Claire MacEvilly
Nutritionist
Food Safety Promotion Board
7 Eastgate Avenue
Little Island
Cork, Ireland

Mrs Kirsti Peltola
Nutritionist, Friend of the
   British Nutrition Foundation
3 Denbigh Gardens
Richmond
Surrey TW10 6EN

Miss Sara Stanner
Senior Nutrition Scientist
British Nutrition Foundation
High Holborn House
52–54 High Holborn
London WC1V 6RQ

Editor:

Dr Gail Goldberg
Senior Nutrition Scientist
British Nutrition Foundation
High Holborn House
52–54 High Holborn
London WC1V 6RQ

Secretariat:

Dr Gail Goldberg
Senior Nutrition Scientist
British Nutrition Foundation
High Holborn House
52–54 High Holborn
London WC1V 6RQ

Miss Kate Deakin
Science Secretary
British Nutrition Foundation
High Holborn House
52–54 High Holborn
London WC1V 6RQ

Mrs Stephanie Hyman
Science Secretary
British Nutrition Foundation
High Holborn House
52–54 High Holborn
London WC1V 6RQ

The British Nutrition Foundation Task Force would like to thank the copyright holders acknowledged in the text for permission to reproduce data and figures in this book.

1
Introduction: Plant Foods and Health

1.1 Historical perspective

There is now a considerable body of evidence that shows that people who follow particular dietary patterns are at reduced risk of a range of chronic diseases. Diets rich in fruits and vegetables, whole grain cereals and complex carbohydrates are generally associated with lower disease risk. It has been more difficult for researchers to identify the specific component(s) of these diets that may identify the 'protective' agent(s). There are at least three possible explanations (not necessarily mutually exclusive): that the key critical components have not been identified; and/or that it is only in a complex combination of substrates and cofactors that the optimal nutrient profile emerges; and/or that confounding is obscuring the findings, and that attempts to identify key components by a reductionist approach are likely to be unsuccessful.

It is clear that humans eat foods in complex patterns that cannot easily be disaggregated. What may be considered protective or beneficial in one context may not in another because other aspects of diet may also differ, or the burden of disease or other risk factors may differ. There may be a threshold of effect and, depending on what the range and shape of the distribution of intakes is within a particular population, an effect may or may not be seen. Of particular relevance, when considering an apparent protective effect of diets rich in plant foods, is the possibility that intakes of potentially harmful substances may be reduced in these diets, and that the protective effect ascribed to plant foods themselves may in fact be due to this lower level of harmful substances in the diet, rather than to components in the food *per se*.

Despite these difficulties in interpretation, a considerable amount of expense and effort has been invested in attempting to identify active components within plant foods and their mechanisms of action. To date much of the work has concerned animal studies and *in vitro* experiments, and there are recognised difficulties and limitations in the extrapolation of this type of data to the human situation.

In attempting to explore mechanisms of action, much of the focus has been on the potential of substances within plant foods to act as antioxidants. It has also been recognised for some time that living organisms have developed complex and multi-faceted defence systems to protect themselves against the harmful effects of free radicals, such as are formed from oxygen as a result of oxidative metabolism. This defence system is fundamental to the organism's survival because free radicals can damage and affect the function of critical molecules such as DNA, proteins and lipids. The search for biomarkers of oxidative damage that might be suitable for human intervention studies has been the major thrust of the UK government's research programme concerning antioxidants in food, formerly funded through MAFF and now under the auspices of the Food Standards Agency. A critical appraisal of this programme has recently been conducted by the British Nutrition Foundation on behalf of the Agency (Buttriss *et al.*, 2002).

1

In the context of the present review, emphasis is placed on exploring the possibility that a diversity of substances found in food, particularly plant-derived foods and drinks, that are yet to be recognised as nutrients in the conventional sense but to which have been attributed a wide array of properties, including antioxidant function, may underlie the protective effect attributed to a diet high in fruits, vegetables and other plant foods. Potential mechanisms are discussed in Chapter 4.

The recently completed EU-funded concerted action EUROFEDA (European Research on Functional Effects of Dietary Antioxidants) has helped to clarify questions such as: whether or not dietary antioxidants are capable of preventing oxidative damage; what research is needed to determine meaningful dose–response relationships; and what is likely to be an optimal intake of the various bioactive compounds (Astley & Lindsay, 2002). To answer these questions, the project aimed to identify the most useful, reproducible and reliable biomarkers of oxidative damage; assess what is known about the bioavailability of dietary antioxidants (including how best to determine this, and what factors influence uptake, metabolism and tissue distribution); determine the role of dietary antioxidants in the minimisation of oxidative damage in tissues (particularly those with a high metabolic energy requirement); and ascertain the role of dietary antioxidants in gene expression (see www.ifr.bbsrc.ac.uk/EUROFEDA). A summary of what is currently known about the bioavailability of plant derived substances can be found in Chapter 6.

1.2 Definitions and terminology

1.2.1 Plant foods

In this report we consider the health effects of plant foods. We include under this definition:

- fruits, vegetables, cereals, pulses, nuts, seeds, herbs and spices
- plants which have been processed in some way to yield foods and drinks whose origin is primarily plant-based (*e.g.* oils and other sub-

stances derived from cereals and seeds, hot and cold beverages, chocolate, condiments).

1.2.2 Categorisation of plant-derived foods and drinks adopted in this report

The categories adopted in this report and examples of foods and drinks are illustrated in Table 1.1 and summarised below. The different food groups and their constituents are discussed in detail in Chapters 7 (fruit and vegetables), 8 (cereals, nuts and pulses), 9 (beverages), 10 (plant lipids) and 11 (miscellaneous: chocolate and herbs, spices and condiments).

(i) Fruit and vegetables

The COMA report on cancer (Department of Health, 1998b) makes the point that the term 'fruit and vegetables' is used in most studies in a culinary rather than a botanical sense, and covers a wide variety of plants and parts of plants. In many studies, it is often not clear which are included or excluded in the analysis. However, it is generally assumed that potatoes are excluded and regarded as starchy foods. It is often unclear whether or not pulses are included in the studies' categorisation. In this report, the term fruit and vegetables (see Chapter 7) excludes cereals and grains, seeds and nuts, and pulses.

(ii) Cereals and grains

This category covers all cereal grains eaten as food, *e.g.* wheat, oats, barley, rice, maize (corn). Foods derived from these plants are generally consumed as staple items within the diet. The terms 'wholegrain' and 'wholemeal' are commonly used to describe minimally processed grains. It should be noted that although these terms are useful for comparative purposes, in reality virtually all grains undergo some processing to make them palatable, *e.g.* removal of the husk from brown rice (see Chapters 8 and 12).

(iii) Nuts

This category includes all forms of nuts, with the

Table 1.1 Categorisation of plant-derived foods and drinks adopted in this report.

Group	Examples
Fruits	
Tree fruits	Apples, pears, plums, apricots, peaches, cherries, citrus fruits, dates, pineapple, mango, papaya, fig, olive
Soft fruits	Strawberries, raspberries, blackberries, cranberries, currants
Other	Melons, grapes, rhubarb, kiwi, bananas
Vegetables	
Root crops*	Carrot, turnip, swede, parsnip
Cabbage family	Cabbage, broccoli, Brussels sprouts
Onion family	Onions, leeks, garlic
Salad vegetables	Lettuce, celery, cucumber
Tomato family	Tomato, sweet peppers, chilli peppers, aubergine
Mushrooms and fungi	Mushroom varieties, Quorn™
Other	Squashes, sprouted seeds, sea vegetables
Cereals (grains)	Wheat, barley, maize (corn), millet, oats, rice, rye
Tree nuts and seeds	Walnuts, cashew nuts, almonds, chestnuts, pecan nuts, brazil nuts, hazelnuts, pistachio, pine kernels, sesame seeds, sunflower seeds, pumpkin seeds
Pulses (legumes)	Soya beans and products, *e.g.* tofu, red kidney beans, butter beans, chick peas, lentils, peanuts (groundnuts)
Beverages	Tea, coffee, cocoa, wine, spirits, beer
Oils and lipids	Seed oils, olive oil, sterols, CLA, sphingomyelin
Chocolate	Dark chocolate, milk chocolate
Herbs, spices, condiments	Sage, rosemary, thyme, ginger, pepper, cumin, mustard, tomato-based sauces

*Potato, sweet potato and yam are classified as starchy foods, rather than vegetables, in many food guide systems, *e.g.* the UK's *Balance of Good Health* (Food Standards Agency, 2001).

exception of peanuts, which, despite their name, are in fact a legume (see Chapter 8).

(iv) Pulses

The term pulses is used to describe the seeds of legumes, *e.g.* beans and lentils, that are typically dried (to allow storage) and then rehydrated and soaked and cooked before use (see Chapters 8 and 12).

(v) Beverages

The hot beverages commonly consumed in the UK are tea, coffee, cocoa and herbal teas (see Chapters 9 and 11). Cold beverages commonly consumed in the UK are fruit juice, wines, spirits and beers (see Chapters 7 and 9).

(vi) Oils and other plant lipids

Seeds and nuts and some pulses, *e.g.* soya, are rich sources of unsaturated oils, as are olives (see Chapter 10). This report also includes reference to plant sterols and stanols, and other dietary lipids with proposed health benefits which are derived from plant sources but found in foods of animal origin, namely conjugated linolenic acid (CLA) and sphingolipids (Chapter 10).

(vii) Miscellaneous (chocolate, herbs, spices and condiments)

In Chapter 11, information can be found about chocolate, derived from cocoa and hence rich in polyphenols. The category herbs, spices and condiments (Chapter 11) includes terpenoids, particularly aromatic compounds, and sulphur-containing compounds.

(viii) Composite dishes

Many plant foods discussed in this report are neither eaten on their own nor eaten raw. Many are consumed in combination with others, for example eaten as soups, sauces and pies, in the case of fruit, vegetables and cereals; as baked products (*e.g.* pies, cakes, bread, pizzas and biscuits); consumed with milk in the case of breakfast cereals and hot beverages. Composite dishes are included in survey data and are sometimes categorised separately or included together with other foods. There are known and potential interactions, both positive and negative, between different constituents. These may affect their properties and functions (see Sections 1.5.1 and Table 1.9) and bioavailability (see Chapter 6). Furthermore, the effects of preparation, cooking and processing of foods on the properties of the constituents discussed in Chapters 6–11 have to be considered (see Chapter 12).

1.2.3 Classification

The botanical (Latin) names and classes of the plants and other organisms discussed in this report can be found in the relevant chapters (see Chapters 5 and 7–11). The bioactive compounds discussed in this report are members of a number of families of compounds defined on the basis of their structure and biochemistry. In turn, most of these families are comprised of many sub-classes and derivatives. The terminology adopted in this report can be found in Chapter 2.

1.2.4 Substances in food that have an effect on health

Benders' Dictionary of Nutrition and Food Technology (Bender & Bender, 1999) defines nutrients as *essential dietary factors such as vitamins, minerals, amino acids and fatty acids.* Essentiality is a common theme of most conventional definitions. Nutrients have traditionally been viewed as food components that either cannot be synthesised in

the body (*e.g.* vitamin C, ascorbic acid), or whose synthesis requires a specific factor that may in certain circumstances be absent or inadequate (*e.g.* sunlight exposure in the case of vitamin D). Therefore, they need to be supplied in the diet. For example, if the supply of vitamin C in the diet is inadequate, the deficiency disease scurvy results.

Nutrients have also been regarded as necessary for normal structure and function, beyond the avoidance of clinical deficiency disease, and hence contributors to healthy growth and development. However, in contrast to their essential functions, these properties may be shared by a number of other substances in foods and drinks that have not been conventionally regarded as 'nutrients'. Consequently, there is now recognition that many other components of food, particularly plant foods, may have a biological activity that may influence structure and/or function. In general, absorption into the bloodstream in a bioavailable form will be a prerequisite (see Chapter 6), although dietary fibre is an example where benefits are accrued (*e.g.* helps prevent constipation) in the absence of absorption of the fibre itself.

In this report, we have not attempted to redefine the term 'nutrient'. However, we do believe it is useful to take into account that whilst a 'nutrient' is essential in order to prevent a life-threatening deficiency disease (*e.g.* scurvy, beriberi or pellagra), the same nutrients may have other health effects, perhaps via different mechanisms. Furthermore, similar effects may also be derived from consumption of other biologically active substances in food, which do not meet the traditional definition of a nutrient. In other words, food components may be categorised as being either specific to a particular deficiency disease (*i.e.* a condition that is only caused by inadequate provision of the relevant substance) or non-specific (the biological functions affected may be influenced by a number of factors via the same or different mechanisms). Vitamin C, for example, would have both specific activity (in relation to scurvy) and non-specific activity (in relation to its antioxidant functions). Other nutrients may have only specific (*e.g.* thiamin) or non-specific activity (*e.g.* non-provitamin A carotenoids or flavonoids).

To elaborate this, again using vitamin C as an example, prolonged absence from the diet over a period of 3–6 months results in scurvy (Department of Health, 1991). Clinical disease can be prevented by regular consumption of small amounts (10 mg/day or less) of the vitamin, which permits collagen synthesis and the maintenance of the integrity of connective tissue. The UK Reference Nutrient Intake (RNI) is 40 mg/day in adults, which further allows for detectable plasma levels to act as an effective means of transfer between body pools. Plasma levels approach a plateau at daily intakes of between 70 and 100 mg (Department of Health, 1991); however, tissue levels are not saturated until daily intakes reach 200 mg/day or more. At intakes above the RNI, interest has grown in the potential for vitamin C to have positive health effects beyond its traditionally recognised functions. Vitamin C also acts as an antioxidant, a facet not directly related to its function in collagen synthesis, and the suggestion is that this function may be responsible for its putative effects at higher intakes (see Section 1.4.2). Equally plausible is the potential of other antioxidant substances in foods to contribute to the body's overall antioxidant defences. The recent review of vitamin C recommendations in the USA (National Academy of Sciences Food and Nutrition Board, 2000) has attempted to take into account the available evidence for 'optimising' intakes, although the relation to health of the criteria used to define 'optimum' are not clear. It is also important to recognise that these same nutrients may be detrimental in excess. Upper safe levels for a range of nutrients have now been established by the Scientific Committee for Foods and values have been reported by the UK's Expert Vitamins and Minerals Group (www.food-standards.gov.uk, Oldreive, 2003).

1.3 Consumption patterns of plant-derived foods and drinks

1.3.1 Sources of information

At a national level, information on consumption of foods, including plant foods, comes from a variety of sources. The principal surveys are conducted for Government:

- The National Food Survey (now the Expenditure and Food Survey, EFS)
- The National Diet and Nutrition Survey
- Health Survey for England.

The National Food Survey (NFS) (which has recently merged with the Family Expenditure Survey to become the Expenditure and Food Survey) has been conducted annually for the population of Great Britain as a whole since 1950. Some 7000 households record food purchases. More recently, information on food eaten outside the home has also been collected. Although not a direct measure of consumption by individuals, data from the NFS provide valuable information about trends, and regional and socio-economic variations. The National Diet and Nutrition Survey (NDNS) is a rolling programme of cross-sectional surveys of 1500–2000 individuals in one of four age groups selected for simplicity of access (see Section 1.3.3). The Health Survey for England is a rolling annual survey of health status and reported behaviours in around 17 000 individuals and intermittently collects qualitative information in relation to dietary habits [*e.g.* cardiovascular disease (Department of Health, 1999a)]. Within this series, additional surveys of diet and/or nutrition status have also been performed in various population groups, *e.g.* ethnic minorities, young people (Department of Health, 1998a, 2001a). All such sources can provide useful information.

Not all countries conduct such detailed population surveys. Nevertheless, data are available from other countries that enable comparisons to be made (see Section 1.3.4 and Table 1.5), *e.g.* food supply statistics, sometimes referred to as 'food balance sheets' or 'food disappearance statistics', such as those produced by the Food and Agriculture Organisation.

1.3.2 Trends in household consumption in the UK

Information on trends in consumption of fruit, vegetables and other plant-derived foods in the home in the UK can be found in the annual NFS/EFS reports. Some data collected during the

Plants: Diet and Health

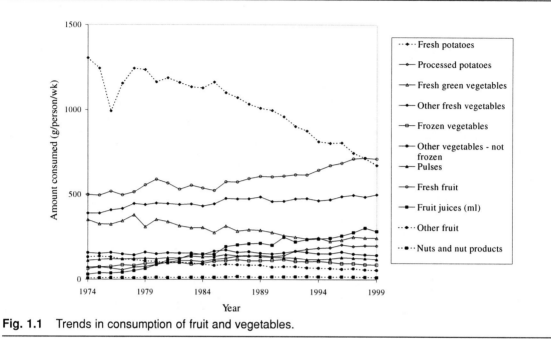

Fig. 1.1 Trends in consumption of fruit and vegetables.

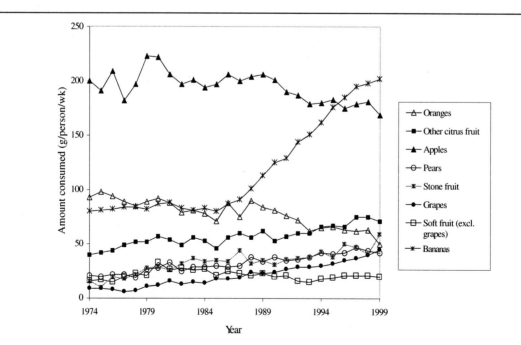

Fig. 1.2 Trends in fresh fruit consumption.

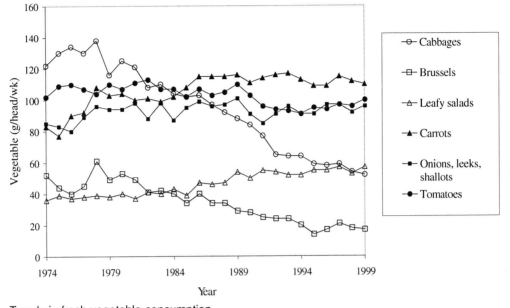

Fig. 1.3　Trends in fresh vegetable consumption.

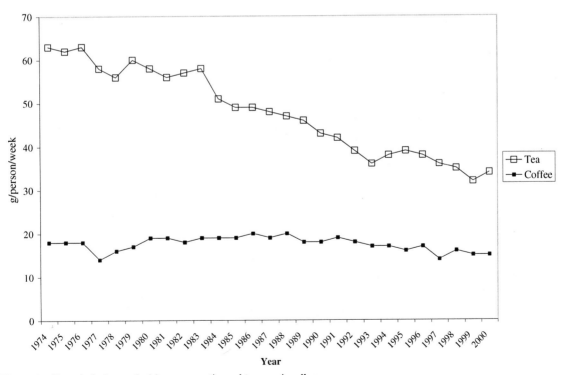

Fig. 1.4　Trends in household consumption of tea and coffee.

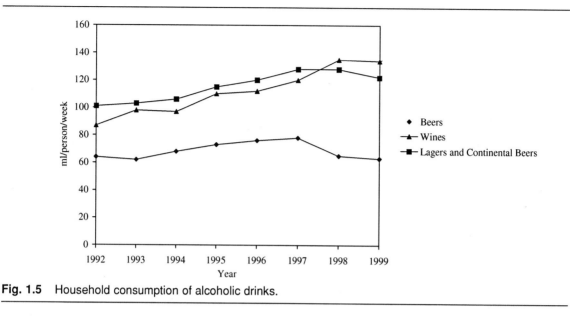

Fig. 1.5   Household consumption of alcoholic drinks.

period 1974–99 are presented in Figs 1.1–1.5. Figure 1.1 illustrates overall trends in household consumption of different categories of plant foods in Britain. Although in food grouping systems, such as the *Balance of Good Health* (Food Standards Agency, 2001), potatoes are classed as starchy foods (such as bread), and do not count towards the recommended five servings a day of fruit and vegetables, they are included in Fig. 1.1 for information. This figure shows that the biggest change is the fall in potato consumption that has not been compensated by a rise in consumption of processed potato products. There has also been a substantial rise in household fruit juice consumption. This began to rise in the 1970s and by 1980 had increased to 87 g/person/week. By 1990 the average intake was 202 g/person/week and in 2000 was 303 g/person/week.

Figures 1.2 and 1.3 illustrate the changes in the consumption of individual fruits and vegetables during 1974–99. A notable change has been the rise in banana consumption from around 100 g/person/week during the period 1974–85 to over 200 g in 1999. There has been a substantial decline in consumption of vegetables such as Brussels sprouts and cabbage and a rise in leafy salad vegetables and carrots. The contribution made to total household vegetable consumption by frozen vegetables in 1974 was 6.5% (63 g/person/week); intake peaked in 1991 at 117 g/week (12%), falling again and reaching 9% (87 g/week) by 1999.

Table 1.2 illustrates trends in consumption of vegetables (fresh and frozen, but excluding potatoes and pulses), fruit (fresh, frozen, canned and dried) and fruit juice. Data are presented for 5-yearly intervals between 1974 and 1999. It is also interesting to note the changes that have occurred in dietary staple consumption during this period, with reductions in potatoes and bread and increases in rice and breakfast cereals, although the total amount of starchy staple food has fallen progressively. It is likely that pasta consumption has risen too, although specific consumption data have only very recently been collected and reported separately. During this period there has been little change in total vegetable consumption, with per capita average daily consumption (excluding potatoes and pulses) in 1999, within the home, being just 142 g/day. Fruit consumption has risen slightly during the 25-year period, with average household daily consump-

Table 1.2　Household consumption trends in Britain for categories of plant foods, 1974–99 (g/person/week).

	1974	1979	1984	1989	1994	1999
Total vegetables (all types, excluding potatoes and pulses)	962	1004	937	1041	968	993
Total fruit (all types)	632	665	628	692	712	766
Fruit juice	30	63	150	214	240	284
Pulses	111	125	133	135	117	119
Nuts and nut products	7	11	12	13	16	13
Potatoes (fresh and frozen products)	1375	1311	1233	1151	997	872
Bread	946	890	865	833	758	717
Rice	16	21	28	30	37	68
Breakfast cereals	81	96	117	126	134	134
Pasta	–	–	–	–	–	79

Source: National Food Survey (MAFF, 1975, 1980, 1985, 1990, 1995, 2000b). The NFS reports also provide data on the contribution of levels of consumption of foods to the intakes of various nutrients (see Tables 1.7 and 1.8).

tion reaching 109 g/day in 1999. This combined figure falls well short of the recommended minimum of 400 g/day (see Chapter 13), although it has to be acknowledged that some fruit and vegetable consumption is likely to take place outside the home. NFS data for 1999 (MAFF, 2000b) indicate that average weekly per capita consumption of vegetables (excluding potatoes), salad and fruit outside the home was 74, 22 and 20 g, respectively.

1.3.3　Intakes in different age and gender groups in the UK

The National Diet and Nutrition Surveys (NDNS) provide detailed information for specific population groups. Data are now available for children aged 1½–4½ years (Gregory *et al.*, 1995), young people aged 4–18 years (Gregory *et al.*, 2000), adults aged 19–64 years (Henderson *et al.*, 2002) and people aged 65 years and older (Finch *et al.*, 1998). A separate Food Standards Agency-funded study of the diets of low-income families is also under consideration. Scrutiny of all these data from individuals not only gives an overview of estimated consumption levels in the UK but also helps to identify population groups that may be at risk because of a low status of one or more nutrients. Table 1.3 shows selected data on intake

levels of plant foods from each of these major surveys.

It is apparent from Table 1.3 that all age groups fall below the 400 g recommendation for fruit and vegetable daily intake. For 19–64 year olds, the daily intake of fruit and vegetables averages 213 g/day, and if fruit juice is included this rises to 261 g/day. For older adults (65 years and above) who are not in a home or a hospital, the respective figures are 202 and 226 g/day. For children, even older children, intakes fall far short of the target. For example, in 15–18 year olds, average daily intakes of fruit, fruit juice and vegetables are, respectively, 44, 62 and 65 g for boys and 54, 61 and 83 g for girls (Gregory *et al.*, 2000), *i.e.* totalling less than 200 g per day, even with the inclusion of fruit juice. Excluding fruit juice, the average daily intakes of fruit and vegetables for 15–18 year olds are 108 and 136 g for boys and girls, respectively.

1.3.4　Variations in intake within and between populations

It is important to note the heterogeneity of diets within and between populations that have to be taken into account when examining epidemiological data (see Chapter 3).

Plants: Diet and Health

Table 1.3 Average weekly consumption (g) of plant-based foods and drinks by various age groups in the UK.

	1½–4½ years*	4–18 years*†			19–64 years*‡			65 years plus§
	Male & female	Male	Female	Average	Male	Female	Average	Male & female
Vegetables	188	346	411	379	818	842	830	738
Fruit	348	366	410	388	608	719	664	674
Fruit juice	258	380	381	381	340	327	334	171
Pulses	84	155	114	135	144	84	114	60
Nuts/products	5	10	6	8	17	12	15	5
Potatoes/products (excluding snacks)	388	769	664	717	821	651	736	699
Bread	281	592	476	534	855	566	711	642
Rice	35	153	127	140	226	168	197	32
Breakfast cereals	138	251	160	206	222	186	204	262
Pasta	127	185	187	186	212	174	193	52
Chocolate	75	138	115	127	73	60	67	24

Data are from whole samples (*i.e.* including non-consumers).
Sources: *Gregory *et al.* (1995); †Gregory *et al.* (2000); ‡Henderson *et al.* (2002); §Finch *et al.* (1998). Data for free-living individuals used.

Table 1.4 Socio-economic and regional differences in household consumption of selected plant foods (g/person/week) in 2000.

	Households with an earner, under £180/week	Households with earnings over £1070/week	South East England	North West England	Scotland	National average
Total vegetables (excluding potatoes)	937	1201	1159	954	878	1077
Fresh green vegetables	190	277	265	196	158	240
Other fresh vegetables	391	601	535	427	414	492
Processed vegetables	357	324	359	331	306	345
Total fruit, including fruit juice	837	1670	1267	946	924	1120
Fruit juice	211	631	364	237	246	303
Fresh fruit	573	968	821	652	615	745
Total Bread	751	601	716	724	756	720
Breakfast and other cereals	383	506	432	389	414	434
Potatoes	1000	671	865	879	810	909

Source: National Food Survey 2000 (DEFRA, 2001).

(i) Differences within the UK population

From data provided by the NFS, it is evident that for fruit and vegetable consumption, for example, differences exist in intakes when socio-economic variables (Table 1.4) and to a lesser extent region are taken into account. The differences in fruit juice consumption are particularly noteworthy. Intakes of most vitamins and minerals tended to be lower in Scotland and to a lesser extent in the north of England than elsewhere, although this was sometimes the result of lower total energy intakes.

Differences are also apparent in the NDNS surveys; for example, children in families in receipt of benefits or classified as in manual or low-income households were less likely to eat a range of fruit and vegetables or to drink fruit juice (Gregory *et al.*, 2000). All these findings tend to be reflected in the intakes of those micronutrients for which these foods are good sources, *e.g.* vitamin C.

(ii) International comparisons

Table 1.5 shows data on national supplies of fruit and vegetables in selected countries, between 1961 and 1998 (Food and Agricultural Organisation, 2000). This type of population level data is relatively easy to collect compared with information based on the dietary records of individuals (*e.g.* in the NDNS surveys), which requires meticulous attention to detail. However, there are also important drawbacks: data exist only for basic commodities, and they cannot show patterns in different sectors of the population. The data also substantially over-estimate the amounts of food actually eaten (as is evident from the differences in apparent energy supply) for example, because they do not account for wastage.

The data in Table 1.5 illustrate these points. For example, the per capita consumption of vegetables appears to have increased in the UK over the past 10 years, whereas information on the food consumed by individual households shows this not to be the case.

Naska and colleagues (Naska *et al.*, 2000) have compared the mean and median fruit and vegetable intakes in 10 European countries, using data derived from household budget surveys retrieved from the Data Food Networking (DAFNE) databank. With the exception of Greece and Spain, average daily intakes in the countries studied fell short of the WHO recommendation (World Health Organisation, 1990) of 400 g/day. Intakes of vegetables were more likely to be low than were intakes of fruit, using targets of 250 and 150 g/day respectively. These data are discussed in more detail in Chapter 13.

1.4 Sources, intakes and properties of constituents of plant-derived foods and drinks

1.4.1 Sources and intakes

A diversity of nutrients and other potentially bioactive substances is to be found in plant-derived foods and drinks (Table 1.6). For some of these constituents, plant foods are major sources in the UK diet (see Tables 1.7 and 1.8). A brief explanation of the function of those particularly relevant to this report is given below.

1.4.2 Properties of antioxidants

The human diet contains a diversity of compounds that possess antioxidant activity, some of which have already been recognised to be important for health, *e.g.* vitamins E and C (see Section 1.4.3). However, many other substances with antioxidant properties are present in foods (see Section 1.4.9), most of which are phenolic compounds (see Chapters 2, 7 and 9). A theme running throughout this report is the considerable attention that has been focused on the potential health effects of antioxidants found in plant-derived food and drinks. It should be noted, however, that in addition to being antioxidants, some of these substances also possess other properties which may prove influential [see Chapter 4 and the literature (Buttriss *et al.*, 2002)].

Antioxidants are considered important because they can protect against the harmful effects of free radicals, or reactive oxygen species (see Chapter 4) which are formed as a result of oxida-

Table 1.5 Trends in national supplies of fruit and vegetables in selected countries 1965–2000 (kg/head/year).

Country	Total fruit									Total vegetables								
	1965	1970	1975	1980	1985	1990	1995	1999	2000	1965	1970	1975	1980	1985	1990	1995	1999	2000
Mediterranean countries																		
Greece	128.0	126.5	113.3	122.3	138.1	165.3	152.4	172.7	162.1	145.9	224.0	275.4	240.8	301.0	259.3	280.5	283.5	293.1
Italy	111.1	128.0	111.9	112.3	115.3	129.1	119.1	138.9	141.0	151.9	170.8	166.3	169.2	172.2	172.5	177.4	183.8	185.5
Portugal	85.1	71.4	72.0	50.7	51.0	100.6	122.0	138.6	133.1	118.6	130.1	168.6	108.9	150.2	180.7	170.1	188.3	176.7
Spain	60.1	66.6	85.1	91.0	99.7	115.9	89.1	119.1	116.9	149.1	149.0	181.2	175.0	168.3	210.1	148.2	163.7	157.1
Other European countries																		
UK	58.7	61.2	55.0	58.4	64.6	75.8	78.0	85.5	83.9	64.4	75.5	70.6	78.1	81.1	87.7	78.1	87.0	83.9
Eire	48.0	53.1	50.9	61.9	63.7	79.8	61.7	70.8	87.5	41.5	46.7	63.3	79.8	62.7	70.6	69.7	73.2	73.1
France	73.2	83.9	65.1	63.3	68.6	80.4	93.7	89.7	94.4	143.5	134.7	114.9	115.0	125.8	126.8	129.1	130.4	131.3
Belgium/Luxemberg	62.7	81.7	68.5	84.0	72.7	122.7	114.7	114.2	120.9	81.3	87.9	83.7	75.1	94.7	94.0	124.1	148.1	146.9
Netherlands	74.2	90.6	84.2	111.7	93.5	136.6	151.2	136.4	127.4	65.6	88.7	73.9	63.7	76.9	78.0	72.2	88.6	83.7
Germany	87.6	110.2	111.8	107.4	107.5	122.5	106.4	115.8	131.7	49.1	60.9	62.3	67.5	74.4	74.5	72.2	74.1	73.9
Denmark	65.0	68.8	64.3	57.9	61.0	76.3	68.0	91.8	103.2	35.2	52.9	41.5	57.6	79.0	78.4	81.9	103.0	104.9
Finland	40.7	51.5	83.4	88.7	61.4	78.9	52.8	86.4	85.0	15.5	20.1	25.9	35.2	45.0	55.9	63.5	71.8	71.1
Norway	72.1	78.1	78.7	85.2	97.9	98.4	97.4	107.3	108.0	47.6	50.2	46.3	61.6	51.8	57.3	60.1	61.7	58.6
Sweden	72.4	86.6	85.6	80.4	78.3	96.6	81.8	98.4	98.6	36.0	38.2	41.7	47.7	54.8	65.9	64.7	73.8	71.9
Other countries																		
USA	76.2	88.4	100.6	110.3	108.8	119.3	111.7	112.1	124.8	90.6	94.7	105.7	102.1	111.2	116.5	122.5	134.1	125.8
Canada	88.4	83.8	102.3	116.8	114.1	112.2	120.3	128.4	125.1	83.9	83.0	94.4	96.4	109.6	117.0	118.2	122.5	119.8
Australia	82.9	91.1	90.0	90.4	94.2	94.2	85.5	88.5	91.9	63.1	64.2	66.3	68.9	80.0	87.7	86.4	89.7	98.9
New Zealand	64.9	72.5	66.8	83.3	99.3	98.7	117.3	112.4	115.7	93.9	80.7	88.4	95.2	92.4	102.7	197.9	140.0	141.2
Japan	38.4	53.5	61.5	55.2	51.5	49.7	52.9	52.5	51.0	117.6	126.0	120.4	121.6	118.6	115.4	115.6	112.4	111.6

Source: Food and Agriculture Organisation (2003): see FAOSTAT Database (www.fao.org).

Table 1.6 Nutrients and other constituents of plant-derived food and drinks.

Plant constituent	Main plant-derived sources in the UK diet	Established/putative functions
Calcium	Milk and milk products are a major provider; other sources include bread, pulses, green vegetables (and, if eaten regularly, dried fruit, nuts and seeds, and the soft bones found in tinned fish)	Primary structural role in bones and teeth; also essential for cellular structure, inter- and intra-cellular metabolic function, signal transmission
Carotenoids		
α-Carotene	Carrots, butternut squash, oranges, tangerines; other sources include passion fruit, kumquats	See Chapters 2, 3, 6, 7
β-Carotene	Orange vegetables (*e.g.* carrots), green leafy vegetables (*e.g.* spinach), tomato products; other sources include apricots, guava, mangoes, melon (orange), passion fruit	
Lycopene	Tomatoes and tomato products	
Chromium	Foods rich in chromium include brewer's yeast, meat products, cheese, whole grains, condiments (and legumes and nuts). Cereals and meat are among the largest contributors to intake	Chromium seems to be necessary for potentiating the action of insulin. It may also be involved in lipoprotein metabolism, in gene expression and in maintaining the structure of nucleic acids
Copper	Although shellfish and liver are particularly rich in copper, the main sources in the British diet are meat, bread and other cereal products, and vegetables. Water can also be a source	Copper is a component of a number of enzymes including cytochrome oxidase, superoxide dismutase and enzymes involved in the synthesis of neuroactive peptides
Fibre	All cereals (especially wholegrain), vegetables, fruit, pulses	See Chapters 3, 7, 8
Flavonoids	Tea, wine, onions, apples are major sources. Other sources are listed in Table 6.1	See Chapters 3, 6, 7, 9
Fluoride	Tea is a major source in the British diet. Other sources include fish and water	Fluoride forms calcium fluorapatite in teeth and bone. It protects against tooth decay and may have a role in bone mineralisation
Folate	Folates (naturally occurring forms) are present in green leafy vegetables (raw or lightly boiled), especially sprouts and spinach; green beans and peas; potatoes; fruit, especially oranges; yeast extract; milk and milk products. Liver is also a good source but should not be consumed by pregnant women or women hoping to conceive. In addition, a number of foods contain the synthetic form of the vitamin, folic acid, *e.g.* breakfast cereals and some bread	Folates are involved in a number of single-carbon transfer reactions, especially in the synthesis of purines, pyrimidines, glycine and methionine. Therefore deficiency affects blood cell development and growth. Also see Section 1.4.4 for more recently identified functions
Glucosinolates	Brassica vegetables, *e.g.* sprouts, cabbage, broccoli	See Chapters 5, 6, 7

(cont'd overleaf)

Table 1.6 (cont'd)

Plant constituent	Main plant-derived sources in the UK diet	Established/putative functions
Iodine	Fish and sea vegetables, *e.g.* kelp, are rich sources, but milk and milk products are a major source of iodine in the UK. Beer can also be a significant source, as can meat products	Iodine forms part of the hormones thyroxine and triiodothyronine, which help control metabolic rate, cellular metabolism and integrity of connective tissue. In the first 3 months of gestation, iodine is needed for the development of the immune system
Iron	Meat and meat products are a rich source of well-absorbed iron. Other important sources are cereal products, particularly bread and breakfast cereals, but also other products made from fortified flour, and vegetables. (Iron is also found in eggs, beans, *e.g.* baked beans and lentils, potatoes and dried fruit.) To help iron absorption, a source of vitamin C should be consumed at the same meal as the iron-containing food; on the other hand tea and phytate-rich cereal products (*e.g.* bran) reduce absorption	Component of haemoglobin, myoglobin and many other enzymes, *e.g.* cytochrome P450 (important in Phase 1 hydroxylation reactions, *e.g.* of drugs and other foreign substances). Deficiency causes defective red cell synthesis and hence anaemia. Adverse effects on work capacity, intellectual performance and behaviour can also occur

Lipids

Plant constituent	Main plant-derived sources in the UK diet	Established/putative functions
Monounsaturated fatty acids	Rich plant sources are olive oil and rapeseed oil. Also found in other nut and seed oils and in meat and milk	See Chapter 10
Polyunsaturated fatty acids (*n*-6)	Rich plant sources of *n*-6 polyunsaturated fatty acids are sunflower, safflower and corn oils	
Polyunsaturated fatty acids (*n*-3)	Present in marine plankton and so fish oils are a rich source of long-chain *n*-3 fatty acids. The essential *n*-3 fatty acid α-linolenic acid is found in large amounts in linseed, grapeseed and rapeseed oils, walnut oil and walnuts. It is also present in green leafy vegetables, soya beans and hazelnuts	
CLA	Main dietary sources are milk and ruminant meat (beef and lamb), derived from fermentation of grass and related fodder	
Sphingolipids	Sphingolipids are present as minor components in most foods; soya beans have the highest concentration but other sources include eggs, milk, cheese and meat. The greatest contribution to intake is milk	
Sterols	Major dietary sources are plant stanol/sterol-enriched spreads and other foods. Naturally present in vegetable oils, *e.g.* soya oil. Less important sources are cereals, nuts and vegetables	

Table 1.6 (cont'd)

Plant constituent	Main plant-derived sources in the UK diet	Established/putative functions
Magnesium	Main sources are cereals, cereal products, *e.g.* bread (particularly wholegrain/wholemeal), and green vegetables. Some magnesium is also found in milk, and a small amount is contributed by meat and potatoes. (Nuts and seeds are fairly rich in magnesium)	Involved in skeletal development (intimately involved in calcium metabolism) and in the maintenance of electrical potential in nerve and muscle membranes. Acts as a cofactor for enzymes requiring ATP, in the replication of DNA and the synthesis of RNA
Manganese	Tea is a major source. Other sources include wholegrain cereals, bread, vegetables, nuts and seeds	Manganese is a component of a number of enzymes and is necessary for the activation of others
Molybdenum	Molybdenum is widely distributed but found particularly in vegetables, bread and other cereals. Other sources include milk and milk products, eggs (and pulses)	Molybdenum is essential for the functioning of a number of enzymes involved in the metabolism of DNA and sulphites
Niacin	Meat and meat products, bread, fortified breakfast cereals, potatoes, milk and milk products are the main sources. It is also provided by fish.	Nicotinamide is the reactive part of the co-enzymes, NAD and NADP, and so is very important in intermediary metabolism; requirement is related to energy metabolism
Phytoestrogens	Soya, seeds, *e.g.* linseed, other pulses, grains, nuts	See Chapters 5, 6, 8
Potassium	Particularly abundant in vegetables, potatoes, fruit (especially bananas) and juices. It is also found in bread, fish, nuts and seeds. Meat and milk also contribute to intake, but these foods, particularly processed meat products and cheese, also provide some sodium (thus reducing the potassium to sodium ratio)	Potassium is principally an intracellular cation and, like sodium, is involved in acid–base regulation, generation of trans-membrane concentration gradients and electrical conductivity in nerves and muscles
Riboflavin	Milk and milk products, especially milk, and fortified breakfast cereals are the main sources in the British diet. Smaller quantities are provided by meat and meat products	Required for oxidative processes; there are a number of flavin-dependent enzymes
Selenium	Cereals, meat and fish contribute the bulk of the selenium in the British diet	Selenium is an integral part of the enzyme glutathione peroxidase, one of the enzymes which protects against oxidative damage. A number of other selenoproteins exist, including one involved in thyroid hormone synthesis
Sulphur-containing compounds	Onions, leeks, garlic, chives, also see Glucosinolates	See Chapters 2, 3, 7, 11

(cont'd overleaf)

Table 1.6 *(cont'd)*

Plant constituent	Main plant-derived sources in the UK diet	Established/putative functions
Terpenoids (other than carotenoids)	Herbs and spices, *e.g.* mint, sage, coriander, rosemary, ginger	See Chapters 2 and 11
Thiamin	All cereals, especially bread and breakfast cereals, potatoes, are the main sources. Smaller quantities are provided by a wide range of foods, including meat and meat products, milk and milk products, vegetables	Involved in the metabolism of fat, carbohydrate and alcohol
Vitamin B$_6$	Widely distributed in foods. Particular sources are potatoes and breakfast cereals	Vitamin B$_6$, as pyridoxal phosphate, is a cofactor for a large number of enzymes associated with amino acid metabolism
Vitamin C	Richest sources are citrus fruit, citrus fruit juices, kiwi fruit and soft fruits. Other sources include green vegetables, other fruit, peppers, potatoes, especially new potatoes	Vitamin C prevents scurvy and aids wound healing. It also assists in the absorption of non-haem iron and is an important antioxidant. It can also act as a pro-oxidant in the presence of certain metal ions and oxygen
Vitamin E	Vegetable oils, margarine, wholegrain cereals, eggs, vegetables, especially dark-green leafy types, and nuts provide most of the vitamin E in the British diet	It is the major lipid-soluble antioxidant in membranes. Immune function is influenced by vitamin E
Vitamin K	Green leafy vegetables are the richest source, but it is also found in other vegetables, fruit, dairy produce, vegetable oils, cereals and meat	The main function is synthesis of pro-coagulant factors. Also involved in bone health
Zinc	Meat, meat products and milk and its products, bread and other cereal products (especially wholemeal) are the major providers. Other sources include eggs, beans and lentils, nuts, sweetcorn and rice. Absorption is relatively poor from phytate-rich cereals	Either directly or indirectly (through effects on a series of enzymes), zinc is involved in the major metabolic pathways contributing to the metabolism of proteins, carbohydrates, energy, nucleic acids and lipids. Hence inadequate intakes are reflected in growth retardation, and in adverse effects on tissues with rapid turnover, *e.g.* skin and the intestinal mucosa, and the immune system

Table 1.7 Contribution of plant foods to the intake from household food of selected vitamins, 1999 (calculated % contribution to total in parentheses).

	Vitamin C (mg/person/day)	β-Carotene (µg/person/day)	Vitamin E (mg/person/day)	Folate (µg/person/day)	Vitamin B$_6$ (mg/person/day)
Total fruit	28 (45)	39 (2)	0.47 (5)	16 (7)	0.13 (7)
Fresh	13 (21)	29 (2)	0.29 (3)	7 (3)	0.09 (5)
Fruit juice	14 (23)	6 (0.3)	0.06 (1)	7 (3)	0.03 (2)
Total vegetables	19 (31)	1385 (79)	0.97 (10)	48 (20)	0.19 (10)
Fresh green	3 (5)	93 (5)	0.14 (1)	18 (8)	0.04 (2)
Other fresh	6 (10)	1018 (58)	0.34 (3)	15 (6)	0.09 (5)
Frozen	3 (5)	157 (9)	0.06 (1)	7 (3)	0.02 (1)
Other, not frozen	1 (2)	117 (7)	0.43 (4)	8 (3)	0.04 (2)
Bread	–	–	0.05 (1)	18 (8)	0.06 (3)
Breakfast cereals	2 (3)	0	0.27 (3)	33 (14)	0.24 (12)
Rice	0	0	0.03 (0.3)	2 (0.8)	0.02 (1)
Nuts and nut products	0	0	0.09 (0.9)	1 (0.4)	0.01 (0.5)
Pulses	0	12 (0.7)	0.07 (0.7)	5 (2)	0.02 (1)
Potatoes (including frozen products	7 (11)	0	0.92 (9)	29 (12)	0.46 (23)
Tea	–	0	0	9 (4)	0.02 (1)
Total intake (from all foods and drinks)	62	1751	9.74	238	1.98

Source: MAFF (2000) and personal communication.

tive metabolism (*i.e.* as a result of the many chemical reactions and metabolic processes that occur in the body). Reactive species are capable of modifying important molecules such as DNA, lipids and proteins, affecting their ability to function or causing them to function abnormally, processes often referred to as oxidative damage (see Chapters 4 and 9). Antioxidants have the ability to scavenge and/or neutralise free radicals, or are necessary to enable other molecules to perform such a function.

A major risk factor for coronary heart disease is an elevated LDL (low-density lipoprotein) cholesterol level in the blood. High levels of LDL cholesterol predispose to the formation of atherosclerotic plaques in arteries, *e.g.* coronary arteries. It is now recognised that an important step in this process is the prior oxidation of LDL, which results in it being scavenged by macrophages in the artery walls (Witztum, 1994; Ferns & Lamb, 2001). This causes the macrophages to develop into the cholesterol-laden foam cells characteristic of fatty streaks, which are precursors of atherosclerotic plaques. It has been proposed that certain dietary patterns, such as a diet rich in fruit, vegetables and other plant foods, may help protect against heart disease and other circulatory diseases by providing antioxidants which in some way inhibit this process (see Chapter 4 for more details).

From this has stemmed an interest in whether an imbalance between the production of free radicals and the body's antioxidant defence system provides the basis for mechanisms involved in the initiation and development of chronic disease states, such as cardiovascular disease and various

Table 1.8 Contribution of some plant foods to the intake from household food of selected minerals, 1999 (calculated % contribution to total in parentheses).

	Calcium (mg/person/day)	Iron (mg/person/day)	Zinc (mg/person/day)	Magnesium (mg/person/day)	Potassium (g/person/day)
Total fruit	18 (2)	0.4 (4)	0.2 (3)	19 (8)	0.27 (10)
Fresh	10 (1)	0.2 (2)	0.1 (1)	11 (5)	0.17 (7)
Fruit juice	4 (0.5)	0.1 (1)	–	4 (2)	0.07 (3)
Total vegetables	42 (5)	1.0 (10)	0.5 (7)	19 (8)	0.33 (13)
Fresh green	11 (1)	0.2 (2)	0.1 (1)	3 (1)	0.07 (3)
Other fresh	13 (2)	0.3 (3)	0.1 (1)	5 (2)	0.14 (5)
Frozen	4 (0.5)	0.1 (2)	–	2 (1)	0.03 (1)
Other, not frozen	14 (2)	0.4 (4)	0.3 (4)	9 (4)	0.09 (3)
Bread	60 (7)	1.2 (12)	0.6 (8)	24 (10)	0.09 (3)
Breakfast cereals	11 (1)	1.7 (17)	0.4 (5)	13 (6)	0.06 (2)
Rice	1	0.1 (1)	0.1 (1)	2 (1)	0.01
Nuts and nut products	1	0	0.1 (1)	3 (1)	0.01
Pulses	8	0.3 (3)	0.1 (1)	6 (3)	0.06 (2)
Potatoes (including frozen products)	8 (1)	0.6 (6)	0.3 (4)	20 (9)	0.44 (17)
Alcoholic drinks	4 (0.5)	0.1 (1)	0	4 (2)	0.03 (1)
Tea	1 (0.1)	–	0.1 (1)	5 (2)	0.08 (3)
Total intake (from all foods)	811	9.9	7.5	229	2.59

Source: MAFF (2000) and personal communication.

cancers. The function of dietary antioxidants in the body is referred to in Chapter 4. Thus, many studies involving *in vitro* and animal models have been conducted. However, to address properly any relationship in humans, it has been considered necessary to develop biomarkers of oxidative damage. Progress has been slow, in part because of the challenging analytical problems associated with measurement of DNA oxidation, in particular, and also because of the general lack of information about important aspects such as intra- and inter-individual variability in the levels of oxidised DNA present in normal healthy individuals or the impact of ageing. These issues are discussed in more detail in Chapter 6. When considering the potential benefits of antioxidants, it should not be forgotten that whilst there is evidence that antioxidants can protect against damage induced by reactive oxygen species (ROS), it is now recognised that they have a role as signalling molecules, under the influence of the redox potential of the cell (see Chapter 4). Interference with this process might be harmful. It is speculated that ROS production in healthy cells is under tight regulation, but under circumstances of acute oxidative stress, this regulation may break down, compromising the cells if antioxidant capacity is inadequate.

Furthermore, issues relating to bioavailability have to be considered. Just because bioactive compounds give promising results *in vitro* and in animal studies does not mean that they can perform similar functions in humans, or even be effectively absorbed, let alone reach target tissues. Also, the doses and forms of the compounds used in experimental studies may not be physiologically and/or nutritionally relevant. Despite these caveats the results of such studies are often extrapolated to attempt to explain epidemiological relationships between diet and health. Similarly, the results of epidemiological studies are often used as the rationale for exploring the properties of individual foods and their constituents in more detail.

1.4.3 Antioxidant vitamins

(i) Carotenoids

β-Carotene is a member of a family comprising more than 600 different carotenoids (carotenoids are terpenoids, see Chapter 2). The predominant carotenoids present in the diet are α-carotene, β-carotene, cryptoxanthin, α-cryptoxanthin, lutein, lycopene and zeaxanthin. The dietary sources of each of these can be found in Table 1.6 and information on their bioavailability in Chapter 6. It is recognised that carotenoids can function in a number of ways (*e.g.* as antioxidants) and only some possess provitamin A activity (*e.g.* β-carotene). In addition to antioxidant capacity, a number of functions have been ascribed to this group of plant constituents. These are discussed in more detail in Chapters 6 and 8. Table 1.6 shows the foods that contribute to the intakes of these substances in the UK. The NFS for 2000 (DEFRA, 2001) indicated that average intake of β-carotene from household food and drink was 1793 μg/person/day. Table 1.7 shows the proportions of intake provided by different plant foods. The NFS does not publish data on intakes of carotenoids other than β-carotene but some of these data are now being collected in the NDNS programme. To date, data are available for older people (Finch *et al.*, 1998) and school children (Gregory *et al.*, 2000). In free-living (non-institutionalised) subjects over the age of 65 years (not taking supplements), median intakes in men and women, respectively, were for β-carotene 1486 and 1093 μg/day; for α-carotene 257 and 154 μg/day; and for β-cryptoxanthin 19 and 18 μg/day. Among school children, median intakes in boys and girls, respectively, of β-carotene were 1011 and 1016 μg/day; for α-carotene 139 and 163 μg/day;

and of β-cryptoxanthin 23 and 24 μg/day. For all three carotenoids there were wide variations in intake within age and gender groups, and some subjects in the school children survey had zero intakes of some carotenoids during the 7-day dietary recording period.

(ii) Vitamin C

Dietary reference intakes exist in the UK (Department of Health, 1991) and elsewhere, *e.g.* the USA (National Academy of Sciences Food and Nutrition Board, 2000) for vitamin C (40 mg/day for adults in the UK and 90 mg/day for men and 75 mg/day for women in the USA). The NFS for 2000 (DEFRA, 2001) indicated that average intake from household food and drink was 65 mg/person/day. Table 1.7 shows the proportions of intake provided by different plant foods. For a long time now it has been recognised that vitamin C prevents scurvy. More recently, it has been recognised that it is necessary for effective wound healing. It also assists in the absorption of non-haem iron by converting Fe^{3+} to Fe^{2+}. Vitamin C can act as an antioxidant; however, it can also act as a pro-oxidant in the presence of certain metal ions (*e.g.* free copper and iron) and oxygen. There are also interactions between the metabolism of vitamins C and E [see (*iii*) below].

(iii) Vitamin E

Vitamin E is the term used to describe all tocols and tocotrienol derivatives that exhibit the biological activity of α-tocopherol. This group of compounds is highly lipophilic and functions within membranes and lipoproteins (see Chapters 4 and 10). Vitamin E is the major lipid-soluble antioxidant in membranes, able to break the sequence of events resulting from the transfer of a free electron from one molecule to another, by quenching it. There is evidence from *in vitro* studies that vitamin C [see (*ii*) above] is capable of regenerating the tocopheroxyl radical which is formed on inhibition of lipid peroxidation by vitamin E (Hamilton *et al.*, 2000). In turn the vitamin C may be regenerated by glutathione. It must be noted, however, that there are limitations in the extent to which *in vitro* data can be extrapolated to humans. When Dietary Reference Values were established by COMA (Department of Health, 1991), it was considered that there were insufficient data available to establish a reference nutrient intake. Thus currently in the UK there is a 'safe' intake of above 3 mg/day in women and above 4 mg/day in men; the USA has a dietary reference intake of 15 mg/day for adults. Table 1.6 shows the foods that contribute to vitamin E intake in the UK. Green leafy vegetables (Chapter 6) and vegetable oils (Chapter 9) are the richest sources. The NFS for 2000 (DEFRA, 2001) indicated that average intake from household food and drink was 10.15 mg/person/day. Table 1.7 shows the proportions of intake provided by different plant foods.

1.4.4 Folate and other B vitamins

The main dietary sources of folate in Britain are cereals and cereal products (especially fortified breads and breakfast cereals), leafy green vegetables and milk products. The contribution of plant foods to folate intake is illustrated in Table 1.7. Current interest in folate is twofold (Department of Health, 2000a): first, the evidence that it is protective against the development of neural tube defects during pregnancy (all women who might become pregnant are advised to take a daily 400 µg supplement and to continue this practice for the first 12 weeks of pregnancy); second, that low intakes are associated with raised plasma levels of homocysteine. The latter is recognised to be independently associated with risk of atherosclerosis of coronary, cerebral and peripheral vessels (Clarke *et al.*, 1991; Stampfer & Malinow, 1995). In addition to promoting oxidative modification of LDL cholesterol, homocysteine can influence clotting mechanisms (see Chapter 4) and reduce the production of endothelium-derived nitric oxide, which has vasodilatory effects (Department of Health, 2000a).

In the Physicians Health Study, a prospective study which included 15 000 men, plasma levels of homocysteine were higher in cases of myocardial infarction than in controls, and those in the top 5% of plasma levels were at 3.1 times the risk over a 5-year period compared with the 90 subjects with the lowest levels. This risk rose to 3.4 after correction for other risk factors (Stampfer *et al.*, 1992). In the British Regional Heart Study, serum homocysteine was also shown to be higher in stroke cases than in controls (Perry *et al.*, 1995). A meta-analysis of 27 studies (mainly of middle-aged men) indicated that plasma homocysteine levels increase with age, and elevation of total homocysteine showed a graded and linear association with risk of vascular disease in most, but not all, studies. It was estimated that if plasma homocysteine levels were reduced by 5 µmol/L, the mortality from coronary artery disease would be reduced by 10% in US men aged 45 years and by over 6% in women (Boushey *et al.*, 1995; Department of Health, 2000a). Since then there have been further studies, some supportive and others not. In the UK, COMA concluded that there is still a need to determine the strength of the association and the existence of any dose–response relationship with risk, and to take account of all potential confounding factors, particularly within-individual variation in homocysteine levels over time. The results of intervention studies addressing whether or not folic acid supplementation can result in reduced risk of cardiovascular disease are awaited.

Plant foods such as green vegetables are an important source of natural folate, but given current patterns of consumption, cannot be relied upon to provide sufficient intakes for some sections of the population. Consequently, in the USA, all grain products are now fortified with folic acid (140 µg/100 g grain). Fortification of flour has also been advocated by COMA, at the level of 240 µg/100 g in food products as consumed (Department of Health, 2000a). Whether this should go ahead has been the subject of a public consultation, and for the time being at least, fortification has been rejected by the UK government (see Chapter 13).

Several other B vitamins, particularly vitamins B_6 and B_{12}, are also closely involved in homocysteine metabolism, and it has been shown recently that combined supplementation with both folic acid and vitamin B_{12} is effective in lowering plasma homocysteine levels (Department of Health, 2000a).

1.4.5 Other vitamins and minerals

Table 1.6 lists many of the other vitamin and minerals present in plant foods, and their functions and properties where known. The role of iron in human nutrition can be found in another Task Force report (British Nutrition Foundation, 1995a). Information about copper has also been published recently (Hughes & Buttriss, 2000). Selenium is a mineral that is a crucial component of a number of enzymes, *e.g.* glutathione peroxidase, which is part of the body's defence against oxidative damage (see Chapter 3). The Total Diet Study indicates that average intake of selenium from household food was 39 μg/day in 1997 (MAFF, 1999). The sources of selenium are shown in Table 1.6. In 1997, 22% of selenium intake was derived from cereals and cereal products. Selenium is discussed in more detail in Chapter 8 and in a Briefing Paper devoted to the topic (British Nutrition Foundation, 2001a). Magnesium and potassium are also the subjects of much recent interest. Suter has identified potassium, magnesium (and fibre) as significant modifiers of stroke risk in men, particularly those with hypertension (Suter, 1999). The Nurses Health Cohort Study (Ascherio *et al.*, 1996) reported an inverse association between intakes of magnesium and potassium (and dietary fibre, fruit and vegetables) with self-reported systolic and diastolic blood pressure, but found that magnesium, potassium and fibre were not significantly associated with risk of diagnosed hypertension.

1.4.6 Unsaturated fatty acids

Unsaturated fatty acids in plant foods (see Chapter 10) can be broadly categorised as mono-unsaturated (*e.g.* the 18-carbon oleic acid), *n*-3 polyunsaturated (*e.g.* the 18-carbon essential fatty acid α-linolenic acid) or *n*-6 polyunsaturated (*e.g.* the essential 18-carbon fatty acid linoleic acid). Rich plant sources of oleic acid are olive oil and rapeseed oil. Plant seed oils, such as sunflower, safflower and corn oils, are rich sources of linoleic acid (*n*-6). α-Linolenic acid (*n*-3) is found in large amounts in linseed, grapeseed and rapeseed oils,

walnut oil and walnuts. Other sources include green leafy vegetables (particularly purslane), soya bean products and hazelnuts. A number of health benefits, particularly in relation to blood lipids and other cardiovascular disease risk factors such as clotting have been attributed to these types of fatty acid (see Chapters 4 and 10). Indeed, the risk of dying following a heart attack has been shown to be reduced by a diet rich in long-chain *n*-3 fatty acids. Detailed discussion of these aspects can be found in a BNF Task Force Report and a Briefing Paper on the topic (British Nutrition Foundation, 1992, 1999).

1.4.7 Dietary fibre

Dietary fibre (sometimes referred to as non-starch polysaccharide, NSP), found naturally only in plant foods, is not conventionally regarded as a nutrient (see Section 1.2.4) but is recognised as being important for health. Differences in terminology are discussed in Section 3.3.6. Current intakes of fibre (NSP) in the UK average about 12 g/day, which falls short of the dietary reference value of 18 g/day for adults (Department of Health, 1991). Data for the UK indicate that the main sources are vegetables (38%), fruit (12%) and cereals (45%), particularly bread, which contributes 13%, and breakfast cereals (12%) (MAFF, 2000b). Recent data for children aged 4–18 years paint a similar picture, with approximately 40% of dietary fibre coming from fruit and vegetables and approximately a further 40% from cereals and cereal products (Gregory *et al.*, 2000).

Evidence from a number of sources suggests that consumption of fibre-rich foods, in general, is beneficial to health, *e.g.* heart health (see Section 3.3.6), and in reducing the risk of developing certain cancers (see Section 3.4.9 and Chapters 3 and 8).

Soluble forms of dietary fibre (sometimes referred to as viscous fibres) are abundant in fruits (Chapter 7), beans, legumes, gums, *e.g.* guar and gum arabic, barley, psyllium and oats (Chapter 8). Such types of fibre have been shown to lower blood lipid levels in a number of studies in subjects with mild to moderate hypercholesterolaemia, particularly total and

LDL cholesterol, when consumed as part of a reduced-fat diet (Anderson *et al.*, 1992, 2000). They have also been shown to influence glucose metabolism and insulin release in a positive manner (Jenkins *et al.*, 2000). To some extent, these findings overlap with benefits attributed to other forms of dietary fibre found predominantly in cereals (see Chapter 8). This highlights the need to be mindful of the fact that plant foods may indeed have multiple effects on health and more needs to be understood about the interplay between these various influences (Jenkins *et al.*, 2000). See also Chapter 3.

1.4.8 Alcohol

Chapter 9 discusses the bioactive compounds found in alcohol-containing drinks such as wine, beer and spirits, and their potential effects on health. However, there is considerable evidence for positive health benefits of consumption of small to moderate amounts of the alcohol itself. In the past 20 years, numerous studies have found that moderate drinkers have lower total mortality and less coronary heart disease, cholelithiasis (gall stones), diabetes and dementia than either abstainers or heavy drinkers (Macdonald, 1999). The dose–response curve relating mean daily intake of alcohol to morbidity or mortality is therefore U-shaped or J-shaped. This relationship seems to be independent of beverage type (Grobbee *et al.*, 1999), as it has been found in wine drinkers (*e.g.* Renaud *et al.*, 1998) and in consumers of other types of drink, mainly beer drinkers (*e.g.* Keil *et al.*, 1997; Bobak *et al.*, 2000). Although there is evidence from a number of prospective studies, conducted predominantly among wine-drinking populations, that moderate wine consumption is associated with lower cardiovascular disease risk, its superiority over other beverages, or a superiority of red compared with white wine, has not yet been satisfactorily established (see Chapters 3 and 9).

The most recent UK government guidelines on alcohol advocate daily rather than weekly upper limits on intake to avoid the problems associated with 'binge drinking': men up to 4 units daily, women up to 3 units daily (Department of Health, 1995). One unit is equivalent to approximately 10 g of pure alcohol. Whilst moderate intakes appear to be beneficial in terms of heart disease in middle-aged and older people, excessive intakes can cause considerable harm, both physically (*e.g.* cancer) and psychologically. A detailed discussion of all aspects of alcohol and health can be found in Macdonald (1999).

1.4.9 Other plant-derived bioactive substances

There are a number of biologically plausible mechanisms of anti-carcinogenesis, for example, that might involve components of fruits and vegetables other than the currently recognised nutrients. Many of these compounds have previously been regarded only as natural toxicants (*e.g.* quercetin in cell culture can result in cell death) because they form part of the protective mechanisms of plants (see Chapters 7 and 9). However, if their biological activity contributes to the probable protective effect of fruits and vegetables against chronic conditions, such as cancer, a balance of risk and benefits must be considered. These issues are discussed in Chapter 13.

To date, most of the evidence for potential health effects of different compounds has been obtained from *in vitro* techniques or using experimental animal models, and the relevance to the human situation remains to be demonstrated (see Chapters 3 and 6). This information is reviewed in Chapters 7–11. However, a brief introduction to the major classes of compound is given below to set the scene.

(i) Phenolic compounds

Most naturally occurring antioxidants are phenolic compounds. These all possess at least one aromatic ring with one or more hydroxy groups (see Chapters 2, 6 and 9). Phenols and polyphenols include flavonoids (see Chapters 2, 7, 8, 9 and 11) and phytoestrogens (see Chapter 8). These substances are widely distributed in plants and are responsible for many of the colours, aromas and flavours characteristic of vegetables, fruits, herbs and spices and beverages. Diets rich in plant-derived foods and drinks can provide more than 1 g of phenolic compounds per day, although there are large inter-individual variations. Little is known about the bioavailability of different phenolic compounds (see Chapter 6) and their biological effects vary greatly, in terms of both potency and specificity.

Flavonoids are the most numerous of the phenolics and are found throughout the plant kingdom (see Chapter 2). Sub-classes include flavonols such as quercetin and kaempferol, flavones such as luteolin, flavan-3-ols such as catechins, anthocyanins, coumarins and isoflavones (see Chapters 2, 7, 8, 9 and 11). In addition to their antioxidant properties, flavonoids can modify the expression of phase I and phase II enzymes and can therefore function as blocking agents [see Chapter 4 and the literature (Department of Health, 1998b)]. They have also been shown to inhibit the arachidonic acid cascade (Chapter 10), inhibit protein kinase C activity and interfere with the expression of the mutated *Ras* oncogene and so could also function as suppressing agents [see Chapter 4 and the literature (Department of Health, 1998b)]. This wide range of effects shown mainly *in vitro*, in addition to the relatively high intakes of flavonoids, has led to suggestions that phenolic compounds might potentially be the most important source of anticarcinogenic activity in the diet (Department of Health, 1998b). Associations have also been reported with heart health (Chapter 3).

Phytoestrogens (Chapter 8) are structurally similar to mammalian oestrogen, oestradiol, and possess weakly oestrogenic activity. The principal phytoestrogens are the isoflavones and lignans. Linseed is a rich source of lignans and soya protein products contain high concentrations of isoflavones. The average intake of isoflavones in the UK is estimated to be less than 1 mg/day whereas that in Asian countries is approximately 50 mg/day (Department of Health, 1998b).

(ii) Terpenoids

Herbs are a source of antioxidants known as terpenoids (see Table 1.6 and Chapters 2 and 11) for which cancer-protective and other properties have been proposed (Craig, 1999). Carotenoids are also in this category (see Sections 1.4.3(i) and 2.4).

(iii) Sulphur-containing compounds and their derivatives

Glucosinolates (see Table 1.6 and Chapters 2, 5, 6 and 7) are found almost entirely in brassica vegetables (*e.g.* broccoli, cabbage, cauliflower, Brussels sprouts, kale), although there are some cruciferous sources (*e.g.* mustard); about 120 compounds have been isolated. The average intake in the UK is about 46 mg/day (Department of Health, 1998b). Glucosinolates are broken down by cooking and food preparation (Chapter 12) and in the gut (Chapter 5) to a number of products including isothiocyanates and indole compounds. These give rise to the characteristic flavour and also appear to be responsible for the bioactive properties of glucosinolates (Department of Health, 1998b) (Chapters 5–7). In 1998, the COMA Working Group on cancer concluded that there was insufficient evidence to draw conclusions at the time (Department of Health, 1998b), although further studies have since been published (see Section 5.4.3). Concerns have also been expressed about possible adverse effects (see Chapter 5) from these or other components of brassica vegetables and more research is clearly required to assess risk versus benefit.

Plants of the genus *Allium*, *e.g.* onions, garlic and leeks (Chapter 7), are a major source of sulphur compounds (see Section 2.6.2) in the diet. The metabolism of these compounds is complex and they undergo enzymically mediated reactions during processing and cooking (Chapter 12). The end products of these reactions contribute to the smell, flavour and lachrymatory effects of onions and garlic (Fenwick & Hanley, 1985). The most important compounds are the sulphur-substituted cysteine sulphoxides.

There is some evidence that onions, garlic and compounds derived from them can exhibit health-promoting effects (see Chapters 3 and 7), for example in relation to garlic and CVD and some forms of cancer (Fleischauer *et al.*, 2000; Ackermann *et al.*, 2001).

(iv) Chlorophyll and its derivatives

Chlorophyll is ubiquitous in green plants and is the plant pigment central to photosynthesis. It contains the metal ion magnesium. *In vitro* studies have provided suggestions that chlorophyll or its derivatives may have anti-cancer properties. However, the COMA Working Group on cancer (1998) concluded that the relevance to cancer induction in humans of the antimutagenic and anticlastogenic effects of chlorophyll seen in experimental systems is unclear.

1.5 Bioavailability and interactions

Whether or not a nutrient is provided in a bioavailable form in a food is crucial to the food's nutritional value. For example, spinach is relatively rich in iron and calcium but interactions with oxalic acid prevent their absorption and subsequent utilisation. Similarly, iron uptake is inhibited by polyphenols present in a number of plant foods. The bioavailability, where known, of the compounds covered in this report is discussed in detail in Chapter 6.

1.5.1 Interactions between dietary constituents

When composing or choosing a meal, it is foods that are selected, not nutrients, and most individuals make a consistent selection of a range of foods that may be described as a dietary pattern (Jacques & Tucker, 2001). A technique known as principal components analysis has been used to summarise dietary patterns in a number of studies, including the Dietary and Nutritional Survey of British Adults (Gregory *et al.*, 1990). This showed that the first principal component contrasted people who ate more wholemeal bread, high-fibre breakfast cereals, low-fat spreads, salad vegetables, other vegetables and fruit with people who ate more white bread, butter, whole milk, potato and sugar. Those who ate more of the first group of foods were more likely to be better educated and of higher social class. The adult survey data also showed that people who eat more plant-based foods, perhaps not surprisingly, also eat less animal-derived foods. The

effect these dietary patterns have on nutrient intakes is complex, but there is strong collinearity between the nutrients (vitamins and minerals) found in plant-based foods, and it is difficult to attribute disease causality to any individual nutrient. Although it is possible to adjust statistically for other nutrients, this adjustment is not robust with such strongly correlated data.

The combination of foods and drinks eaten and the way in which foods are prepared (Chapter 12) will also affect the biological effects of the individual constituents of the food. The functional availability depends on the amount of a nutrient that can get to the site of its biological action; the uptake, absorption, transport and eventual metabolic role can all be affected by other nutrients. Examples of interactions through which absorption is increased or decreased are given in Table 1.9.

1.5.2 Interactions with other factors

Social, cultural and biological factors interact and influence food patterns and people's behaviour (Jacques & Tucker, 2001). As mentioned above, social class and education are strongly linked to dietary patterns; dietary patterns are linked to other aspects of lifestyle, such as smoking, alcohol and physical activity. An example of an interaction is the finding concerning β-carotene supplementation in smokers (ATBC, 1994; Omenn *et al.*, 1996). See also Chapter 3.

Indeed, the experience with β-carotene indicates the importance of using data from the whole range of studies to estimate both the efficacy and safety of supplements of single nutrients (see Chapter 13). Plasma β-carotene levels in the usual range are inversely correlated with lung cancer incidence. According to COMA (Department of Health, 1998b), 14 out of 18 case-control studies found a lower risk with higher intakes of β-carotene and/or vitamin A, and six prospective studies found lower lung cancer risk associated with higher serum levels of β-carotene. The risk of lung cancer among those with the lowest serum levels of β-carotene was generally about twice that of those with the highest concentrations. Smokers tend to have lower intakes of β-carotene

Table 1.9 Examples of interactions through which the absorption of food constituents are increased or decreased.

Nutrient	Absorption increased by	Absorption decreased by
Iron	Vitamin C, meat, poultry and fish, alcohol	Zinc, calcium, tannins (*e.g.* in tea), flavonoids, phytate
Calcium	Vitamin D	Iron, zinc, phytate, oxalate, oligosaccharides
Magnesium		Phytate
Folate		Alcohol
Carotenoids	Fats and oils	Stannol and sterol esters
β-Carotene and α-carotene	Alcohol	
Lutein and zeaxanthin		Alcohol

and lower serum levels for the same intake. Given these fairly consistent findings, the benefit of supplementation with β-carotene (20 mg/day) was tested in a randomised controlled trial of Finnish men at high risk of lung cancer (50–69 years old and smokers) (ATBC, 1994). The trial found no benefit of β-carotene and the data raised the possibility that the risk of lung cancer in this group was actually increased by the supplementation. The risk of lung cancer was significantly greater (by 18%) in those receiving the supplement compared with those who were not. Similar interim findings of non-significantly increased rates of lung cancer and total mortality have been reported in another study (CARET) in smokers, causing the investigators to discontinue the trial after 4 years of intervention (Omenn *et al.*, 1996). An implication of these results is that perturbation in carotenoid metabolism might modulate the risk of lung cancer. However, similar results were not obtained in a US trial of 22 000 healthy men (physicians; 11% current smokers, 39% ex-smokers at the beginning of the study)

who received β-carotene supplementation for 12 years (Hennekens *et al.*, 1996). There was neither benefit nor harm in terms of the incidence of cancer, cardiovascular disease or death from all causes. COMA (Department of Health, 1998b) concluded that the findings among smokers emphasise the need to be aware of the possibility of adverse effects of high doses of single nutrients.

1.6 Summary

Eating patterns characterised by an abundance of fruit, vegetables and other plant foods are associated with a reduced risk of chronic disease, *e.g.* cardiovascular disease and cancer. The evidence to support this is presented in Chapter 3. The search for the active components in these foods has met with limited success. Research has been focused on the antioxidant vitamins C and E and β-carotene, although a few studies have also looked at other carotenoids and some of the polyphenols (*e.g.* flavonoids) that are the main subject of this Task Force report.

1.7 Research recommendations

To move knowledge forward, there is a need for the following:

- comprehensive information on the quantities of the various plant constituents of interest that are present in a diverse selection of foods
- studies of the bioavailability of these plant constituents and the factors that influence absorption, distribution and tissue uptake, and the likely impact of these substances on metabolic processes
- a better understanding of the interaction of these substances with disease processes
- understanding of nutrient gene interactions and other factors that influence inter-individual variation
- information about interactions and adverse effects.

1.8 Key points

- In this report, the term plant foods is used to describe fruits, vegetables, cereals, pulses, nuts, seeds, herbs and spices, and also plants that have been processed in some way to yield foods and drinks whose origin is primarily plant-based (*e.g.* oils, various hot and cold beverages, chocolate, condiments).
- Information on national food consumption patterns is available from a variety of sources, *e.g.* the UK's National Food Survey (now Expenditure and Food Survey) and the National Diet and Nutrition Survey Programme. From these sources, it is evident that UK fruit and vegetable consumption, for example, varies with socio-economic group (being lower in the lowest social classes) and to a lesser extent with region.
- Information is also available on intakes of the various nutrients provided by plant foods (*e.g.* vitamins C and E; folate; minerals, *e.g.* iron, calcium, selenium, potassium, magnesium; and unsaturated fatty acids) and to a lesser extent there is information available on other substances such as carotenoids and flavonoids.
- There is now a considerable body of evidence that shows that diets rich in plant foods are generally associated with lower disease risks. In the search for the specific constituents that confer this benefit, attention has to date been focused on constituents with anti-oxidant properties, initially vitamins E and C and the carotenoids, but increasingly other plant-derived antioxidants, such as flavonoids have become the focus.
- Whether or not a plant constituent is provided in a bioavailable form in a food is crucial to the food's nutritional value. Interactions can also occur between the constituents present in foods, for example polyphenols present in plant-derived foods can inhibit uptake of iron from the same or other foods.

2
Classification and Biosynthesis of Secondary Plant Products: An Overview

2.1 Introduction

Plants synthesise a vast range of organic compounds that traditionally are classified as primary and secondary metabolites, although the precise boundaries between the two groups can in some instances be somewhat blurred. Primary metabolites are compounds that have essential roles, being associated with photosynthesis, respiration and growth and development. The compounds include phytosterols, acyl lipids, nucleotides, amino acids and organic acids. Other compounds, many of which accumulate in surprisingly high concentrations in some species, are referred to as secondary metabolites. They are diverse structurally and many secondary metabolites are distributed among a very limited number of species within the plant kingdom and so can be diagnostic in chemotaxonomic studies. Although long ignored, the function of these compounds in plants is now attracting attention. Some appear to have a key role in protection against herbivores and microbial infection, as attractants for pollinators and seed-dispersing animals, as allelopathic agents, as UV protectants and as signal molecules in the formation of nitrogen fixing root nodules in legumes. Secondary metabolites are also of interest because of their use as dyes, fibres, glues, oils, waxes, flavouring agents, drugs and perfumes and they are viewed as potential sources of new natural drugs, antibiotics, insecticides and herbicides (Croteau *et al.*, 2000).

In recent years the role of some secondary metabolites as potential protective dietary constituents has become an increasingly important area of human nutrition research. Unlike the 'traditional' nutrients (see Chapter 1), they appear not to be essential for short-term well being, but there is increasing evidence that long-term intakes may have favourable impacts on the incidence of cancers and many chronic diseases, including cardiovascular disease, which are occurring in Western populations with increasing frequency.

Based on their biosynthetic origins, plant secondary metabolites can be divided into three major groups:

- flavonoids and allied phenolic and polyphenolic compounds
- terpenoids
- nitrogen-containing alkaloids and sulphur-containing compounds.

2.2 Classification of phenolic compounds

Phenolics are secondary plant metabolites, characterised by having at least one aromatic ring with one or more hydroxyl groups attached. In excess of 8000 phenolic structures have been reported and they are widely dispersed throughout the plant kingdom (Strack & Wray, 1994; Strack, 1997). The nature and distribution of phenolics can vary depending on the plant tissue, with many of the phenolics synthesized from carbohydrates via the shikimate and phenylpropanoid pathways (Fig. 2.1). Phenolics range from simple, low molecular weight, single aromatic-ringed compounds to the large and complex tannins. They can be classified by the number

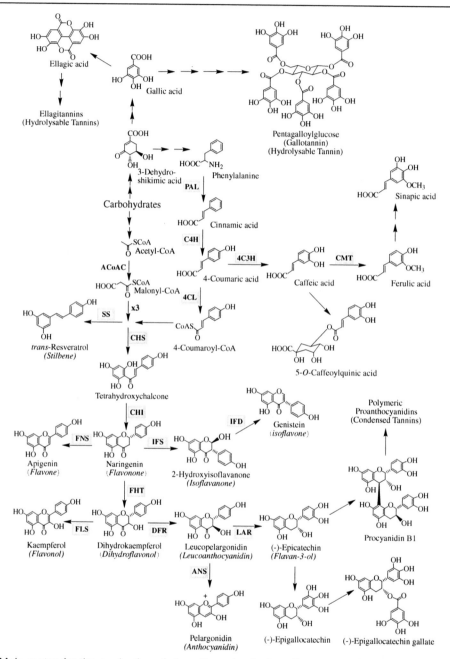

Fig. 2.1   Main routes for the production of phenolic and polyphenolic compounds via the shikimic acid, phenylpropanoid and flavonoid biosynthesis pathways. Enzyme abbreviations: PAL, phenylalanine ammonia-lyase; C4H, cinnamate 4-hydroxylase; 4C3H, 4-coumarate 3-hydroxylase; CMT, caffeate methyl transferase, 4CL, 4-coumarate:CoA ligase; SS, stilbene synthase; CHS, chalcone synthase; CHI, chalcone isomerase; IFS, 2-hydroxyisoflavone synthase; IFD, 2-hydroxyisoflavanone dehydratase; FNS, flavone synthase; FHT, flavanone 3-hydroxylase; FLS, flavonol synthase; DFR, dihydroflavonol 4-reductase; ANS, anthocyanidin 4-reductase; LAR, leucoanthocyanidin 4-reductase.

Table 2.1 Basic structures of phenolic and polyphenolic compounds.

Carbon No.	Skeleton	Classification	Example	Basic structure
7	C_6–C_1	Phenolic acids	Gallic acid	
8	C_6–C_2	Acetophenones	Xanthoxylin	
8	C_6–C_2	Phenylacetic acid	*p*-Hydroxyphenyl-acetic acid	
9	C_6–C_3	Hydroxycinnamic acids	Caffeic acid	
9	C_6–C_3	Coumarins	Esculetin	
10	C_6–C_4	Naphthoquinones	Juglone	
13	C_6–C_1–C_6	Xanthones	Gentisin	
14	C_6–C_2–C_6	Stilbenes	Resveratrol	
15	C_6–C_3–C_3	Flavonoids	Quercetin	

and arrangement of their carbon atoms (Table 2.1) and are commonly found conjugated to sugars and organic acids. Phenolics can be classified into two groups, the flavonoids and the non-flavonoids.

2.3 Flavonoids

Flavonoids are polyphenolic compounds comprising 15 carbons, with two aromatic rings connected by a three carbon bridge (Fig. 2.2). They are the most numerous of the phenolics, and are found throughout the plant kingdom. They are present in high concentrations in the epidermis of leaves and the skin of fruits and have important and varied roles as secondary metabolites. In plants, flavonoids are involved in such diverse processes as UV protection, pigmentation, stimulation of nitrogen-fixing nodules and disease resistance (Koes *et al.*, 1994; Pierpoint, 2000).

The C_6–C_3–C_6 flavonoid structure is the product of two separate biosynthetic pathways (Figs 2.1 and 2.3). The bridge and one aromatic ring, ring B, constitute a phenylpropanoid unit synthesised from phenylalanine, which itself is a product of the shikimic acid pathway. The six carbons of ring A originate from the condensation of three acetate units via the malonic acid pathway. The fusion of these two parts involves the stepwise condensation of a phenylpropanoid, 4-coumaryl CoA, with three malonyl CoA residues, each of which donates two carbon atoms, in a reaction catalysed by chalcone synthase. Tetrahydroxychalcone, the product of this reaction, gives rise to all the other types of flavonoids via the flavonoid biosynthesis pathway (Fig. 2.1).

The main sub-classes of flavonoids are the flavones, flavonols, flavan-3-ols, isoflavones, flavanones and anthocyanidins (Fig. 2.2). Other flavonoid groups, that are of less importance from a dietary perspective, are dihydroflavones, flavan-3,4-diols, coumarins, chalcones, dihydrochalcones and aurones (Fig. 2.4). The basic flavonoid skeleton can have numerous substituents. Hydroxyl groups are usually present at the 4-, 5- and 7-positions. Sugars are very common, with the majority of flavonoids existing naturally as glycosides. Whereas both sugars and hydroxyl groups increase the water solubility of flavonoids, other substituents, such as methyl and isopentyl groups make flavonoids lipophilic.

2.3.1 Flavonols

Flavonols are arguably the most widespread of the flavonoids, being dispersed throughout the plant kingdom with the exception of fungi and algae (see in particular Chapters 7 and 9). The distribution and structural variations of flavonols

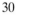

Fig. 2.2 Generic structures of the major flavonoids.

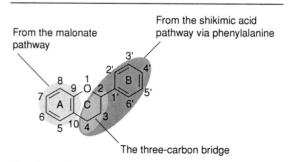

Fig. 2.3 Basic structure and biosynthetic origin of the flavonoid skeleton.

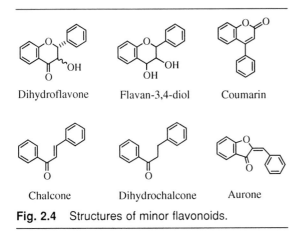

Dihydroflavone　　Flavan-3,4-diol　　Coumarin

Chalcone　　Dihydrochalcone　　Aurone

Fig. 2.4　Structures of minor flavonoids.

are extensive and have been well documented (Williams & Harborne, 1992; Wollenweber, 1992). Flavonols such as myricetin, quercetin, isorhamnetin and kaempferol (Fig. 2.5) are most commonly found as *O*-glycosides. Conjugation occurs most commonly at the 3-position of the C ring, although 5, 7, 4′, 3′ and 5′ substitutions also occur (Herrmann, 1976). Although the number of aglycones is limited, there are numerous flavonol conjugates, with more than 200 different sugar conjugates of kaempferol alone (Strack & Wray, 1994). There is extensive information on the levels of flavonols found in commonly consumed fruits, vegetables and beverages (Hertog *et al.*,

1992, 1993c). However, sizeable differences are found in the amounts present in seemingly similar produce, possibly due to seasonal changes and varietal differences (Crozier *et al.*, 1997, 2000).

2.3.2　Flavones

Flavones have a very close structural relationship to the flavonols (see Fig. 2.2). Although flavones such as luteolin and apigenin have A and C ring substitutions, they lack oxygenation at C3 (Fig. 2.6). A wide range of substitutions is also possible with flavones, including hydroxylation, methylation, *O*- and *C*-alkylation and *O*- and *C*-glycosylation. Most flavones occur as 7-*O*-glycosides (Bohm, 1998). Unlike flavonols, flavones are not widely distributed. The only significant occurrences of flavones are in celery, parsley and some other herbs (see Chapter 11). In addition, polymethoxylated flavones, such as nobiletin and tangeretin, have been found in citrus species (Ooghe *et al.*, 1994).

2.3.3　Flavan-3-ols

Flavan-3-ols (sometimes referred to as flavanols) are the most complex subclass of flavonoids, ranging from the simple monomers (+)-catechin and its isomer (−)-epicatechin, to the oligomeric and polymeric proanthocyanidins, which are also known as condensed tannins (Fig. 2.7).

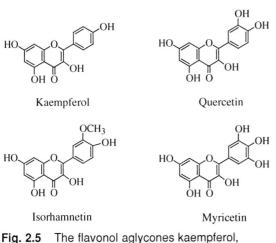

Kaempferol　　Quercetin

Isorhamnetin　　Myricetin

Fig. 2.5　The flavonol aglycones kaempferol, quercetin, isorhamnetin and myricetin.

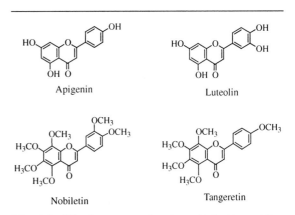

Apigenin　　Luteolin

Nobiletin　　Tangeretin

Fig. 2.6　The flavones, apigenin and luteolin and the polymethoxylated flavones nobiletin and tangeretin.

Proanthocyanidins are formed from (+)-catechin and (–)-epicatechin with oxidative coupling occurring between the C4 of the heterocycle and the C6 or C8 positions of the adjacent unit. Proanthocyanidins can occur as polymers of up to 50 units. In addition to forming such complexes, flavan-3-ols are hydroxylated to form gallocatechins, and also undergo esterification with gallic acid (Fig. 2.7).

Red wines (see Chapter 9) contain oligomeric proanthocyanidins derived mainly from the seeds of black grapes. Green tea (Chapter 9) is also a rich source of flavan-3-ols, principally (–)-epigallocatechin, (–)-epigallocatechin gallate and (–)-epicatechin gallate (Fig. 2.7). The levels of catechins decline during fermentation of the tea leaves and the main components in black tea are

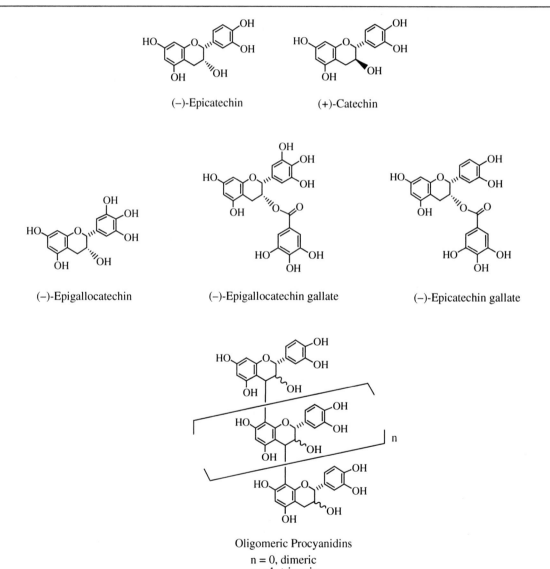

(–)-Epicatechin

(+)-Catechin

(–)-Epigallocatechin

(–)-Epigallocatechin gallate

(–)-Epicatechin gallate

Oligomeric Procyanidins
n = 0, dimeric
n = 1, trimeric
n = 2, tetrameric

Fig. 2.7   Flavan-3-ol structures.

high molecular weight thearubigins (Balentine *et al.*, 1997; Davies *et al.*, 1998). Whilst these can reasonably be described as flavonoid derived, their structures are unknown.

2.3.4 Anthocyanidins

Anthocyanidins, principally as their conjugated derivatives, anthocyanins, are widely dispersed in the plant kingdom being particularly evident in fruit (Chapter 7) and flower tissues where they are responsible for the red, blue and purple colours. In addition, they are also found in leaves, stems, seeds and root tissue (Strack & Wray, 1994). They are involved in the protection of plants against excessive light by shading leaf mesophyll cells. In addition, they have an important role to play in the attraction of pollinating insects.

The most common anthocyanidins are pelargonidin, cyanidin, delphinidin, peonidin, petunidin and malvidin (Fig. 2.8). In plant tissues

Anthocyanidin	R_1	R_2	Colour
Pelargonidin	H	H	orange-red
Cyanidin	OH	H	red
Delphinidin	OH	OH	pink
Peonidin	OCH_3	H	bluish purple
Petunidin	OCH_3	OH	purple
Malvidin	OCH_3	OCH_3	reddish purple

Fig. 2.8 Structures of major anthocyanidins.

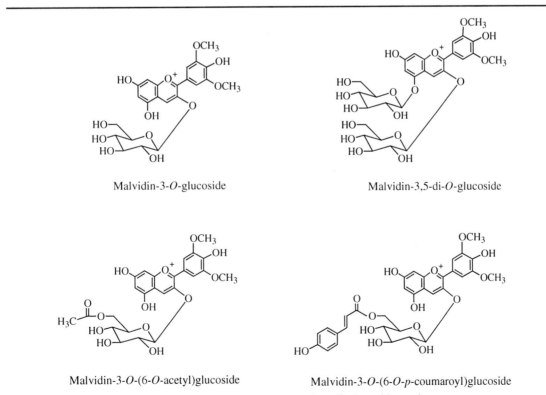

Malvidin-3-*O*-glucoside

Malvidin-3,5-di-*O*-glucoside

Malvidin-3-*O*-(6-*O*-acetyl)glucoside

Malvidin-3-*O*-(6-*O*-*p*-coumaroyl)glucoside

Fig. 2.9 Anthocyanin structures: different types of malvidin-3-*O*-glycoside conjugates.

these compounds are invariably found as sugar conjugates that are known as anthocyanins. They also form conjugates with hydroxycinnamates and organic acids such as malic and acetic acid. Although conjugation can take place on carbons 3, 5, 7, 3′ and 5′, it occurs most often on C3 (Fig. 2.9).

2.3.5 Flavanones

The flavanones are the first flavonoid products of the flavonoid biosynthetic pathway (Fig. 2.1). They are characterised by the absence of the C2–C3 double bond and the presence of a chiral centre at C2 (Fig. 2.2). In the majority of naturally occurring flavanones, ring C is attached to the B ring at C2 in the α-configuration. The flavanone structure is highly reactive and flavanones have been reported to undergo hydroxylation, glycosylation and *O*-methylation reactions. Flavanones are present in especially high concentrations in citrus fruits. The most common flavanone glycoside is hesperidin (hesperetin-7-*O*-rutinoside), which is found in citrus peel (Fig. 2.10). Flavanone rutinosides are tasteless. In

contrast, flavanone neohesperidoside conjugates such as neohesperidin (hesperetin-7-*O*-neohesperidoside) from bitter orange (*Citrus aurantium*) and naringin (naringenin-7-*O*-neohesperidoside) (Fig. 2.10) from grapefruit peel (*Citrus paradisi*) have an intensely bitter taste (Bohm, 1998).

2.3.6 Isoflavones

Isoflavones are also derived from the flavonoid biosynthetic pathway, with naringenin being converted to genistein via 2-hydroxyisoflavanone (Fig. 2.1). Hydroxylation of genistein at C5 then yields daidzein (Fig. 2.11). Isoflavones are characterised by having the B ring attached at C3 rather than the C2 position (Fig. 2.3). They are found throughout the plant kingdom, but the principal source is legumes such as soya bean (*Glycine max*) (see Chapter 8). As with the rest of the flavonoid family, isoflavones such as genistein undergo hydroxylation and methylation reactions, in addition to prenylation, yielding a range of isoflavonoids including coumestans, rotenoids and pterocarpins (Fig. 2.11) (Dewick, 2002).

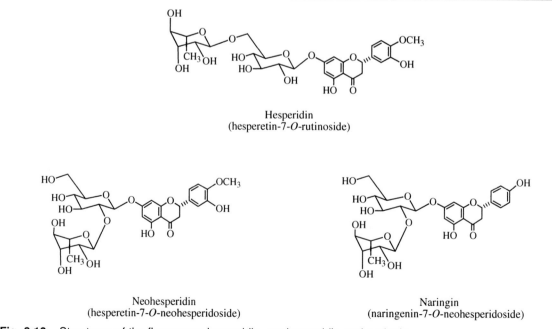

Hesperidin
(hesperetin-7-*O*-rutinoside)

Neohesperidin
(hesperetin-7-*O*-neohesperidoside)

Naringin
(naringenin-7-*O*-neohesperidoside)

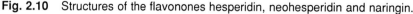

Fig. 2.10   Structures of the flavonones hesperidin, neohesperidin and naringin.

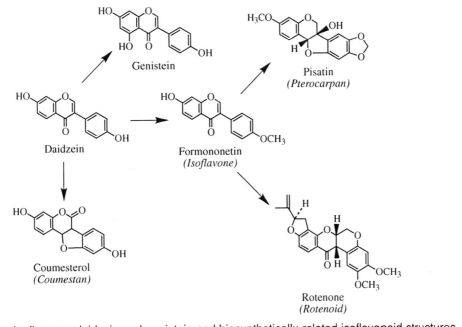

Fig. 2.11   The isoflavones daidzein and genistein and biosynthetically-related isoflavonoid structures.

The soya-derived isoflavones genistein and daidzein and the coumestan coumestrol, from lucerne and clovers (*Trifolium spp.*), have sufficient oestrogenic activity to affect seriously the reproduction of grazing animals such as cows and sheep and are termed phytoestrogens. The structure of these isoflavonoids is such that they appear to mimic the steroidal hormone oestradiol (Fig. 2.12), which blocks ovulation. The consumption of legume fodder by animals must therefore be restricted or low isoflavonoid producing varieties selected.

Dietary consumption of genistein and daidzein from soya products is thought to reduce the incidence of prostate and breast cancers in humans. However, the mechanisms involved are different. Growth of prostate cancer cells is induced by and dependent upon the androgen testosterone (Fig. 2.12), the production of which is suppressed by oestrodiol. When natural oestradiol is insufficient, the isoflavones can lower androgen levels and, as a consequence, inhibit tumour growth. Breast cancers are dependent upon a supply of oestrogens for growth especially during the early stages. Isoflavones compete with natural oestrogens, restricting their availability thereby suppressing the growth of the cancerous cells.

2.4 Non-flavonoids

The main non-flavonoids of dietary significance are the C_6–C_1 phenolic acids, most notably gallic acid and its dimer ellagic acid, which are the source of the hydrolysable tannins, the C_6–C_3 hydroxycinnamates and their conjugated derivatives, and polyphenolic C_6–C_2–C_6 stilbenes (Fig. 2.1, Table 2.1). See Chapter 6 for further information.

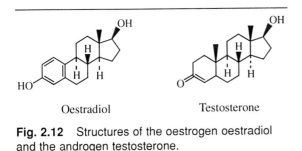

Fig. 2.12   Structures of the oestrogen oestradiol and the androgen testosterone.

2.4.1 Phenolic acids

Phenolic acids are also known as hydroxybenzoates, the principal component being gallic acid. Its name comes from *galle*, the French term for a swelling in the tissue of a plant after attack by parasitic insects. The swelling is from a build-up of carbohydrate and other nutrients that support the growing insect larvae. It has been reported that the phenolic composition of the gall consists of up to 70% gallic acid esters (Gross, 1992).

Although alternative routes exist from hydroxybenzoic acids, gallic acid appears to be formed primarily via the shikimic acid pathway from 3-dehydroshikimic acid (Fig. 2.1). Gallic acid is converted to ellagic acid and to pentagalloylglucose and a range of gallotannins. Ellagic acid is the basic unit of the ellagitannins, which together with the gallotannins are referred to as hydrolysable tannins (Fig. 2.1). Hydrolysable tannins, as their name suggests, are more readily hydrolysed by treatment with dilute acid than condensed tannins (see Section 2.3.3).

Condensed tannins and hydrolysable tannins are capable of binding to and precipitating the collagen proteins in animal hides. This changes the hide into leather, making it resistant to putrefaction. Plant-derived tannins have therefore formed the basis of the tanning industry for many years (Bohm, 1998).

Tannins bind to salivary proteins, producing a taste which humans recognise as astringency. Mild astringency enhances the taste and texture of a number of foods and beverages, most notably tea and red wines. Many tannins are extremely astringent and render plant tissues inedible. Mammals such as cattle, deer and apes characteristically avoid eating plants with high tannin contents. Many unripe fruits have a very high tannin content, typically concentrated in the outer cell layers. Tannin levels decline as the fruits mature and the seeds ripen. This may have been an evolutionary benefit, delaying the eating of the fruit until the seeds were capable of germinating.

It has been suggested that lack of tolerance to tannins may be one reason for the demise of the red squirrel. The grey squirrel is able to consume hazelnuts before they mature, and to survive on acorns. In contrast, the red squirrel has to wait until hazelnuts are ripe before they become palatable, and is much less able to survive on a diet of acorns, which are the only thing left after the grey squirrels have eaten the immature hazelnuts (Haslam, 1998).

Tannins can bind to dietary proteins in the gut and this process can have a negative impact on herbivore nutrition. The tannins can inactivate herbivore digestive enzymes creating aggregates of tannins and plant proteins that are difficult to digest. Herbivores that regularly feed on tannin-rich plant material appear to possess some interesting adaptations to remove tannins from their digestive systems. For instance, rodents and rabbits produce salivary proteins with a very high proline content (25–45%) that have a high affinity for tannins. Secretion of these proteins is induced by ingestion of food with a high tannin content and greatly diminishes the toxic effects of the tannins (Butler, 1989).

2.4.2 Hydroxycinnamates

Cinnamic acid is a C_6–C_3 compound produced by phenylalanine ammonia lyase-catalysed deamination of the amino acid phenylalanine (Fig. 2.1), a reaction believed to be common to all plants. 4-Coumaric acid (alias *p*-coumaric acid) is then produced by hydroxylation of cinnamic acid. The most common hydroxycinnamates are caffeic, 4-coumaric, ferulic and sinapic acids, which are produced by a series of hydroxylation and methylation reactions (Fig. 2.1) and often accumulate as their respective tartarate esters, coutaric, caftaric and fertaric acids (Fig. 2.13). The quinic acid conjugate of caffeic acid, 5-*O*-caffeoylquinic acid (chlorogenic acid) (Fig. 2.13), is a common component of fruits and vegetables. Cinnamic acid and its hydroxycinnamate derivatives are products of the phenylpropanoid pathway and are referred to collectively as phenylpropanoids.

2.4.3 Stilbenes

Members of the stilbene family have a C_6–C_2–C_6 structure (Table 2.1) and, thus, like flavonoids are polyphenolic compounds. Stilbenes are

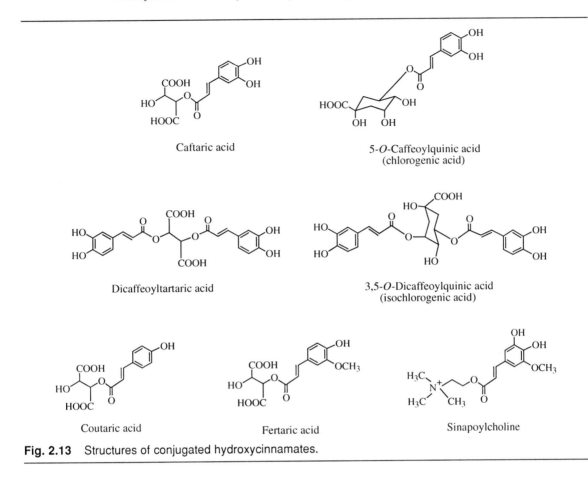

Fig. 2.13 Structures of conjugated hydroxycinnamates.

phytoalexins, compounds produced by plants in response to attack by fungal, bacterial and viral pathogens. *trans*-Resveratrol (see Chapter 8) is synthesised by condensation of 4-coumaroyl CoA with three units of malonyl CoA, each of which donates two carbon atoms, in a reaction catalysed by stilbene synthase (Fig. 2.1). The same substrate yields tetrahydroxychalcone, the immediate precursor of flavonoids, when catalysed by chalcone synthase. Stilbene synthase and chalcone synthase have been shown to be structurally very similar and it is believed that both are members of a family of polyketide enzymes (Soleas *et al.*, 1997). Chalcone synthase is constitutively present in tissues, while stilbene synthase is induced only by a range of stresses including UV radiation, trauma and infection. Resveratrol is found as both the *cis* and *trans* isomers and is present in plant tissues primarily as *trans*-resveratrol-3-*O*-glucoside, which is known as piceid and polydatin (Fig. 2.14).

2.5 Terpenoids

There are more than 25 000 terpenoids, which are structurally very diverse and are classified according to the number of C_5 isoprenoid units incorporated. The main groups include hemiterpenes (C_5), monoterpenes (C_{10}), sesquiterpenes (C_{15}), diterpenes (C_{20}), sesterterpenes (C_{25}), triterpenes (C_{30}), tetraterpenes (C_{40}) and higher terpenoids. Many of the compounds involved are medicinal, therapeutic and flavouring agents. Within the category are the carotenoids, which are C_{40} terpenoids (*i.e.* tetraterpenes).

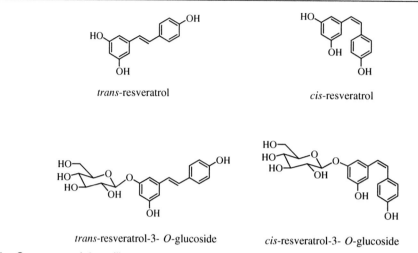

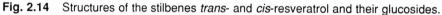

trans-resveratrol-3- *O*-glucoside   *cis*-resveratrol-3- *O*-glucoside

Fig. 2.14   Structures of the stilbenes *trans*- and *cis*-resveratrol and their glucosides.

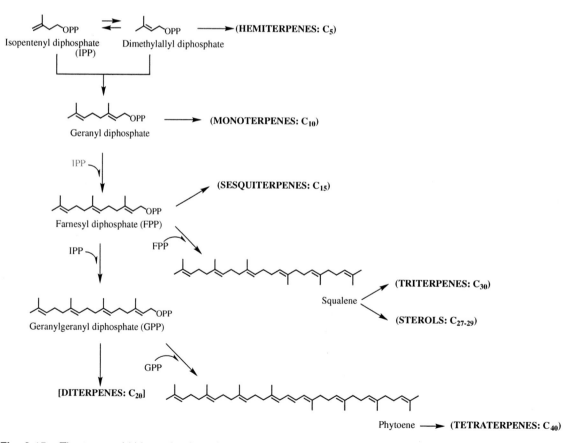

Fig. 2.15   The terpenoid biosynthesis pathway.

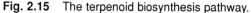

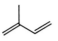

Isoprene

Fig. 2.16 Structure of isoprene, one of a limited number of naturally occurring hemiterpenoids.

All terpenoids are derived from the five-carbon isoprenoid precursor isopentenyl diphosphate (IPP) as outlined in Fig. 2.15. It has recently been discovered that there are two biosynthetic routes to IPP: the classical mevalonate pathway in the cytosol and the deoxyxylulose pathway in plastids. Sesquiterpenoids and sterols are predominantly synthesised in the cytosol by the mevalonate pathway, whereas monoterpenoids, diterpenoids and carotenoids (tetraterpenes) are synthesised in plastids via the deoxyxylulose pathway. There is, however, evidence of a small amount of cross-talk between the pathways, implying that they are not totally autonomous.

2.5.1 Hemiterpenes (C₅)

There are relatively few hemiterpenes in nature, with isoprene (Fig. 2.16), a volatile compound that is released by many plants, being an exception. Dimethylallyl diphosphate (DMAPP) and IPP are reactive hemiterpene intermediates leading to more complex terpenoid structures (Fig. 2.15).

2.5.2 Monoterpenes (C₁₀)

The prenyl transferase-catalysed condensation of DMAPP and IPP leads to the production of the monoterpene geranyl diphosphate which, depending upon the species, is the source of a range of monoterpenes that are components of volatile oils used in flavouring and perfumery. Typical examples include geranial (lemon oil, *Citrus limon*), β-myrcene (hops, *Humulus lupulus*), nerol (rose oil, *Rosa* spp.), linalool (coriander oil, *Coriandrum sativum*), (–)-menthol (peppermint, *Mentha* × *piperita*) and (+)-limonene and (–)-limonene, which have the fragrance of oranges (*Citrus sinensis*) and lemons, respectively. Limonene is the

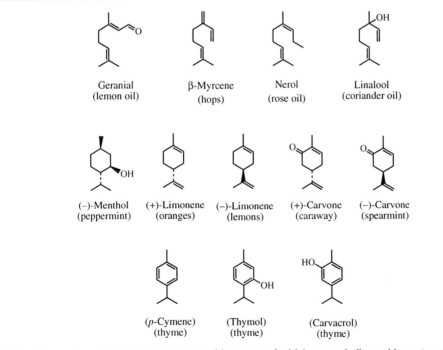

Geranial (lemon oil)   β-Myrcene (hops)   Nerol (rose oil)   Linalool (coriander oil)

(–)-Menthol (peppermint)   (+)-Limonene (oranges)   (–)-Limonene (lemons)   (+)-Carvone (caraway)   (–)-Carvone (spearmint)

(*p*-Cymene) (thyme)   (Thymol) (thyme)   (Carvacrol) (thyme)

Fig. 2.17 Structures of selected monoterpenoids, many of which are volatile and impart a characteristic smell.

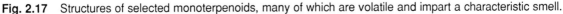

precursor of carvone; (+)-carvone provides the characteristic odour of caraway (*Carum carvi*) while (−)-carvone smells of spearmint (*Mentha spicata*). Thyme (*Thymus vulgaris*) contains *p*-cymene, thymol and carvacrol (Fig. 2.17).

2.5.3 Sesquiterpenes (C₁₅)

A further condensation involving the C_5 IPP and geranyl diphosphate results in the formation of the farnesyl diphosphate (Fig. 2.15), which is the precursor of numerous cyclic sesquiterpenes in the cytosol including γ-bisabolene and (−)-zingiberene, which contribute to the aroma of ginger (*Zingiber officinale*). Sesquiterpenoids are less volatile than diterpenoids. Other C_{15} compounds include α-bisabolol, which is a major component in German chamomile (flowers of *Matricaria chamomilla*), and α-cadinene, which is one of many terpenoids found in juniper berries (*Juniperus communis*), used in making gin. Further cyclisations lead to ring systems larger than six carbons as exemplified by α-santonin from wormseed (*Artemisia cinia*) and related species, which are used for the removal of roundworms. Additional modifications lead to the production of more complex structures such as the

dimeric sesquiterpene gossypol, which is found in immature flower buds and seeds of cotton (*Gossypium* spp.). Gossypol is a male infertility agent and is used in China as a male contraceptive. The structures of these sesquiterpenoids are illustrated in Fig. 2.18.

2.5.4 Diterpenes (C20)

Diterpenes are synthesised from geranylgeranyl diphosphate, which is produced by the addition of IPP to farnesyl diphosphate (Fig. 2.15). Cyclisation of geranylgeranyl diphosphate facilitates the synthesis of many diterpenoid derivatives. The common yew (*Taxus baccata*) contains 11 compounds based on the taxadene skeleton, a structure that features in paclitaxel (taxol), the anticancer agent from Pacific yew (*Taxus brevifolia*) (Fig. 2.19). The side-chains of taxol containing aromatic rings originate from shikimate via phenylalanine (see Fig. 2.1). Other modifications of the diterpenoid skeleton are involved in the synthesis of highly oxidised diterpene trilactones such as ginkgolide A (Fig. 2.19) in *Ginkgo biloba*, extracts of which are marketed extensively as a remedy against a variety of ailments including a decline in cognitive function and memory processes.

ent-Kaurene is a cyclic diterpene and the precursor of gibberellins which regulate a number of key processes in higher plant growth and development, including germination and stem elongation. In *Stevia rebaudiana*, *ent*-kaurene is converted to the triglycoside conjugate stevioside (Fig. 2.19) which accumulates in the leaf in concentrations of up to 10%. Stevioside is more than 100 times sweeter than sucrose and is used commercially as a sweetening agent.

2.5.5 Triterpenoids (C₃₀)

Two molecules of farnesyl diphosphate join tail-to-tail to yield squalene (Fig. 2.15) the precursor of triterpenoids, such as cucurbitacin E, which is found in members of the Cucurbitaceae, and sterols (see Chapter 10), including sitosterol and stigmasterol, which are produced commercially from soya beans (*Glycine max*) and used to produce medicinal steroids (Fig. 2.20). Other C_{30}

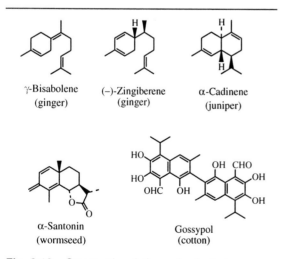

γ-Bisabolene
(ginger)

(−)-Zingiberene
(ginger)

α-Cadinene
(juniper)

α-Santonin
(wormseed)

Gossypol
(cotton)

Fig. 2.18 Structural variations of selected sesquiterpenoids.

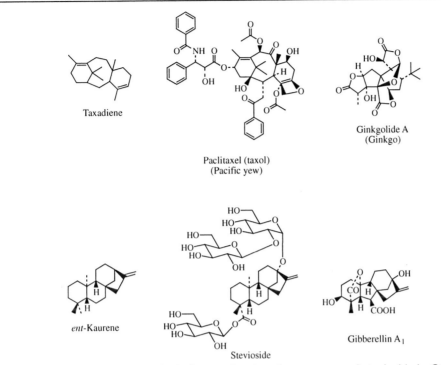

Fig. 2.19 Diterpenoid structures, including *ent*-kaurine, the precursor of stevioside in *Stevia rebaudiana* and, more typically in other plants, gibberellins such as giberellin A$_1$.

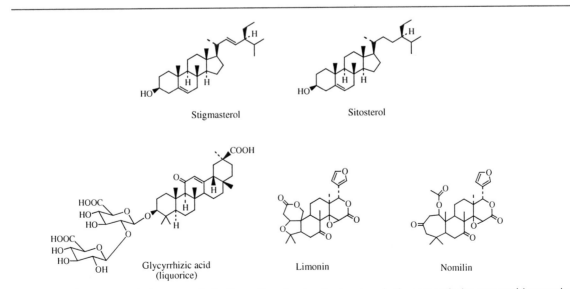

Fig. 2.20 Structures of triterpene derivatives: the sterols sitosterol and stigmasterol; the terpenoid saponin glycyrrhizic acid from liquorice root; and the limonoids limonin and nomilin, which are modified triterpenoids.

derivatives include triterpenoid saponins, such as glycyrrhetic acid, which is found as a diglucuronide conjugate, glycyrrhizic acid (Fig. 2.20), in liquorice root (*Glycyrrhiza glabra*). Modified triterpenoids include limonoids such as limonin and nomilin, which occur in *Citrus* species (Fig. 2.20)

2.5.6 Tetraterpenoids (C_{40})

Carotenoids are the sole tetraterpenoid group although numerous variations on the basic structure occur in nature (see Chapters 6 and 7). In plants, carotenoids have a role along with chloro-

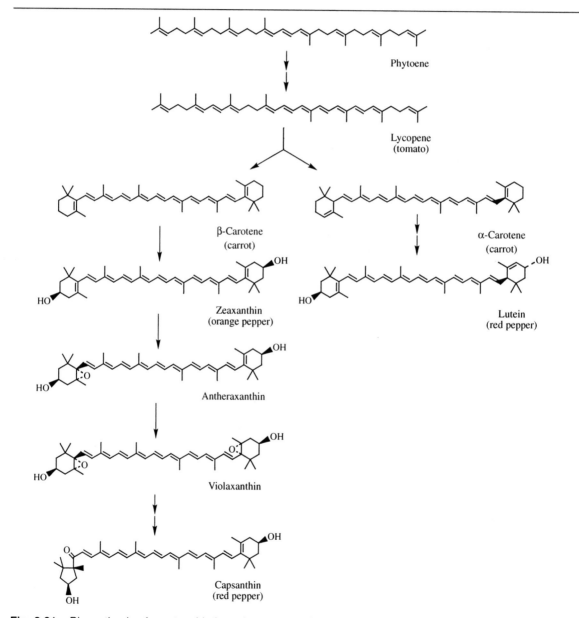

Fig. 2.21 Biosynthesis of carotenoids from the tetrapenoid precursor phytoene.

phyll in photosynthesis as accessory light-harvesting pigments, extending the range of light absorbed by the photosynthetic apparatus. There is also evidence that in humans they are important dietary antioxidants, scavenging free radicals and minimising cell damage, and so might provide protection against some forms of cancer (see Chapter 4). Some carotenoids, *e.g.* β-carotene, are precursors of vitamin A (retinol) (see below and Chapters 1 and 3).

Synthesis of the tetrapene skeleton phytoene involves a tail-to-tail condensation of two molecules of geranylgeranyl diphosphate (Fig. 2.15). Phytoene undergoes structural modification and

is converted to lycopene, which occurs widely in plants and is a significant dietary component because of its presence as the red colorant in tomatoes (*Lycopersicon esculentum* Mill) and tomato-based products. Lycopene is the precursor of both β- and α-carotene, which are responsible for the orange colour of carrots. Lutein, the colorant of yellow peppers (*Capsieum annuum*), is derived from α-carotene, while β-carotene is oxidised via a zeaxanthin → antheraxanthin → violaxanthin → capsanthin pathway (Fig. 2.21). Zeaxanthin accumulates in orange pepper, while capsanthin, the bright red pigment of peppers, is a metabolite of violaxanthin (Fig. 2.21). The pink–red colour of crustaceans, shellfish and salmon is due to astaxanthin (Fig. 2.22). These animals are unable to synthesise carotenoids, and astaxanthin is produced by metabolism of dietary plant carotenoids such as β-carotene.

The A vitamins are metabolites of dietary carotenoids. Vitamin A_1 (retinol), is produced in mammals primarily by oxidative metabolism of β-carotene in the mucosal cells of the intestine. Retinal is produced, which is reduced yielding retinol, which can undergo reduction to form dehydroretinol (Vitamin A_2) (Fig. 2.23). Retinol and its derivatives are found only in animals and animal-based products. Cod-liver oil and halibut-liver oil are rich sources used as dietary supplements.

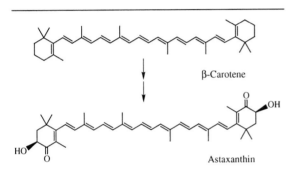

Fig. 2.22 Astaxanthin is produced in crayfish, shellfish and salmon from dietary carotenoids such as β-carotene.

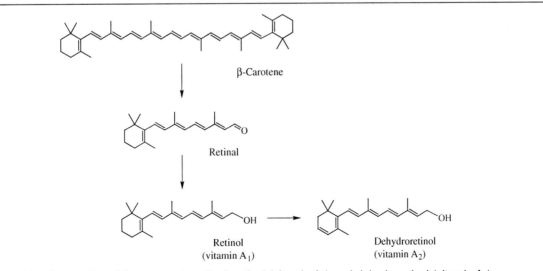

Fig. 2.23 Conversion of β-carotene to retinal, retinol (vitamin A_1) and dehydroretinol (vitamin A_2).

2.5.7 Higher terpenoids

Terpenoid fragments containing several isoprene units are found as alkyl substituents in shikimate-derived quinones. Ubiquinones (co-enzyme Q), which are found in all organisms and function as electron carriers for the electron transport chain in mitochondria, typically have C_{40}–C_{50} side-chains (Fig. 2.24). Even longer polyisoprene side-chains are encountered in rubber (Fig. 2.24), a natural polymer from *Hevea brasiliensis*.

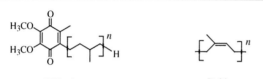

Ubiquinone-n
(Coenzyme Qn)

Rubber
($n = 10^3$–10^5)

Fig. 2.24 Structures of the higher terpenoids ubiquinone and rubber.

2.6 Alkaloids and sulphur-containing compounds

2.6.1 Alkaloids

There are 12 000 or so alkaloids, which contain one or more nitrogen atoms. We now know that alkaloids were the active ingredients in numerous potions and poisons that humans have used for thousands of years. In the last century BC, Cleopatra used extracts of henbane (*Hyoscyamus niger*), which contains atropine (Fig. 2.25), to dilate her pupils and appear more alluring to her male political rivals. During his execution in 339 BC, Socrates drank an extract of hemlock (*Conium maculatum*), which contains coniine (Fig. 2.25), an alkaloid that is extremely toxic, causing paralysis of motor nerve endings. Alkaloid-containing plants were mankind's original '*materia medica*'. Many, including codeine (Fig. 2.25) from the opium poppy (*Papaver somniferum*), are still in use today as prescription drugs. In addition to

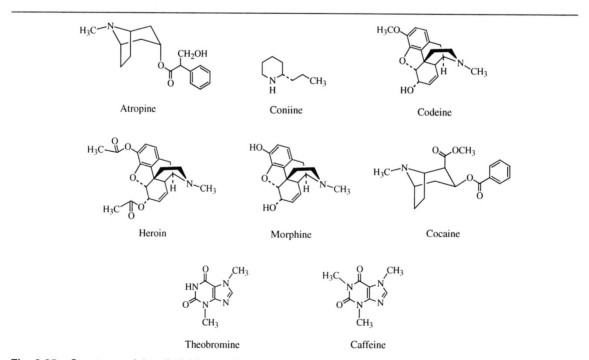

Atropine

Coniine

Codeine

Heroin

Morphine

Cocaine

Theobromine

Caffeine

Fig. 2.25 Structures of the alkaloids atropine, coniine, codeine, opium, morphine and its acetylated derivative heroin and cocaine and the purine alkaloids caffeine and theobromine.

having a strong influence on modern medicine, alkaloids have also influenced world politics. Notorious examples include the opium wars between China and the Britain in the 19th century and the efforts currently under way to eradicate illicit production of heroin, a semi-synthetic compound produced by acetylation of morphine, also a constituent of the opium poppy, and cocaine (Fig. 2.25), a naturally occurring alkaloid of coca (*Erythroxylon coca*).

The biosynthesis of most alkaloids is not understood, although early studies in the 1950s established that in most cases they are formed from the L-amino acids tryptophan, tyrosine, phenylalanine, ornithine, lysine and arginine, either alone or in combination with a steroidal or other terpenoid moiety. However, not all alkaloids are derived from an amino acid core. The well-known purine

alkaloids caffeine and theobromine (Fig. 2.25), which are key components in beverages from coffee beans (*Coffea arabica*), tea leaves (*Camellia sinensis*) and cocoa (*Theobroma cacao*), are synthesised from purine nucleotides (see Chapter 9).

2.6.2 Sulphur-containing compounds

Glucosinolates are found in members of the Brassicaceae. They are nitrogen- and sulphur-containing glucosides which in damaged tissues come into contact with myrosinase and are hydrolysed releasing the aglycone. Glucosinolates of interest include sinalbin in white mustard (*Sinapsis alba*) and sinigrin in black mustard (*Brassica nigra*), as well as the indole glucosino-late glucobrassicin (see Chapter 7), which is found in a number of Brassica species including

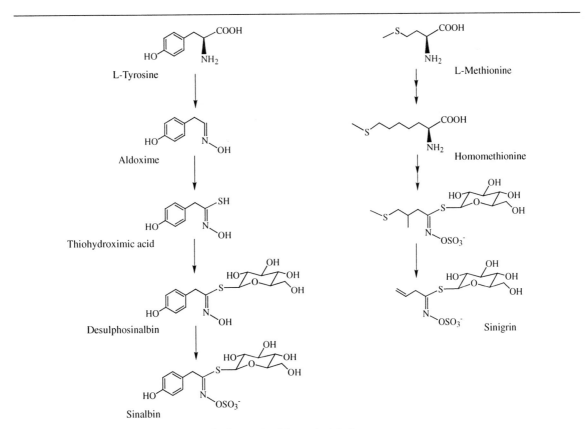

Fig. 2.26 Biosynthesis of the glucosinolates sinalbin and sinigrin.

horseradish (*Armoracia rusticana*) and canola (*Brassica napus*). Sinalbin is synthesised from L-tyrosine. The amino acid first forms aldoxime, which incorporates sulphur from methionine yielding thiohydroximic acid, which is *S*-glycosylated before being sulphonated to produce sinalbin (Fig. 2.26). L-Methionine, which first undergoes chain extension to form homomethionine, is the precursor of sinigrin (Fig. 2.26). L-Tryptophan is the precursor of glucobrassicin. The usefulness of canola seed as an animal feed has been limited in part by the bitter taste of glucobrassicin. Genetically engineered canola has been produced that has been transformed with a gene encoding tryptophan decarboxylase, which redirects the L-tryptophan pool away from glucobrassicin and into tryptamine (Fig. 2.27). The tryptamine is further metabolised and so does not accumulate, and the mature canola seeds contain less glucobrassicin, making them more suitable as an animal feed and a potentially more economically useful product.

Allium species are rich in sulphur-containing compounds. Chives contain *S*-propylcysteine sulphoxide, *S*-1-propenylcysteine sulphoxide is found in onions and garlic accumulates *S*-allylcysteine sulphoxide (alliin), while *S*-methylcysteine sulphoxide is present in all *Allium* species. The amino acid cysteine is the precursor of all these *S*-alkylcysteine sulphoxides (Fig. 2.28).

2.7 Further reading

Further details about not only alkaloids and sulphur-containing compounds but also flavonoids, phenolics and terpenoids can be found in a well-illustrated textbook chapter on natural products (Croteau *et al.*, 2000) and an extremely readable, seminal book entitled *Medicinal Natural Products: A Biosynthetic Approach* (Dewick, 2002). Both of these sources provided valuable information included in sections of this chapter.

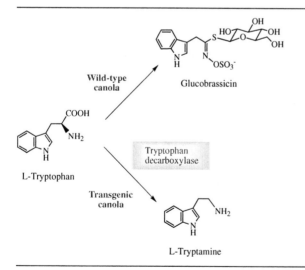

Fig. 2.27 Canola (*Brassica napus*) has been genetically modified using a gene encoding tryptophan decarboxylase from *Catharanthus roseus* so the L-tryptophan is converted to tryptamine rather than the bitter-tasting indole glucosinolate glucobrassicin. The mature seed, which is used as an animal feed, is therefore more palatable.

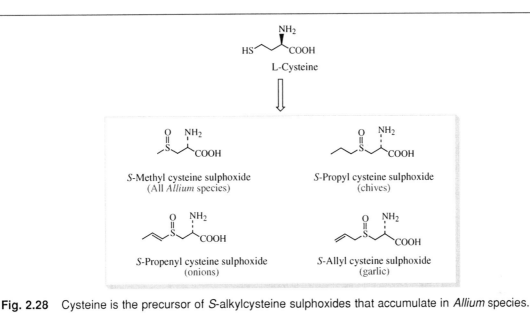

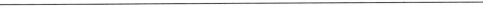

Fig. 2.28   Cysteine is the precursor of *S*-alkylcysteine sulphoxides that accumulate in *Allium* species.

2.8 Key points

- A diverse variety of organic compounds are to be found in edible plants. Some (primarily metabolites) have essential roles in the plant, being associated with photosynthesis, respiration and growth and development. Others (secondary metabolites) protect against herbivores and microbial infection, act as attractants for pollinator and seed-dispersing animals, as allelopathic agents, as UV protectants or as signal molecules in the formation of nitrogen-fixing root nodules in legumes.
- In recent years, the potential for some secondary metabolites to carry health benefits for humans has attracted considerable interest.
- Plant secondary metabolites can be divided into three major groups: flavonoids and allied phenolic and polyphenolic compounds (about 8000 compounds); terpenoids (about 25 000 compounds); and alkaloids (about 12 000 compounds) and sulphur-containing compounds.
- Flavonoids are the most numerous of the phenolics and are found throughout the plant kingdom, concentrated mainly in the epidermis of leaves and the skin of fruits. The group includes flavonols (*e.g.* myricetin and quercetin), flavones (*e.g.* luteolin and apigenin), flavan-3-ols (*e.g.* catechin, epicatechin, proanthocyanidins), anthocyanidins (*e.g.* cyanidin), flavanones (*e.g.* hesperidin, narigen) and isoflavones (*e.g.* genistein and daidzein). The principle non-flavonoid phenolic compounds are hydroxycinnamates (*e.g.* caffeic acid and ferulic acid), stilbenes (*e.g.* *trans*-resveratol) and phenolic acids (*e.g.* tannins).
- Carotenoids (tetraterpenoids) are the best-known members of the terpenoid family.

However, there are more than 25 000 terpenoids in all, many of which have recognised medicinal effects or are flavouring agents. Plant sterols are triterpenoids.

- There are 12 000 or so alkaloids, which contain one or more nitrogen atoms. It is now known that alkaloids were the active ingredients in numerous potions and poisons used over the centuries, and many alkaloids (*e.g.* codeine) are still in use today as prescription drugs. Most alkaloids are synthesised from certain amino acids. However, two well-known alkaloids, caffeine and theobromine, are derived from purine nucleotides.

- A variety of sulphur-containing compounds are also present, including the glucosinolates found in plants of the Brassica family and all the derivatives of the sulphur-containing amino acid cysteine, found in members of the onion family.

3
Epidemiology Linking Consumption of Plant Foods and their Constituents with Health

3.1 Introduction and methodology

Historically, much of the interest in health effects has concerned fruits and vegetables, although as will be apparent elsewhere in this report, substances reported to have protective properties are to be found in most of the food groups that form part of the human diet.

Before reviewing the evidence, it is important to recognise the strengths and weaknesses of data derived from epidemiological studies, in general, and from specific types of study. Trials of individual dietary components in isolation need to be interpreted with caution because they are unlikely to reflect the real-life situation in which these components are consumed. Experiments using laboratory animals, where large amounts of isolated substances may be seen to evoke a strong response, may not evoke the same response under more realistic conditions in humans. Evidence from different types of epidemiological studies should not be combined without careful thought regarding the validity of the data collected and after considering the effects of chance, bias and confounding.

The methods section of any scientific paper should provide essential information about who was studied and how the study was carried out, and is a vital guide to the quality of a paper. The first factor to consider is the type of study conducted and whether this is appropriate to address the objectives.

Attention needs to be paid to the timing of any change in dietary exposure as this may influence the impact of the change, *e.g.* the impact of dietary change during childhood may differ compared with late adulthood when disease is already present. Such effects will be dependent on the way in which the food component exerts its influence (see Chapter 4), *e.g.* via an effect on atherosclerosis (a relatively chronic process) versus an effect on clotting activity (a potentially acute process).

(i) Study design

Ultimately, to interpret the effects of diet, food patterns and nutrients on human health, data from human epidemiological studies must be considered. Animal and human experiments *in vivo* or animal experiments *in vitro* will always be difficult to interpret unless placed in the context of a level of consumption. Nutritional epidemiological studies have to be performed to provide information about the relationships between nutrition and health in human populations consuming usual amounts of foods and nutrients. Such studies aim to explore the relationships between what people eat (the exposure) and their health (the outcome), which can be assessed either as increased risk of disease (*e.g.* a high cholesterol level) or presence of disease (*e.g.* a heart attack). The main purpose is to identify causes so that these can be changed in order to reduce the health burden (see Chapter 13). For a dietary factor to be the cause of ill health an effect must be demonstrated to occur before the onset of an illness or disease, and this must not be the result of a chance association or due to some other factor (such as a confounder).

(ii) Randomised double blind controlled trials

The strongest evidence for efficacy comes from carefully conducted randomised double blind controlled trials in which the investigator attempts to change only one dietary factor, whilst keeping all other aspects of diet constant, and looks at the effect on the outcome of interest. Even in this case, an effect cannot necessarily be extrapolated outside the experimental setting: such an inference can only come from collation of all the relevant data. Furthermore, in many dietary experimental studies it is not possible to change one component of the diet in isolation and it is also difficult for both the observer and the subject to be truly blinded (*i.e.* unaware of the nature of the intervention). Experimental studies provide the most robust conclusions, but it is difficult to study causality as opposed to reversibility.

(iii) Observational studies

In many circumstances an experimental approach is not possible and much of the evidence we use to draw causal inferences comes from observational studies. In these the investigator does not intervene but assesses the differences in the exposure and outcome of interest to see if the two might be related. While such studies cannot individually provide evidence of causality, they can be used to identify dietary factors that might be involved in the onset of disease and together contribute to the overall body of evidence. There are four main types of observational study:

- An *ecological* study compares patterns of disease in different populations or groups with very different diets. For example, this type of study might measure the average amount of fat in the diet in populations and relate this to the incidence or prevalence of coronary heart disease.
- A *cross-sectional* study investigates individuals, rather than populations, and measures both the outcome and the exposure at the same time, without prior knowledge of either. For example, a study may measure the amount of fat in the diet of individuals and their cholesterol levels at the same time point.

- A *case-control* study compares past exposure to a dietary factor between groups of individuals with and without the disease of interest. For example, people with heart disease may be asked about their past fruit and vegetable intake and this is compared with information from individuals without the disease but matched for criteria such as age, gender, smoking habits or blood pressure.
- A cohort (or *prospective*) study measures the exposure of interest in a group of individuals and follows this group over time, recording the incidence of the outcome of interest. For example, a study might assess fruit and vegetable intakes in a group of individuals and follow them over time to compare subsequent cancer incidence rates. Dietary measurements are best made at several points during the follow-up period.

(iv) Measurement error

The size, direction and effect of measurement error need to be considered in all study designs; the impact of measurement error on the measure of effect will depend on the type of study being undertaken. One critical issue is that the method of assessing exposure is fit for the purpose: can it be measured with the accuracy and/or precision required for that design? It is incorrect that there is only one 'true' method of measuring dietary exposure. It is also important to accept that no method can measure 'true' diet perfectly. In many studies, such as case-control and cohort studies, very often the measure of intake used is a ranking measure where subjects are simply divided into thirds of the distribution. As long as there is no differential measurement error, the measure of effect will be correct. Absolute intakes are not required, and therefore an absolute measure is not required. If the study aims to define the proportion above a cut-off, and allowing for underreporting, then an absolute measure is required.

(v) Advantages and disadvantages of different study designs

The primary concern with ecological studies, comparing different populations, is that there are many potential determinants of disease other than the dietary factor under consideration. They include genetic predisposition, other dietary factors, environmental factors and lifestyle practices which may vary in prevalence between different parts of the world with a high or a low incidence of disease. In cross-sectional studies of individuals, because the dietary factor and the disease, or risk of disease, are measured at the same time, it is not possible to assess whether any difference in diet occurred before, or as a consequence of, the disease. Another problem with this study design is that current diet may not be the most appropriate measure, for example people who are aware that they have high cholesterol levels may have already changed their diet. However, recalling past diet is not very reliable either, which is also a problem for case-control studies. Recall bias can also occur because subjects who know they have an illness are more likely to recall the exposure. This would give an erroneous relationship between exposure and disease.

Cohort (prospective) studies do not have these problems and findings are generally considered to be more reliable. However, such studies are expensive and take a long time. Furthermore, they cannot be performed for rare diseases because an excessive amount of time would be required before any cases of the disease occurred in the study population. For this reason, cohort studies often rely on surrogate markers (such as cholesterol levels as an indicator of heart disease risk).

(vi) *A framework for assessing the strengths and weaknesses of individual studies*

The problems presented by each design must be considered when assessing the validity of a study and how its results may be generalised to other populations or circumstances. Many reviews of the epidemiological literature linking diet and disease have been published, but few have used a systematic approach to judge the impact of the scientific quality of the information on the conclusions drawn from the review. An example of a systematic approach is the COMA report on diet and cancer (Department of Health, 1998b). The COMA Working Group used a systematic review

method for scoring case-control and cohort studies, developed by the Nutritional Epidemiology Group, an informal group of researchers from across the UK. The Group has developed a scoring system that enables the relative merits of different studies to be judged, based on a checklist of aspects that should be addressed in a good study. The emphasis of the scoring system is on the quality of the information provided by the study with respect to diet, such that a study primarily investigating non-dietary factors will tend to gain a low score, regardless of the effectiveness of the study as a whole. Separate scoring systems are used for case-control and cohort studies (Margetts *et al.*, 1995). Margetts *et al.* also described the outcome of an inter-observer variation study conducted to test the robustness of their approach. This revealed that the scoring system can reliably rank studies, but that this requires careful attention to the details provided in each study.

(vii) *Relative risks and odds ratios*

The results of studies are often presented as relative risks (RR). This is a measure of the magnitude of the association between an exposure and a disease. For a cohort study, the relative risk (or risk ratio) is calculated as the ratio of the incidence of disease in the exposed group to the incidence of disease in the non-exposed group. A relative risk of 1.0 indicates the rates of disease are the same in the exposed and unexposed groups. A value greater than 1.0 indicates a positive association or an increased risk among those exposed to a risk factor. In a case-control study, where participants are selected on the basis of disease status, an indirect measure of the relative risk, the odds or rate ratio, is used. This is defined as the ratio of the exposure to a particular factor among those with the disease compared to the exposure among the controls.

3.2 Evidence for health effects of plant foods

There are data to suggest that people who consume diets rich in fruit, vegetables and other plant-based foods are at reduced risk of various chronic diseases, such as coronary heart disease and stroke (Section 3.3) and cancer (Section 3.4). Beneficial effects of such dietary patterns have also been reported in diabetes, eye conditions, such as cataract and macular degeneration, and lung function (Section 3.5). Considerable time and effort have been invested in attempts to identify whether specific substances are responsible for the health effects attributed to plant foods. Analysis of these data is the focus of this report.

There are several plausible reasons why there may be an association between fruit and vegetable consumption and reduced risk of chronic disease, apart from possible confounders associated with other factors such as non-smoking and physical activity (Lampe, 1999). These include modulation of detoxification enzymes; stimulation of the immune system; reduction of platelet aggregation; an effect on cholesterol synthesis, blood pressure or hormone metabolism; and antioxidant effects. These are discussed in more detail in Chapters 4, 7, 8 and 10. Plant foods may also play a role in reducing risk factors for chronic diseases, for example raised serum cholesterol (Section 3.3.1) and hypertension (Section 3.3.1), both risk factors for CVD, and in secondary prevention (Section 3.3.1).

3.3 Coronary heart disease and stroke

3.3.1 Risk factors for CVD and secondary prevention

Two of the most important risk factors for CVD are raised serum cholesterol and hypertension. Many experimental studies have explored the effects of changing diet on these two risk factors, although there are relatively fewer trials that have assessed the effects of changing food patterns. The most widely quoted study that has changed dietary patterns is the DASH trial (Appel *et al.*, 1997). This study showed that a diet rich in fruits and vegetables, low in fat and incorporating low-fat dairy products, without changes in salt or weight loss, could lower blood pressure. Reducing salt had an additional benefit (Sacks *et al.*, 2001). Other trials have broadly supported the

results from DASH showing that moving dietary patterns towards a more plant-based food intake is associated with lower blood pressure.

A trial by Hodgson *et al.* (Hodgson *et al.*, 1999) showed that giving isoflavones did not reduce blood pressure compared with response to a placebo, again highlighting a need for caution in extrapolating from the effects of foods to specific compounds and *vice versa*.

The Lyon Diet Heart Study (de Lorgeril *et al.*, 1999) showed that various modifications to a 'Mediterranean'-type diet, in patients who survived a first myocardial infarction, led to a statistically significant reduction in the occurrence of subsequent cardiac death and non-fatal myocardial infarction over a 4-year period. The dietary changes included fruit and vegetable intakes and the type of fat consumed. The percentage energy from fat in the diet of the control group was 33.6% compared with 30.4% in the experimental group; these fat intakes are well below current UK levels. No details on the exact dietary differences or the increase in plant based food intake were given, but the authors noted that there appeared to be good compliance with dietary advice over the 4 years of follow-up.

3.3.2 Fruit and vegetables

Although there is a vast literature on the effects of changing the type and amount of fat in the diet on serum cholesterol concentration, there is less published research on the effects of increasing fruit and vegetable intakes on risk factors for disease. There have been many studies that have looked at the effects of functional foods with plant stanols and sterols added (see Chapter 10), but the direct relevance to plant-based diets and effects on cholesterol is less clear.

Armstrong and Doll were among the first to draw associations between population food patterns, based on UK NFS data, and mortality from CHD data (Armstrong & Doll, 1975). CHD rates were higher in areas where fruit and vegetable consumption was lowest. Across Europe, countries whose populations consumed the most fruits and vegetables have been shown to have lower rates of CHD, and analyses of trends over time suggest an inverse relationship between declines in fruit and vegetable consumption and increasing rates of CHD. Bobak *et al.* compared men in the Czech Republic, Bavaria and Israel and suggested that differences in fruit and vegetable intakes may explain differences in risk factors between Eastern and Western Europe (Bobak *et al.*, 1999). Ness and Powles reviewed the literature linking fruit and vegetable consumption with CHD (Ness & Powles, 1997) and stroke (Ness & Powles, 1999). They found that in nine of 10 ecological studies, two of three case-control studies and six of 16 cohort studies there was a significant inverse association between coronary heart disease and intake of fruit and vegetables (or a nutrient used as a marker of intake) (Ness & Powles, 1997). For stroke, three of five ecological studies, none out of one case control study and six of eight cohort studies showed an association of this type (Ness & Powles, 1999). The authors concluded that although studies showing no effect may be under-reported, the results were consistent with a strong protective effect of fruit and vegetables for stroke and a weaker protective effect for coronary heart disease.

Key *et al.* studied a cohort of health-conscious men and women, 43% of whom said they were vegetarian. They found that daily consumption of fresh fruit was associated with significantly lower deaths from ischaemic heart disease after adjustment for smoking (rate ratio 0.76), deaths from cerebrovascular disease (rate ratio 0.68) and in all-cause mortality (rate ratio 0.79) (Key *et al.*, 1996). In a subsequent study, Key *et al.* conducted a pooled analysis of data from five major cohort studies in the USA, UK and Germany. Vegetarians (defined as not eating any fish or meat) had a 24% lower mortality from ischaemic heart disease than non-vegetarians. This reduction in risk was greatest for the younger age groups; for example, the rate ratio for premature death from ischaemic heart disease (under the age of 65 years) was 0.55 and for those aged 65–79 years it was 0.69 (Key *et al.*, 1998).

The Women's Health Study in the USA has shown that women who eat more fruit and vegetables have a lower cardiovascular risk, particularly in relation to myocardial infarction (Liu

et al., 2000). Strandhagen *et al.*, in a cohort study of Swedish men, reported similar results (Strandhagen *et al.*, 2000). A recent factor analysis using data from the Health Professionals Follow-up Survey (Hu *et al.*, 2000) showed that men following a 'prudent diet', characterised by higher intake of vegetables, fruit, legumes, whole grains, fish and poultry, were less likely to develop coronary heart disease. Knekt *et al.* found that intake of apples and onions and intake of flavonoids were inversely linked to coronary mortality in a Finnish cohort (Knekt *et al.*, 1996). A more recent analysis from this study has shown that apples remain protective against thrombotic or embolic stroke, after adjustment for intake of quercetin. This suggests that there may be other bioactive substances in apples that need further investigation (see Chapter 7).

In their meta-analysis of cohort studies investigating the relationship between ischaemic heart disease and markers of fruit and vegetable consumption (both the foods themselves and related nutrients), Law and Morris concluded that the risk of ischaemic heart disease is about 15% lower at the 90th than at the 10th centile of fruit and vegetable intake (Law & Morris, 1998).

van't Veer and colleagues carried out a review of 250 observational studies (case-control and prospective) on cardiovascular disease and cancer, in which measurements were made of fruit and vegetable intake (excluding potatoes) (van't Veer *et al.*, 2000). The authors noted that overall, testing the efficacy of fruits and vegetables in population trials is hampered by methodological factors such as blinding (that is, it is not possible to mask the true exposure in either subjects or researchers), compliance and study duration. Relative risks (RR) or odds ratios (OR) (depending on the type of study) for high versus low intake of fruit and vegetables were calculated. The proportion of cases attributable to low consumption was estimated using three scenarios: best guess, optimistic (using stronger RRs) and conservative (using weaker RRs and eliminating the contribution of smoking and/or drinking). These RRs usually represented risk for subjects in the highest versus the lowest category of intake, typically a difference of about 150 g day of fruit and vegetables. These estimates represent the overall effect of beneficial and adverse properties of fruits and vegetables. The researchers calculated the proportion of cases of CVD that could be prevented in the Dutch population if current average intakes of 250 g/day were increased to 400 g/day (the World Heath Organisation recommendation, see Chapter 13). The 'best guess' estimate for cardiovascular disease was 16% (8000 cases annually), ranging from 6% (conservative) to 22% (optimistic).

Joshipura *et al.* examined intakes of specific fruits and vegetables, as well as overall fruit and vegetable intake, in two large cohorts of US men and women, followed for 8 and 14 years, respectively, and free of cardiovascular disease, cancer and diabetes at baseline (Joshipura *et al.*, 1999). After controlling for standard cardiovascular risk factors, those in the highest quintile of fruit and vegetable intake (median 5.1 servings per day in men and 5.8 in women) had a relative risk for ischaemic stroke of 0.69 compared with those in the lowest quintile. An increment of one serving per day of fruit or vegetables was associated with a 6% lower risk of ischaemic stroke. Green leafy vegetables, cruciferous vegetables, and citrus fruit including fruit juice contributed most to the apparent protective effect.

3.3.3 Pulses

There have been relatively few studies that have looked specifically at the effects of pulses and nuts and risk of CHD and stroke (see also Chapter 8). Participants in the National Health and Nutrition Examination Survey (NHANES) epidemiological follow-up study who ate more legumes (including dry beans, as well as peanuts and peanut butter) had lower risk of CHD and CVD (Bazzano *et al.*, 2001). No association was found between legume consumption and stroke in the two Boston cohort studies (Joshipura *et al.*, 1999).

Legumes, including soya and its products, have been associated in clinical studies with decreased serum cholesterol. Anderson *et al.* reported that their meta-analysis of 38 studies, which provided an average of 47 g/day of soya protein, showed an

average reduction in total and LDL cholesterol of 0.6 and 56 mmol/L, respectively (Anderson *et al.*, 1995). It should be noted that despite a wide range of soya protein intakes (17–124 g/day) in these studies, no dose–response effect was evident. Also, only seven of the studies used intakes of soya protein of 25 g or less. Achievement of an intake of 25 g within the context of the UK diet would require replacement of dietary items at each meal with soya-derived foods, *e.g.* soya drink or tofu (British Nutrition Foundation, 2002c). The Joint Health Claims Initiative's Expert Committee has reviewed the available data for a health claim relating to soya and cholesterol lowering (see www.jhci.co.uk).

3.3.4 Nuts

Kris-Etherton *et al.* have recently reviewed the epidemiological studies linking nut consumption and risk of CHD (Kris-Etherton *et al.*, 2001). They showed that in five large cohort studies (the Adventists Health Study, the Iowa Women's Health Study, the Nurses Health Study, the Cholesterol and Recurrent Events (CARE) Study and the Physicians Health Study), eating nuts more than once a week was associated with a decreased risk of CHD in both men and women (RRs varied from 0.45 to 0.75). They also reviewed 11 clinical trials of the effects of diets containing nuts on lipid and lipoprotein endpoints: they concluded that it was not possible to attribute the lipid-lowering effect to nuts alone because of the complex nature of most of the dietary interventions. Four clinical trials compared the lipid lowering effects of diets with or without nuts, and suggested that the diets with nuts had a greater effect. Kris-Etherton *et al.* concluded that nuts may contain cholesterol-lowering bioactive compounds, but further research is required to identify what these might be.

3.3.5 Cereals

Cereal grains and their products are an important part of most diets around the world. The terminology is confusing, although Truswell has recently tried to clarify this (Truswell, 2002). There are, at the time of preparing this review, only three cohort studies that have specifically explored the association between wholegrain cereals and risk of CVD (Pietinen *et al.*, 1996; Jacobs *et al.*, 1999; Liu *et al.*, 1999). The consensus from those studies is that people who eat a healthy diet, of which wholegrain cereals form a part, have a lower risk of CVD (see www.jhci.co.uk).

There have been many studies that have assessed the association between fibre and CVD or serum lipids in particular (these studies are covered in Section 3.3.6).

3.3.6 Dietary fibre

Before discussing the epidemiological evidence linking dietary fibre intake and disease risk, it is important to highlight the confusion in terminology used in this area. 'Dietary fibre' is a generic term that covers a wide range of different substances and in most epidemiological studies it has not been possible to disentangle whether there are specific components of fibre or particular types of fibre that have effects on health parameters (see also Chapter 1). Some researchers use the term NSP (non-starch polysaccharides), others dietary fibre, and differences between studies may be partly explained by which substances in plant foods have been included to derive the measurements. Worldwide there are differences in the type of methodology used to measure fibre, the Englyst and AOAC methods being the most common. This is of relevance because different methods measure a slightly different range of fibre constituents.

In a prospective cohort study of almost 45000 US male health professionals, followed up for 6 years, the age-adjusted relative risk was 0.59 among men in the highest quintile of total dietary fibre intake compared with men in the lowest quintile (Rimm *et al.*, 1996a). The strongest association (RR = 0.45) was for fatal coronary disease. The Nurses' Health Survey found an apparently protective effect of wholegrain cereal intake on risk of CHD. The relationship was not explained by other risk factors or the contribution to the intakes of dietary fibre, folate, vitamin B_6 or vitamin E (Liu *et al.*, 1999).

A protective effect of dietary fibre was found in the Finnish α-tocopherol, β-carotene (ATBC) cancer prevention study (Pietinen *et al.*, 1996), with cereal fibre showing a stronger association than vegetable or fruit fibre. The relative risk of coronary death in the highest quintile of total dietary fibre intake was 0.69 when compared with the lowest quintile.

3.3.7 Nutrients: vitamin E, vitamin C and carotenoids

As discussed in Section 1.4.3, antioxidants have been the focus of much research interest with respect to CHD (Buttriss *et al.*, 2002). During the 1980s and early 1990s, Gey and colleagues observed that across various European populations there was an inverse relationship between cardiovascular disease risk and diets rich in vitamin C, in particular, and β-carotene and vitamin E, reflected in blood plasma levels (Gey *et al.*, 1987, 1993a,b).

Plasma vitamin C concentration was inversely related to mortality from all causes and from cardiovascular disease and ischaemic heart disease in men and women in the EPIC–Norfolk prospective study (Khaw *et al.*, 2001) (see Section 3.4 for a brief description of the EPIC study). Risk of death during the 4-year study period in the top vitamin C quintile was about half the risk in the lowest quintile, the association being continuous through the whole distribution of concentrations. A 20 μmol/L difference in vitamin C, approximately equivalent to a 50 g/day difference in fruit and vegetable intake, was associated with a 25% fall in the risk of all-cause mortality, which was independent of other risk factors. The authors concluded that a small increase in fruit and vegetables, amounting to an extra daily serving, has encouraging prospects in helping to prevent disease (see Chapter 13).

In their review of relative risks for CHD, Tavani and La Vecchia found that whilst case-control studies and six cohort studies suggested inverse associations between β-carotene and relative risk of coronary heart disease, four more recent cohort studies showed no effect (RR around 1). Four randomised controlled trials of β-carotene supplementation were found to give relative risks close to unity for the association. The authors concluded that the apparent benefit in observational studies may be linked to consumption of foods rich in β-carotene rather than β-carotene itself (Tavani & Vecchia, 1999).

Spencer *et al.* found inconsistent indications for vitamin E supplementation studies, with some studies (particularly those using high dose supplements of 400 or 800 IU/day) showing an inverse association with cardiovascular endpoints and others, often the lower dose studies, showing no benefit or a detrimental effect when vitamin E was combined with β-carotene (Spencer *et al.*, 1999).

Azen *et al.* demonstrated that vitamin E supplements providing greater than 67 α-tocopherol equivalents per day (well in excess of the recommended intakes) reduced the progression of atherosclerosis, assessed by measuring carotid artery wall thickness (Azen *et al.*, 1996).

As discussed in Section 1.5.2, the ATBC trial in heavy smokers (with vitamin E and β-carotene) found no effect on cardiovascular disease among controls but an increased risk of cardiovascular disease or mortality in the β-carotene group (Albanes *et al.*, 1995; Leppala *et al.*, 2000). Similar findings with respect to β-carotene were also observed in the CARET study (Omenn *et al.*, 1996). The Cambridge Heart Antioxidant Study (CHAOS) found a significant reduction in the incidence of non-fatal myocardial infarction in 2002 subjects randomised to 268 or 536 α-tocopherol equivalents a day. However, there was a non-significant excess of cardiovascular deaths in the vitamin E- supplemented group (Stephens *et al.*, 1996). Gaziano *et al.* found a significant 50% reduction in secondary coronary events in subjects randomised to receive β-carotene (Gaziano *et al.*, 1995). A sub-study of the Heart Outcomes Prevention Evaluation (HOPE) trial found no difference in atherosclerosis progression rates (carotid artery) in high-risk patients on vitamin E supplements (400 IU/day) or placebo (Yusuf *et al.*, 2000).

In their meta-analysis of cohort studies, in which a 15% reduction in risk of ischaemic heart disease between the top and bottom deciles of fruit and vegetable consumption was estimated,

Law and Morris concluded that intakes of β-carotene or vitamin E are unlikely to be important. They suggested that the combined effect of potassium, folate and possibly fibre in fruit and vegetables could account for the difference in risk (Law & Morris, 1998).

The US National Academy of Sciences Food and Nutrition Board (NAS) has reviewed reference intakes for vitamins C and E and carotenoids. The Panel looked for scientifically valid experiments, measurements of relevant biomarkers, reliable intake data, *in vivo* rather than *in vitro* experiments, strength of evidence and role in health (National Academy of Sciences Food and Nutrition Board, 2000). The NAS Panel concluded that observational epidemiology is very strong for foods such as fruits and vegetables, but this cannot be used to identify individual nutrients. Intervention studies, which are typically limited to a single dose level and a specific population, have generally provided weak and ambiguous conclusions. On balance, the Panel concluded that the evidence is not supportive of a preventative role in chronic diseases for antioxidants. Because of the quality of the available evidence, the Panel did not use chronic disease as a factor in establishing dietary reference intakes. In reaching this decision they took into account the following criteria for diet–disease relationships: whether there is evidence of the strength of the association, a dose–response relationship, a temporally correct association, consistency of the association, specificity of the association and biological plausibility.

3.3.8 Other plant-derived substances

Several studies have investigated associations between flavonoids and coronary heart disease. For example, the Iowa postmenopausal women's study reported flavonoid intake to be associated with a decreased risk of death from coronary heart disease after adjustment for age and energy intake. Of the foods contributing to flavonoid intake, only broccoli was strongly associated with a decreased risk (Yochum *et al.*, 1999). There was no association between flavonoid intake and stroke. In a review of prospective epidemiological studies, Hollman and Katan found that intake of flavonols and flavones was inversely associated with subsequent coronary heart disease in most but not all studies (Hollman & Katan, 1999). There are many reasons why mechanisms other than those involving antioxidants may be responsible for some of these observations, and these are addressed in detail in Chapters 4, 8 and 10. In addition, non-antioxidant nutrients may be involved. For example, it is also now recognised that dietary folate/folic acid intake is inversely associated with blood levels of homocysteine, a recognised risk factor for coronary heart disease, although it is yet to be demonstrated whether or not this association is causal (see Section 1.4.4). Indeed, Parodi has hypothesised that it is folate, rather than other dietary constituents, that is largely responsible for the cardiovascular benefits attributed to the Mediterranean style of eating (Parodi, 1997).

3.3.9 Summary for CHD and stroke

Plant-based diets are associated with lower risk of cardiovascular disease (*e.g.* CHD and stroke). Fruit and vegetable consumption is generally associated with other health-promoting activities, *e.g.* being physically active and not smoking, as well as higher consumption of wholegrain cereals and lower consumption of animal-derived foods. Adjustment for such factors does not explain the association between high fruit and vegetable intake and lowered risk, although adjustment often attenuates the strength of the association. There is evidence of a dose–response relationship that is consistent with current recommendations to increase intakes of these foods (see Chapter 13). It is difficult to separate out the role of diet in general and of specific nutrients in particular, and so the causal mechanism(s) of this dietary pattern remain to be established. Most epidemiological research has focused on a number of individual antioxidants studied in relative isolation and it is likely that at the very least there is a complex interaction between the many components found in plant foods, and the rest of the diet, that may have an integrated effect on cardiovascular disease risk.

3.4 Cancer

The COMA Working Group on The Nutritional Aspects of Cancer (Department of Health, 1998b) systematically reviewed the data on associations between diet and various forms of cancer. This subject has also been reviewed by the World Cancer Research Fund (World Cancer Research Fund, 1997). The strongest associations were found for fruit and vegetable consumption. The term 'fruit(s) and vegetables' is used in most studies in a culinary, rather than botanical, sense, and covers a wide variety of plants and parts of plants. In many studies it is often not clear which are included or excluded in the analysis. The Working Group followed the original studies' various definitions of fruits and vegetables to include all fresh, canned, frozen and dried fruits and vegetables, *except* potatoes and pulses (see Chapters 1 and 13). Some studies distinguished between cruciferous, salad and green or green/yellow vegetables, and between citrus and non-citrus fruits. However, most studies refer only to fruit or vegetable consumption (or both) in general.

The COMA Working Group concluded that, overall, there is moderate evidence that higher vegetable consumption will reduce the risk of colorectal cancer, and that higher fruit and vegetable consumption will reduce the risk of gastric cancer. There is weak evidence, based on fewer data, that higher fruit and vegetable consumption will reduce the risk of breast cancer. These cancers combined represent about 18% of the cancer burden in men and about 39% of the cancer burden in women in the UK, so even a small reduction in relative risk can have important public health benefits in terms of the reduction in the absolute numbers of people affected. The data generally show a graded reduction in risk associated with higher fruit and vegetable consumption. There are no data to support an increased cancer risk with higher fruit and vegetable consumption. The overall picture supported the hypothesis that the consumption of fruits and vegetables protects against the development of some cancers. On the basis of their conclusions, the COMA Working Group recommended that fruit and vegetable consumption in the UK should increase. They did not specify by how much, but said that any increase would be expected to carry benefits (see Chapter 13). Similar conclusions were reached by the WCRF (World Cancer Research Fund, 1997) which looked at the available data from a global perspective. The findings and conclusions of the COMA working group are briefly summarised in Sections 3.4.1–3.4.6 and 3.4.9–3.4.10, and more details can be found elsewhere (Department of Health, 1998b). The results of studies published since these two major reviews have generally been consistent with their findings. A few notable exceptions are discussed below.

A review of 250 observational studies, most of which concerned cancer (van't Veer *et al.*, 2000) estimated that the incidence of cancer in The Netherlands could be reduced by 19% (12 000 cases annually). This ranged from a 6% reduction (conservative estimate) to 28% (optimistic estimate), if the average intake of fruit and vegetables were to rise from 250 to 400 g/day. Evidence was strongest for gastrointestinal cancers, followed by hormone-related cancers (see Section 3.3.2 for details of the study).

Data are now becoming available from a nine-country collaborative study (EPIC, European Prospective Investigation into Cancer and Nutrition), designed to investigate dietary and other determinants of cancer and other diseases. The study began in 1992 and involves 406 303 subjects including two cohorts in the UK (Oxford and Norfolk) (Stanner, 2001). In the EPIC–Norfolk cohort of the study, additional data have been collected to allow assessment of determinants of chronic disease. Data published to date from the study suggest that plasma ascorbic acid is inversely related to cancer mortality in men but not women (Khaw *et al.*, 2001). Preliminary data have indicated that a high consumption of fruit and vegetables reduced the incidence of gastrointestinal and colorectal cancers. A weak inverse association was found between stomach cancer and intakes of fresh fruit and cereals/cereal products, but no association was demonstrated with vegetable intake. The preliminary findings do not demonstrate any significant associations between fruit and vegetable consumption and either lung or prostate cancer (EPIC, 2002).

3.4.1 Fruits and vegetables and breast cancer

COMA concluded that, for fruits, the evidence from case-control studies was weakly consistent; higher intakes are associated with lower risk of breast cancer. For vegetables, the evidence was moderately consistent. There are few cohort studies in this area, and more recent studies point to a lack of association (Smith-Warner *et al.*, 2001; Willett, 2001a).

One component present in fruits and vegetables that might account for the observed association is dietary fibre. In pre-menopausal but not in post-menopausal women, dietary fibre produced a significant reduction in one or more oestrogen fractions. There is strong and consistent evidence for higher circulating levels of oestrogens in populations at high risk of breast cancer, particularly in postmenopausal women (Department of Health, 1998b) (see Chapter 8).

Data from a recent nested case-control study indicated an inverse relationship between breast cancer risk and serum levels of a range of carotenoids (Toniolo *et al.*, 2001). Blood concentrations of carotenoids have been proposed as a marker of fruit and vegetable intake (see Chapter 6).

3.4.2 Fruits and vegetables and lung cancer

The COMA Working Group concluded that cigarette smoking remains the overwhelming risk for lung cancer. However, there is moderately consistent evidence that higher consumption of fruits and weakly consistent evidence that higher consumption of vegetables are associated with a lower risk of lung cancer. The possibility of confounding cannot be excluded as many studies have failed to characterise adequately the lifetime exposure to tobacco smoking.

One mechanism for a possible protective effect of fruits and vegetables is via their antioxidant capacity to protect against free radical-induced DNA damage. However, β-carotene and α-tocopherol are unlikely to be the mediators of any effect. Although higher dietary intakes and blood levels of β-carotene and α-tocopherol have generally been associated with a lower risk of lung cancer, supplementation with β-carotene and α-tocopherol did not reduce lung cancer rates in three intervention trials after up to 12 years (Hennekens *et al.*, 1996; Omenn *et al.*, 1996). Nevertheless, if these nutrients have an effect at an early stage in the carcinogenic process, the design of these trials might not be capable of demonstrating a protective effect.

A prospective study in China found an inverse association between the level of urinary isothiocyanates (a metabolite of the glucosinolates found in cruciferous vegetables, see Chapter 7) and lung cancer risk (London *et al.*, 2000). The reduction in risk was strongest in those who were genetically deficient in enzymes that rapidly eliminate these compounds. Dietary isothiocyanates have also been shown to inhibit lung cancer in animal models (Hecht, 1999).

3.4.3 Fruits and vegetables and colorectal cancer

The COMA Working Group concluded that there is moderately consistent evidence from case-control studies, especially from those judged to be well conducted, that higher consumption of vegetables is associated with a lower risk of colon cancer. However, the evidence from cohort studies is only weakly consistent (also see Section 3.4.11). Evidence of an effect of fruit consumption is limited and inconsistent.

A number of plausible mechanisms have been postulated to explain why vegetables might reduce the risk of colorectal cancer (see Chapters 4, 5 and 7), and there is some evidence that some of these might operate in humans.

3.4.4 Fruits and vegetables and gastric cancer

The COMA Working Group concluded that there is moderately consistent evidence that higher intakes of fruits and vegetables are associated with lower risk of gastric cancer. A plausible mechanism concerning vitamin C has been proposed, but the evidence that it operates in human gastric carcinogenesis is equivocal. Hypotheses relating diet to gastric cancer have generally not taken account of the aetiological importance of infection with *Helicobacter pylori*. Although it is

possible that confounding by *H. pylori* infection may partly account for these findings, the strength and consistency and dose–response relationship argue against this.

3.4.5 Fruits and vegetables and oesophageal cancer

The COMA Working Group concluded that the evidence that higher consumption of fruits and vegetables reduces the risk of oesophageal cancer is strongly consistent, but the available prospective data cannot be extrapolated directly to the UK population. Smoking, a risk factor for oesophageal cancer, may cause confounding.

Mechanisms have been postulated, and higher dietary intakes of antioxidant nutrients (β-carotene, vitamin C and vitamin E) are associated with lower risk of oesophageal cancer in case-control studies. However, intervention trials using supplements of various combinations of vitamins and minerals have not found any effect on the appearance of precancerous lesions, oesophageal cancer incidence or mortality.

3.4.6 Fruits and vegetables and other cancers

There have been few studies of fruit and vegetable consumption and risk of prostate cancer, cervical cancer, pancreatic cancer or bladder cancer. The limited data for all four cancers are moderately or strongly consistent for reduced risk with higher fruit and vegetable consumption, although the data are too limited to draw firm conclusions (Department of Health, 1998b). The COMA Working Group did not consider skin cancer.

3.4.7 Legumes and nuts

Very few studies have specifically investigated the relationship between the consumption of legumes or nuts and the risk of cancers and the evidence is often difficult to interpret (see also Chapter 8). The World Cancer Research Fund report (1997) identified 58 epidemiological studies that reported results for pulses and cancer risk, either for specific pulses or pulses in general. There was no clear picture: 50% reported a reduced risk of cancer, 38% reported an increased risk and 12%

reported no association. More recently, in Seventh-day Adventists, Fraser has reported that intake of legumes is inversely associated with risk of cancers of the colon and the pancreas (Fraser, 1999).

Very few studies have looked specifically at the association between nut consumption and cancer risk and the WCRF Report concluded that there was no evidence to suggest that nuts might protect against some cancers (World Cancer Research Fund, 1997).

3.4.8 Cereals

The WCRF panel concluded that cereals modify the risk of cancers at various sites or else show no relationship (World Cancer Research Fund, 1997). According to their review, diets rich in wholegrain cereals possibly decrease the risk of stomach cancer (based on evidence from six case-control studies), but they found insufficient evidence to support an inverse association with colon cancer. A recent US prospective study (McCullough *et al.*, 2001) supports a modest role for plant foods (including wholegrain cereals) in reducing the risk of fatal stomach cancer.

3.4.9 Fibre and cancer

The COMA Working Group concluded that there is no evidence that increased fibre intake is associated with increased risk of cancer. However, there is moderately consistent evidence, particularly from case-control studies, that higher intakes of dietary fibre are associated with lower risk of colon cancer, possibly through effects on colonic fermentation and increasing stool weight (see Chapter 5), although this is not sufficient to amount to evidence of a protective effect. Furthermore, it should be recognised that people who consume more dietary fibre also consume more plant foods in general, and typically fewer animal-derived foods. Therefore, some of the effect of dietary fibre on colon cancer risk may be due to the effects of other aspects of diet associated with a high fibre intake.

Since publication of the COMA report, however, results of several studies have cast doubt on the strength of this association. These investigated the impact of fibre on the development of recurrent colorectal adenomas, which are considered to be precursor lesions of colorectal cancer. No effect was found with either a high-fibre diet (18 g/1000 kcal) (Schatzkin *et al.*, 2000) or a wheat bran fibre supplement (Alberts *et al.*, 2000). These results reflected those of the prospective Nurses Health Study (Fuchs *et al.*, 1999). In addition, a soluble fibre supplement was shown to have an adverse effect on recurrence of colorectal adenomas (Bonithon-Kopp *et al.*, 2000), leading Goodlad to question the wisdom of advocating fibre supplements as a means of reducing colon cancer risk, although he acknowledged the apparent benefit of a high-fibre diet for general and cardiovascular health (Goodlad, 2001). Intakes in Britain are currently about 12 g/day and so fall short of the 18 g/day recommendation.

The epidemiological evidence that higher intakes of dietary fibre are associated with lower risk of breast cancer is inconsistent. Whilst most case-control studies show a significantly reduced risk of breast cancer with higher intakes of fibre in post-menopausal women, three out of four prospective studies have failed to find an association between fibre intake and breast cancer (Department of Health, 1998b).

3.4.10 Other plant-derived substances and cancer

Several studies have investigated associations with flavonoids. There was no association found between the intake of five major flavonoids and mortality from total cancer, lung cancer, colorectal cancer or stomach cancer in an analysis of data from the Seven Countries Study after 25 years of follow-up (Hertog *et al.*, 1995), or with mortality from cancer at all sites in the Zutphen Elderly Study (Hertog *et al.*, 1994). Therefore, despite plausible mechanisms, there is little observational evidence for a beneficial effect of flavonoids against cancer.

COMA recommended the avoidance of β-carotene supplements as a means of protecting against cancer (see Section 1.5.2) and to exercise caution in the use of high doses of purified supplements of other micronutrients, as they cannot be assumed to be without risk.

Since publication of the COMA report, several studies have been published showing inverse associations between cancer risk and higher folate/folic acid consumption (see Section 1.4.4), for example in relation to colon (Giovannucci *et al.*, 1998) and breast cancers (Sellers *et al.*, 2001).

3.4.11 Summary for cancer

The strongest association between plant food intake (particularly fruit and vegetable intake) and cancer risk comes from case-control studies and, as indicated in Section 3.1, this type of methodology has a number of limitations. In the light of recent prospective (cohort) studies, which are not subject to the same biases, Willett has suggested that associations may have been over-stated (Willett, 2001b).

3.5 Other age-related diseases

3.5.1 Type 2 diabetes

A recent analysis from the US Health Professional Follow-up study of 42 504 men showed that a prudent dietary pattern was associated with a decreased risk (RR = 0.84 lowest versus highest fifth of intake, 95% CI 0.70–1.00) of type 2 diabetes (van Dam *et al.*, 2002). The prudent dietary pattern was characterised by high consumption of vegetables, legumes, fruit, whole grains, fish and poultry. Another US cohort study found that low consumers of fruits and vegetables were more likely to develop diabetes (Ford & Mokdad, 2001). This study confirmed the results from an early cross-sectional study in the UK that showed that high consumption of fruit and vegetables and low consumption of processed meat and fried foods was inversely associated with previously undiagnosed type 2 diabetes (Williams *et al.*, 2000).

Results from the 10-year follow-up of US nurses showed that women who were in the top fifth of wholegrain cereal intake had a 38% lower risk of developing diabetes than women in the lowest fifth of intake; the effects were not explained by dietary fibre intake or intake of magnesium or vitamin E (Liu *et al.*, 2000).

It is well known that people with diabetes are vulnerable to oxidative stress. There have been a number of short-term clinical trials to assess whether isolated flavonoid compounds could influence lipoprotein vulnerability to oxidation. Results have been mixed, with some studies showing an effect (Lean *et al.*, 1999) and others not (Blostein-Fujii *et al.*, 1999). There have been many studies that have assessed the hypo-glycaemic effect of compounds found in many different foods; the relevance of these studies to humans is not clear.

3.5.2 Age-related macular degeneration and cataract

Age-related macular degeneration (AMD) and cataract are eye disorders which are increasing among older people. Macular degeneration is the leading cause of irreversible blindness in people over the age of 65 years. The macula is the central part of the retina and in the early stages of the disease begins to accumulate lipid deposits known as drusen, ultimately resulting in atrophy associated with distortion and finally loss of vision (especially in the central area of vision). Cataracts result from glycosidation of lens proteins, which leads to opacities forming within the lens. Although the aetiology of cataracts varies and they can develop at any stage of life, the vast majority develop in elderly individuals, and so are sometimes referred to as senile cataracts. Detailed discussions of nutrition and the eye, particularly cataracts, are available (Taylor & Takahama, 2000; Wu & Leske, 2000).

The tissues of the lens and of the retina are subject to oxidative stress throughout life, as a result of the combined exposure to light and oxygen, and it has been proposed that antioxidants may prevent cellular damage by reacting with free radicals produced during the process of light absorption (Christen *et al.*, 1996). It has been shown that lens proteins may be protected against *in vitro* oxidative attack by carotenoids and vitamins E and C (Diplock *et al.*, 1998). See also Chapter 4.

In the first US National Health and Nutrition Examination Survey (NHANES-I), people with a low intake of fruit and vegetables rich in carotenoids had a significantly higher risk of AMD than those with a higher level of consumption (Goldberg *et al.*, 1998). In another study, those with the highest quintile of carotenoid intake had a 43% lower risk of AMD than those in the lowest quintile (Seddon *et al.*, 1994). Among the carotenoids, lutein and zeaxanthin have been most strongly associated with reduced risk of AMD.

These two carotenoids present in the retina, are referred to as macula pigments, and they have been shown to protect against light-initiated oxidative damage. An intervention study has shown that these carotenoids can be significantly increased by dietary supplementation (Johnson *et al.*, 2000). These carotenoids are found in green leafy vegetables, and also fruit and vegetables of other colours, such as orange pepper, kiwi fruit, grapes, spinach, orange juice, courgettes and different kinds of vegetable squash (Sommerburg *et al.*, 1994).

One of the fatty acids that is present at high concentrations in fish oils, docosahexaenoic acid (DHA) (see Chapter 10), is also abundant in the retina of the eye. A recent prospective study of dietary fat and the risk of AMD (Cho *et al.*, 2001) found a modest inverse relation between DHA intake and AMD in those consuming at least four servings of fish a week (the richest source of DHA is oil-rich fish). A positive association was found with the DHA precursor α-linolenic acid, which is a minor fatty acid component of the retina and is found in seeds and other plant foods.

There is also considerable evidence to suggest that increased dietary intakes and plasma concentrations of antioxidants are inversely associated with decreased risk of cataract in elderly subjects. Cataracts of other aetiologies are relatively rare and so are less accessible to study, but to date there is no evidence to show that their incidence can be reduced via antioxidants. Most, but not all, studies have shown an inverse association between fruit and vegetable intake and risk of cataract. Hankinson *et al.* showed an association with spinach, but not carrots (Hankinson *et*

al., 1992). NHANES-II identified an inverse association between serum ascorbic acid and prevalence of cataract, based on a total of 252 women and 164 men with a self-reported history of cataract (Simon & Hudes, 1999).

The Blue Mountains Eye Study (Cumming *et al.*, 2000), based on 2900 subjects aged between 49 and 97 years of age, showed that, after adjusting for other known risk factors, those in the highest fifth of intake of protein, vitamin A, niacin, thiamin and riboflavin had statistically significantly lower risk of nuclear cataract than those in the lowest fifth of intake.

Prospective studies among women (Chasan-Taber *et al.*, 1999a,b), and to a weaker but consistent extent in men (Brown *et al.*, 1999), have reinforced the theoretical and experimental studies in suggesting that both lutein and zeaxanthin and foods rich in these carotenoids (broccoli, spinach and kale) may reduce the risk of cataracts.

The Beaver Dam Eye Study (Lyle *et al.*, 1999) did not show any strong link between five measured carotenoids and risk of cataracts, but did show an inverse association with serum tocopherols. The POLA study of 2584 inhabitants of Sete, France, found that lipid-standardised plasma α-tocopherol levels were also inversely associated with signs of AMD (Delcourt *et al.*, 1999); no associations were found for plasma retinol and ascorbic acid. Jacques *et al.* (1997) showed an inverse association between long-term (>10 years) vitamin C supplement use and prevalence of opacities (Jacques *et al.*, 1997).

In summary, the evidence is suggestive that increased fruit and vegetable intakes are associated with lower risk of AMD and with cataracts in elderly subjects. It is not yet clear which components and which vegetables are protective; confounding cannot be ruled out in explaining some of the associations previously reported.

3.5.3 Chronic obstructive pulmonary disease

Chronic obstructive pulmonary disease (COPD) is an all inclusive and non-specific term that refers to a defined set of breathing-related symptoms, characterised by airflow obstruction. Asthma is defined as a chronic inflammatory airway disorder. The criteria used to define COPDs in general have not always been applied in the same way in all epidemiological studies, thus making review more problematic.

Bearing problems of definition in mind, there have been a number of recent reviews of the links between nutrition and COPDs (Schunemann *et al.*, 2001; Trenga *et al.*, 2001). Schunemann *et al.* concluded that the largest body of literature exists for a protective effect of vitamin C and fresh fruit and vegetable intake. Existing studies cannot distinguish the effect attributed to specific nutrients from that of a 'healthy' diet. It may be that there are other substances in fruits and vegetables, which have not yet been measured, that may be protective, and it would be premature to attribute causality to any measured antioxidants alone. The review concluded that the evidence is insufficient to recommend the use of any supplements, but the data do support the recommendation to eat more fruits and vegetables.

There are too few data to conclude that flavonoids are protective for COPDs (Schunemann *et al.*, 2001). A recent population-based case-control study in south London showed that, after adjusting for potential confounding factors, apple consumption was protective against asthma (odds ratio 0.84, 95% CI 0.75–0.97) (Shaheen *et al.*, 2001). The authors concluded that there is a need for a better understanding of how flavonoids or other constituents of apples influence respiratory health. Shaheen *et al.* also found that a higher intake of selenium was protective and the authors commented on the declining intake of selenium in the UK population, which they speculate may be expected to lead to an increased prevalence of asthma in the future.

3.5.4 Osteoporosis and bone health

There is a limited amount of information that suggests that a diet rich in plant foods is also beneficial to bone health. This area has been reviewed recently (New, 2001).

3.6 Conclusions

Eating patterns characterised by an abundance of fruit, vegetables and other plant foods are associated with a reduced risk of chronic disease, *e.g.* cardiovascular disease and cancer, and to a lesser extent other conditions such as age-related eye defects. Although these findings have been supported by many studies, the association is usually of moderate strength. The search for the active components in these foods has met with limited success. Research has been focused on the antioxidants vitamins C and E and β-carotene, although a few studies have also looked at other carotenoids and some of the polyphenols (*e.g.* flavonoids) that are the main subject of this Task Force report. Promising and generally consistent results have been reported in animal and *in vitro* studies, but to date convincing evidence from human intervention and epidemiological studies is sparse.

3.7 Research recommendations

- Studies of the bioavailability of the constituents of plants and the factors that influence absorption, distribution and tissue uptake, and the likely impact of these substances on metabolic processes.
- Development and validation of biomarkers of intermediate endpoints, both biological response markers and early disease markers, and emphasis on the relevance of the biomarker to the disease end-point.

- Application of the validated biomarkers of intermediate endpoints in randomised controlled trials testing the efficacy of foods containing these bioactive compounds in the maintenance of health and wellbeing.
- There is a need for soundly constructed prospective studies and parallel mechanistic studies, designed to identify active components in plant foods, their mode of action and any interactions that occur between them. Identification of these would enable dietary advice to be more specific.

3.8 Key points

- It is important to recognise the strengths and weaknesses of data derived from epidemiological studies, in general, and from specific types of study.
- Eating patterns characterised by an abundance of fruit, vegetables and other plant foods are associated with a reduced risk of chronic disease, *e.g.* cardiovascular disease (coronary heart disease and stroke) and some cancers. A less extensive amount of information is also available for type 2 diabetes, age-related macular degeneration, cataract, and chronic obstructive pulmonary disease. Although these findings have been supported by many studies, the association is usually of moderate strength.
- The search for the active components in these foods has met with limited success; specific constituents responsible for the association have yet to be identified, and so have not been widely investigated in epidemiological studies.
- Research has been focused on the antioxidants vitamins C and E and β-carotene, although a few studies have also looked at

other carotenoids and some of the polyphenols (*e.g.* flavonoids) that are among the main subjects of this report. Promising and generally consistent results have been reported in animal and *in vitro* studies but, to date, convincing evidence from human intervention and epidemiological studies is sparse. The evidence that antioxidants such as vitamins E and C and β-carotene specifically are responsible for the beneficial effects of fruit and vegetables is at best equivocal.
- The need for caution when it comes to advocating supplements of individual substances provided by plant foods has been clearly underlined by the findings of several intervention studies that demonstrated that large doses of β-carotene may actually be detrimental to the health of certain groups, *e.g.* heavy smokers.
- There is a need for soundly constructed prospective studies and related mechanistic studies, designed to identify active components in plant foods, their long-term health effects and their mode of action. Identification of these would enable dietary advice to be more specific.

4
Potential Mechanisms of Action of Bioactive Substances Found in Foods

4.1 Introduction

There is considerable epidemiological evidence (see Chapter 3) to indicate that populations that consume diets rich in plant foods have a reduced incidence of various cancers and of cardiovascular disease (CVD) (Block, 1992). A great deal of work has been undertaken into understanding why such diets might have this effect. In particular, the nature of the potential bioactive agents present in fruit and vegetables has recently received considerable attention (Rhodes, 1996; Hasler & Blumberg, 1999). More complex epidemiological data have been valuable in focusing attention on specific components of fruit- and vegetable-based diets; see, for example, Gey's studies on the role of vitamins E and C in heart disease (Gey *et al.*, 1993b). However, precise evaluation of their roles requires, in addition to epidemiological associations, that specific substances in the foods are identified which have chemical properties or activities that may help prevention or reduction of the occurrence of cancer and CVD and other conditions. This has involved the testing of individual food components in animal and cellular models of cancers and heart disease to attempt to identify active components and potential mechanisms by which such substances might act.

The substances present in foods that may be bioactive appear to be complex groups of compounds with variable structures and activities and it is therefore unlikely that they all act by common mechanisms. Whilst this initially may appear to be surprising, it should be considered in the light of current knowledge indicating that the pathophysiological processes leading to, *e.g.* cancer or to CVD are very complex. Thus, there are many potential sites and stages, where bioactive substances in food could act to reduce the possibility of formation of cancerous cells, or of the atherosclerotic plaque in CVD. The potential mechanisms of action can therefore only be appreciated in the context of current concepts of the pathogenesis of cancers and CVD, and this approach will be followed here. This chapter will therefore initially provide an overview of the pathogenesis of cancer and CVD, followed by an indication of potential sites where plant bioactive compounds might have protective effects. Other potential effects, for example, on age-related macular degeneration, will also be considered briefly.

Finally, in this introduction it is pertinent to sound a word of caution concerning the interpretation of mechanistic studies in which purified compounds have been examined as putative modifiers of pathophysiological processes. Many such studies have been undertaken by classical biochemical or toxicological methods in which little attention has been paid to the physiological relevance of the concentrations at which the compound has been examined. Consequently, in some situations, effects have been shown at high concentrations which will not be achieved *in vivo* and subsequently been reported as potential mechanisms of action for those compounds (see Chapters 6–11).

4.2 Potential mechanisms by which plant bioactive substances may help protect against cancer

It should be appreciated that the specific mechanisms by which individual constituents of diets affect the cancer process are usually poorly understood. In recent years, a great deal of scientific data have been obtained such that the mechanisms of carcinogenesis are now understood to a degree where specific food constituents can be tested to evaluate their ability to inhibit or promote specific processes which could be predicted to prevent or delay carcinogenesis. A widely appreciated example of this is the ability of specific plant constituents to act as antioxidants, reducing the damage to DNA and other important biomolecules, caused by reactive free radical species (Duthie *et al.*, 2000).

4.2.1 The cancer process

The chief causes of cancer appear to be environmental, with a genetic predisposition playing a relatively small, but important, role in the overall incidence of these diseases. A fundamental feature of tumours is uncontrolled growth of cells in the tissue in question. This lack of control of cell proliferation and differentiation underlies the disorder and a greater understanding of these processes has underpinned our increased understanding of these disorders.

Fundamental studies have indicated that the process of carcinogenesis following exposure to a carcinogen can be envisaged as a series of events (World Cancer Research Fund, 1997). In practice, such events do not always occur as a linear process, but it can be helpful to conceptualise the process as follows:

- exposure of the organism to the carcinogen
- metabolism of the carcinogenic agent
- interaction between the carcinogen and cellular DNA – *initiation*
- repair of the DNA damage, death of the cell or persistence of the damaged cells
- replication and growth of the abnormal cells into definable pre-neoplastic cells – *promotion*
- growth of the tumour and spread to other tissues.

Substances within food, that are potentially bioactive, can interact with this process at all stages.

(i) Exposure of the organism to a potential carcinogen and its metabolism

Humans are continually exposed to numerous substances (as well as radiation) that are theoretically capable of inducing mutations in DNA. These include smoking and some hydrocarbons in exhaust gases. Data indicate that such agents act by a variety of mechanisms of which reactive oxygen species, free radicals and molecules capable of readily generating oxygen radicals produced during normal metabolism, and the generation of alkylating agents, appear to be particularly important.

Many agents, that are potentially carcinogenic to cells are enzymatically metabolised by the cell to make them more water soluble and hence readily excreted. This process is undertaken by so-called *Phase I enzymes* including the cytochrome P450 system. In undertaking this conversion, the agents are also converted to a form that allows them to more readily bind to cell macromolecules such as DNA, RNA, proteins and lipids. This process is known as *metabolic activation* of the carcinogen.

Further metabolism of potentially carcinogenic substances occurs by *Phase II detoxification enzymes*, including enzymes such as the glutathione transferases, which inactivate substances by reaction with the major cellular reducing agent glutathione.

It is important to note that these processes (both the exposure of cells to a carcinogen and its metabolism) can be very site specific, leading to the recognised tissue and cell specificity of certain carcinogens.

The requirement for enzymatic activation and detoxification at these sites means that genetic variations in enzyme activities can influence the susceptibility of individuals to a large number of potentially carcinogenic agents. In addition, substances that modify the activity of Phase I enzymes involved in metabolic activation or the activity of Phase II detoxification enzymes can act to reduce the chance of mutagenic DNA damage.

Some plant-based bioactive agents appear to have these properties and are discussed later.

(ii) Initiation – interaction between the carcinogen and cellular DNA

Initiation of the cancer involves a series of events whereby the carcinogenic agent induces alterations in the DNA of a cell to produce a mutation which can be inherited, and which may confer upon the cell the potential for neoplastic growth.

The structure of DNA can be modified if carcinogenic molecules become chemically bound to it, or react with it. Examples of such adducts include hydroxyl groups, methyl groups and aromatic hydrocarbons. This is potentially an important step in the initiation of the cancer cell because these adducts can distort the shape of the DNA, causing misreplication during DNA replication and a mutation in the new strand. This can cause mistranslation (and hence the potential formation of an abnormal protein), and if sufficiently extensive, can result in DNA breakage.

Events such as those described above appear to be particularly important if they occur in key molecules such as oncogenes or tumour-suppressor genes which are involved in the regulation of cell growth and differentiation in a co-ordinated manner.

There is increasing evidence that hydroxyl radical attack on the guanine (G) and cytosine (C) bases of DNA plays a crucial role in initiation of certain cancers (Guyton & Kensler, 1993). These bases appear to be particularly susceptible to attack by free radical species, and formation of the 8-hydroxylated derivative of G [measured as 8-oxo-dG (attached to deoxyribose) or 8-oxo-G] has been extensively reported in experimental carcinogen treatment protocols (Floyd *et al.*, 1990). It is thought that, if damage is not repaired, the presence of 8-oxo-G in DNA can be mutagenic; DNA polymerases selectively incorporate A with 8-oxo-G rather than C (Shibutani *et al.*, 1991). The result of this will be a G→T transversion (see Fig. 4.1).

In most cases, the most likely result of an interaction of a carcinogen with DNA is that the resulting damage will be repaired by efficient DNA repair systems. All nucleated cells contain multiple enzyme systems involved in DNA repair that are generally still poorly understood. Their function is crucial to the prevention of cancerous changes in cells, and it is now recognised that defects in single enzyme systems, either genetically programmed, or due to damage to the gene coding for that protein can result in increased mutations within cells.

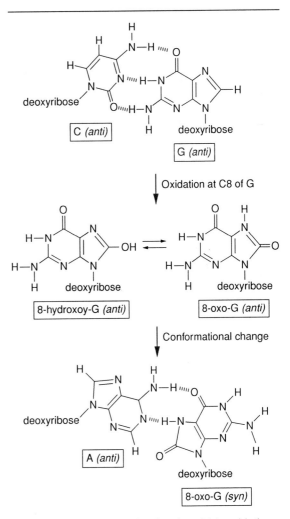

Fig. 4.1 Potential mechanism by which oxidation of guanine at C8 can lead to G→T transversions [redrawn from Guyton, KZ & Kensler KW (1993) Oxidative mechanisms in carcinogenesis. *British Medical Bulletin*, **49**, 523–44, by permission of Oxford University Press].

(iii) Promotion – replication and growth of the abnormal cells into definable pre-neoplastic cells

This process involves alterations in gene expression and cell proliferation that transform the initiated cell into a group of cancer cells. It involves the interaction of a series of tumour promoters with the initiated cells. Such tumour promoters do not necessarily have carcinogenic activity alone, but appear to increase tumour development. Examples of substances that are known to have these effects include chemicals such as the phorbol esters and certain barbiturates, some hormones and some dietary factors. There is also some evidence that reactive oxygen species can act as mediators of many known tumour promoters and that generators of free radicals can act as tumour promoters (Guyton & Kensler, 1993). The mechanisms underlying these effects are currently the subject of extensive research, but they include induction of the expression of a number of genes regulating cellular growth (such as the

proto-oncogenes, c-*fos* and NF$_\kappa$B), and an interaction with intracellular signalling pathways.

The final stage of the cancer process involves growth of the tumour with destruction of surrounding tissue and increased blood vessel formation (angiogenesis) to supply nutrients to the dividing cancer cells and spread to other tissues. Numerous factors are involved in this process and the resulting tumour mass appears to contain increasingly abnormal genetic material. Again there is evidence that reactive oxygen species may play a role in these changes.

An outline of these various steps in the genesis of the cancer cell is presented in Fig. 4.2.

4.2.2 Potential sites where plant bioactive compounds might act

Experimental studies have determined that specific substances present in plant foods (see Chapters 7–9 and 11) can act at a variety of sites relevant to the development of the cancer cell. The mechanisms involved [modified from Hasler & Blumberg (1999)] might include the following:

- inhibition of carcinogen activation
- induction of hepatic detoxification pathways
- antioxidant effects/metal chelation properties
- enhancement of the immune response
- induction of apoptosis/suppression of mitosis
- alterations in hormone metabolism.

4.2.3 Specific examples of actions of plant bioactive compounds

(i) Allium or sulphur compounds

Allium vegetables contain a number of sulphur compounds (see Sections 2.5 and 7.5.2) that may have anti-cancer effects by induction of Phase II detoxification mechanisms. There is also evidence that they may specifically inhibit the bacterial conversion of nitrate to nitrite in the stomach, acting to reduce the potential carcinogenic effects of nitrite.

(ii) Antioxidant vitamins

The antioxidant nutrients (*e.g.* vitamin E, vitamin C and some carotenoids) are likely to have their

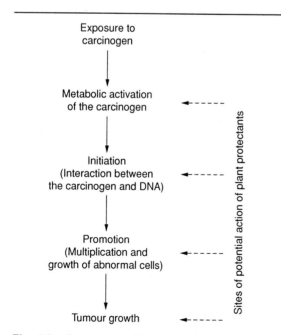

Fig. 4.2 A summary of the steps that are generally thought to be involved in carcinogenesis (for more details, see World Cancer Research Fund, 1997).

potential anti-cancer effect through reducing oxidative damage to DNA, and also by interacting with various other aspects of the above scheme, such as proliferation, by influencing redox-regulated genes involved in cell proliferation.

(iii) Dithiolthiones

These compounds have also been shown to inhibit metabolic activation of some carcinogens *in vitro* and to enhance the ability of cells to detoxify activated carcinogens. This may be achieved by the enhancement of cellular glutathione content and the activation of glutathione transferases (Hasler & Blumberg, 1999).

(iv) Flavonoids

These compounds (see Section 2.2.1) appear to have the potential to interact with the above scheme of cancer induction at a number of different points. These include inhibition of the metabolic activation of carcinogens by modulation of the activity of specific Phase I and II enzymes (Rhodes, 1996), and by acting as antioxidants, reducing oxidative damage to DNA and influencing other redox-regulated aspects of cell proliferation. Many other phenolic compounds (see Section 2.2) found in foods also appear to be capable of induction of detoxification systems and have antioxidant properties in experimental systems.

(v) Isothiocyanates (derived from glucosinolates)

Zhang and Talalay proposed that the putative anti-cancer properties of isothiocyanates (see Sections 5.3 and 7.5.3) are mediated by down-regulation of cytochrome P450 (thus suppressing activation of carcinogens) and by induction of Phase II enzymes such as glutathione-S-transferase and quinone reductase (Zhang & Talalay, 1994).

(vi) Phytoestrogens

These compounds are known to compete with oestradiol to bind with oestrogenic receptors (isoflavones have a stronger binding affinity for

ERβ than ERα), modifying steroid metabolism (see Section 8.6). These and other potential actions [*e.g.* possible inhibition of cell growth through interacting with growth factor receptors (*e.g.* the EGF receptor)] appear to allow them to alter the growth and proliferation of hormone-dependent cancer cells. Some phytoestrogens may also have antioxidant properties (Cassidy, 1996).

(vii) Salicylates

Fruits and vegetables contain salicylates (Swain *et al.*, 1985; Janssen *et al.*, 1996a), but whether they are present in sufficient amounts and/or are bioavailable is still open to question (Janssen *et al.*, 1996b). In addition to the effects on CVD, there is also interest in the possible effects of salicylates in the reduction of certain cancers, *e.g.* colorectal cancer (Paterson & Lawrence, 2001). These issues are discussed in Chapters 3, 6 and 7.

4.3 Potential mechanisms by which plant bioactive substances may protect against CVD

The stimulus for much of this work has derived from epidemiological studies (see Section 3.3), indicating that people who consume diets rich in fruit and vegetables have a lower incidence of CVD (Block, 1992). Research has been primarily focused on the role of the well-recognised antioxidant nutrients vitamin E, vitamin C and some carotenoids, but the publication of a study suggesting that dietary flavonoids might protect against heart disease has widened the range of compounds that receive research interest (Hertog *et al.*, 1993a).

4.3.1 The process of atherosclerosis

A considerable amount of previous work has been concentrated on the role of dietary saturated fatty acids and blood cholesterol as major risk factors for CVD. The recognition of cholesterol as a major risk factor led to dietary intervention trials aimed at reducing blood cholesterol, but in recent years there has been increasing evidence that oxidised low-density lipoprotein (LDL), rather than cholesterol *per se*, may be the atherogenic component (Steinberg *et al.*, 1989). LDL is a cholesterol fraction that contains a high proportion of polyunsaturated fatty acids (PUFA) in the phospholipid layer (see Section 10.4). These PUFA are susceptible to free radical-mediated peroxidation, and there is increasing evidence that this oxidised LDL is important, and possibly obligatory, in the pathogenesis of the atherosclerotic lesion.

Many studies have now indicated that increased risk of CVD in Western countries is associated with a relatively low intake of antioxidant nutrients (Gey *et al.*, 1993b). More specific evidence of associations has also been obtained from epidemiological studies (see Section 3.3), examining the relationship between median plasma concentrations of specific antioxidants in different geographical areas and mortality from CVD. These have indicated that the incidence of CVD is inversely related to the plasma content of vitamins E and C, β-carotene and vitamin A (Gey *et al.*, 1993a). However, intervention studies have not have not shown effects of these specific components (see Chapter 3).

In association with the epidemiological recognition of a potential protective role for antioxidants in preventing CVD, there has been an increasing amount of data supporting a role for free radical species in LDL oxidation as a key step in the development of atherosclerotic lesions. These studies have indicated that the process of atherosclerosis can be considered as a series of events [modified from Rice-Evans *et al.* (1995)]:

- minor damage to the vascular endothelium induces monocyte adherence
- transformation of monocytes to macrophages
- oxidation of fatty acids in LDL
- uptake of oxidised LDL by scavenger receptors on macrophages
- conversion of macrophages into lipid-laden foam cells
- release of factors by the macrophages which stimulate the proliferation of smooth muscle cells

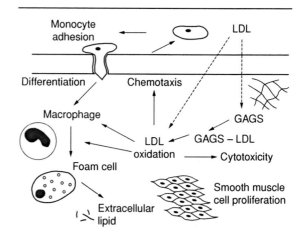

Fig. 4.3 Possible mechanisms involved in the pathogenesis of atherosclerosis (redrawn from Rice-Evans *et al.*, 1995 with permission from Elsevier).

- formation of an atherosclerotic plaque
- reduction in vessel lumen diameter restricting blood flow
- plaque disruption and occlusion of blood flow.

A schematic illustration of the process is shown in Fig. 4.3 (Witztum, 1994; Rice-Evans *et al.*, 1995). The number of sites at which dietary factors might potentially interact is limited in comparison with the process of carcinogenesis, but include the following.

(i) Monocyte adherence to sites of endothelial cell damage

Sites of minor damage to the endothelial cell will induce the release of chemotactic factors to attract monocytes from the circulation, and the up-regulation of adhesion molecules on both white cells and tissue surfaces. Some of the released chemotactic factors (*e.g.* prostanoids and cytokines) may be modified by specific dietary factors.

(ii) Oxidation of LDL

Dietary lipid load and hence circulating levels of lipids are likely to influence this process. The susceptibility of LDL to oxidation, producing an atherogenic form, may also depend on its antioxidant content. For example, when LDL is exposed to a copper-mediated oxidation system, vitamin E in the outer phospholipid layer of the LDL is depleted first, followed by carotenoids such as lycopene and β-carotene. LDL oxidation is delayed if vitamin C is present in the external medium, presumably because vitamin C regenerates vitamin E. Increasing the vitamin E or ubiquinone content of LDL by dietary supplementation of volunteers also inhibits oxidation of LDL to the atherogenic form. This suggests that nutritional antioxidant intakes may be important in inhibiting the pathogenesis of CVD (Esterbauer *et al.*, 1992; Witztum, 1994; Rice-Evans *et al.*, 1995).

The mechanisms by which LDL is oxidised *in vivo* have yet to be clearly characterised. Oxidation is unlikely to occur in plasma where metal ions are safely bound to proteins such as ferritin, transferrin and caeruloplasmin, and where there are adequate antioxidants available to inhibit the process. Thus LDL modification may be restricted to regions of the vascular intima. Although LDL can be modified by lipoxygenases (Rankin *et al.*, 1991), much work has been concentrated on the potential role of oxygen radical reactions catalysed by copper. Copper ions effectively promote oxidation of LDL *in vitro* and the release of copper from caeruloplasmin within the atherosclerotic lesion may lead to peroxidation of preformed fatty acid hydroperoxides formed within the lesion by macrophage-derived superoxide and hydrogen peroxide (Heinecke *et al.*, 1986). Plant-based substances capable of inhibiting the oxidation of LDL or acting as metal chelators, preventing metal catalysed oxidation of LDL, are therefore likely to interfere in this process.

(iii) *Reduction in vascular tone*

Many aspects of the atheroscerotic process lead to a restriction in the lumen of the vasculature. Manipulation of vascular tone is, therefore, a potential way of relieving the functional consequences of the ensuing reduced blood flow. Recent evidence indicates that certain plant-derived compounds have vasodilatory effects, potentially facilitating increased blood flow to affected tissues (Burns *et al.*, 2000).

(iv) *Haemostasis*

The haemostatic system maintains blood in the fluid state by controlling bleeding and playing a role in tissue repair. It is now generally accepted that the majority of acute vascular events (sudden coronary death, acute myocardial infarction, unstable angina and most strokes) are caused by thrombosis (resulting in vessel occlusion), secondary to plaque rupture. Moreover, levels of some components of the haemostatic system are associated with the risk of coronary heart disease (CHD) and stroke, and the contribution of platelets and the coagulation system to the progression of atherosclerosis itself is increasingly recognised. Hence, individuals may be at risk of clinical arterial disease due to an increased thrombotic tendency. Moreover, atherosclerosis is now recognised as a chronic inflammatory disease (see below and Chapter 10) which may contribute to prothrombotic changes, therefore increasing the likelihood of future thrombotic events. Platelets and coagulation factors are primary determinants of blood coagulability (fibrin formation), whereas the fibrinolytic system is responsible for dissolving blood clots. The involvement of platelets, the coagulation cascade and fibrinolysis in haemostasis is summarised in Fig. 4.4 and reviewed elsewhere (Kelly *et al.*, 2001).

(a) Platelet activation

Platelets circulate freely in the blood and do not adhere to intact endothelium. However, in response to vessel wall injury, platelets rapidly undergo the process of adhesion, shape change (from discs to spheres, forming pseudopods), secretion and aggregation resulting in the formation of a precisely localised haemostatic plug. Platelet aggregation by these agonists is mediated in part, through the intracellular formation of thromboxane A_2 ($T \times A_2$), an eicosanoid, produced from arachidonic acid (AA) (see Chapter 10). Stimulated endothelial cells also release nitric oxide (NO) which, in addition to causing vasodilation, inhibits platelet aggregation, promotes disaggregation and inhibits platelet adhesion to the endothelium. The balance between the opposing effects of $T \times A_2$ released by platelets, and prostaglandin I_2 (PGI_2) released by endothelial cells is important in maintaining normal blood vessel function. The central role for platelets in thrombosis and CVD has led many to investigate whether platelet function is modifiable by dietary, as well as pharmacological means (see Section 4.3.4 and Chapters 7 and 10).

(b) Coagulation

There are two major pathways by which prothrombin (factor II) is converted to thrombin, the so-called intrinsic and the extrinsic, although the two systems are not separate and actually activate each other resulting in the generation of thrombin (Kelly *et al.*, 2001). Thrombin converts fibrinogen to fibrin and activates platelets (see above), resulting in the formation of the haemostatic plug. Fibrin is eventually degraded during clot lysis (fibrinolysis) by the enzyme plasmin (see Fig. 4.4). Studies have shown that raised levels of blood clotting factors such as fibrinogen (Ernst & Resch, 1993), FVIII and von Willebrand factor (vWF) (Meade *et al.*, 1994) are positively associated with CHD. Data are more limited for the role of haemostatic factors in stroke, although raised levels of fibrinogen (Smith *et al.*, 1997; Bots *et al.*, 2002), FVIII and vWF (Folsom *et al.*, 1999) have been associated with an increased risk of stroke. Disturbances of the fibrinolytic system, measured via a global test of fibrinolytic activity, degradation products of fibrinolysis (particularly D-dimer) and specific components including plasminogen-activator inhibitor-1 (PAI-1) and tissue-plasminogen activator (t-PA) are also associated with CHD [an overview is available (MacCallum & Meade, 1999)]. In a prospective study, tPA antigen and fibrin D-dimer were independently associated with risk of stroke (Smith *et al.*, 1997).

The effects of dietary components on the coagulation system have been investigated, and this also impacts on platelet function because thrombin is a potent platelet aggregating agent (agonist) and fibrinogen enhances the rate of ADP-induced platelet aggregation (Meade *et al.*, 1985a,b).

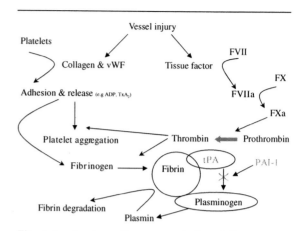

Fig. 4.4 A schematic representation of the extrinsic coagulation pathway, with the involvement of platelets, an ordered series of proteolytic transformations, in which the constituent zymogens of the coagulation pathway are converted to active enzymes (serine proteases) that culminates in the generation of thrombin (courtesy of Dr Colette Kelly, University of Reading).

4.3.3 Potential sites where plant-based bioactive compounds might act

Experimental studies have indicated that specific substances present in plant foods (see Chapters 7–11) can act at a variety of sites relevant to the development of CVD. These might include the following:

- modification of hormonal profile
- modification of lipid profile
- decrease of serum cholesterol
- reduction in lipid oxidation/antioxidant effect
- metal chelation
- anti-inflammatory effects
- haemostasis.

4.3.4 Specific examples of actions of plant-based bioactive compounds

(i) Antioxidant vitamins

The antioxidant nutrients (*e.g.* vitamin E, vitamin C and β-carotene) have a number of effects that are likely to be of relevance in this area. Most important may be their ability to reduce oxidative damage to LDL and other lipids and (in a similar manner to their anti-cancer role, see Section 4.2) influencing smooth muscle cell proliferation by modification of the expression of redox-regulated genes involved in regulation of this process.

(ii) Fatty acids

PUFA and MUFA may exert a number of effects that can help protect against CVD. The effects of these classes of fatty acids on blood cholesterol and lipid profiles are discussed in Chapter 10. Diets rich in MUFA, *n*-6 or *n*-3 fatty acids that decrease platelet phospholipid AA could reduce the synthesis of proaggregatory thromboxanes derived from the latter. Certainly, the potency of eicosanoids derived from long-chain *n*-3 PUFA (*i.e.* EPA and DHA) is less than those derived from *n*-6 PUFA. The effect of EPA in the endothelial cell is to produce PGI_3, which has inhibitory effects similar to those of prostacyclin (PGI_2). Thus interventions (increase in *n*-3 fatty acids) that change the balance are conceived as altering thrombosis risk (see Chapter 10). Although α-linolenic acid (ALNA), the precursor to EPA/DHA, was thought to share some of the beneficial effects of these compounds on thrombotic tendency (de Lorgeril *et al.*, 1994), more recent work suggests it does not appear to reproduce the beneficial haemostatic effects of the long chain *n*-3 PUFA (Wensing *et al.*, 1999) but may possess antiarrhythmic effects (De Deckere *et al.*, 1998).

There is also some evidence to suggest that a change or alteration in platelet membrane composition, via a change in fatty acid composition/lipoprotein concentration that affects membrane fluidity (see Chapter 10), could affect the properties of the surface membrane receptors of platelets (Hornstra & Rand, 1986; Hussein *et al.*, 1997; Huhle *et al.*, 1999).

Diets rich in MUFA have been shown to influence the postprandial activation of FVII (Roche *et al.*, 1998; Zampelas *et al.*, 1998). The possible mechanism for this effect is that the MUFA diet resulted in smaller numbers of larger chylomicrons, which may theoretically provide fewer contact sites for activation of FVII (Silva *et al.*, 2001).

(iii) Flavonoids

These compounds appear to have the potential to act as antioxidants, reducing oxidative damage to LDL and influencing redox-regulated aspects of cell proliferation (Hertog & Hollman, 1996). Some are also reported to act as metal chelators, although whether this reduces metal-catalysed oxidation of LDL is the subject of controversy (Takahama, 1985).

The flavonoids quercetin and rutin are also reported to be inhibitors of platelet aggregation (Gryglewski *et al.*, 1987), and new data indicate that many polyphenols (see Section 2.2) found in foodstuffs, such as red wine (see Section 9.6), have potent vasodilatory effects when tested *in vitro* (Burns *et al.*, 2000). However, the anti-aggregatory effects of flavonoids seen *in vitro* were not observed *in vivo* when onions and parsley were fed to human volunteers (see Chapter 7). No effect on platelet aggregation, thromboxane B2 production, factor VII or other haemostatic variables were observed (Janssen *et al.*, 1998). Furthermore, although black-tea polyphenols (see Chapter 9) inhibit platelet aggregation *in vitro*, neither the chronic (4 weeks) nor the acute consumption of black tea altered platelet aggregation *ex vivo* in human plasma samples (Hodgson *et al.*, 2002). The discrepancy between the results of *in vitro* and *ex vivo* studies may relate to the non-physiological concentrations of polyphenols used in the *in vitro* studies.

(iv) Folate

There has been considerable recent interest in the possibility that folic acid plays a specific role in reducing CHD by lowering plasma homocysteine concentration (see Chapters 1 and 13). It is thought that elevated plasma homocysteine levels may be linked mechanistically to specific processes. For example, homocysteine has been reported to promote the oxidative modification of LDL cholesterol, stimulate the proliferation of vascular smooth muscle cells and have prothrombotic effects by enhancing the activities of factor XII and factor V. In addition, homocysteine appears to have a vasoconstrictive effect by reducing endothelial nitric oxide production. Trials to examine the potential role of folic acid in this area are in progress.

(v) Phytoestrogens

A lowering effect of phytoestrogens (see Section 8.8.4) on blood cholesterol levels has been documented which may contribute to a protective effect against coronary heart disease. These compounds also compete with oestradiol to bind with oestrogenic receptors, modifying steroid metabolism. There is also some evidence that they can block the action of some growth factors, thus modifying the growth and proliferation of some cells. Some phytoestrogens may also have antioxidant properties (Cassidy, 1996). Genistein has also been shown to inhibit thrombin formation and platelet activation *in vitro* (Wilcox & Blumenthal, 1995). There appears to be a lack of evidence/lack of studies investigating soya/genistein-rich diets and their effects on coagulation in humans.

(vi) Plant sterols

These compounds (see Section 10.9) show structural similarities to cholesterol and inhibit absorption of cholesterol from the gut, reducing the circulating levels of both total and LDL cholesterol.

(vii) Salicylates

The principal metabolite of aspirin is salicylic acid, which is found in a number of plant foods (see Chapter 7). There is increasing interest in whether the salicylates in fruits and vegetables have protective effects against CVD. Serum concentrations of salicylic acid have been found to be higher in vegetarians than non-vegetarians (Blacklock *et al.*, 2001). However, whether or not salicylates are present in plant foods in sufficient quantities to have an effect (Chapter 7) and whether they are bioavailable (see Chapter 6) are subjects of debate. The use of aspirin in CVD derives from an effect on blood platelets (see above), but it may have other effects. There is

now overwhelming evidence that aspirin reduces the incidence of major vascular events in those with previous or developing clinical episodes of arterial disease and it is common practice to administer low doses (80–160 mg/day) of aspirin to prevent ischaemic events in patients with coronary artery disease.

(viii) Sulphur compounds

There is growing interest in the sulphur-containing glucosinolates as potential modifiers of carcinogenesis. This is discussed in Chapter 5. There has also been interest in the properties of sulphur-containing members of the *Alliaceae* family (onions and garlic) (Ackermann *et al.*, 2001). Various mechanisms of action have been proposed (see Section 7.4.2) but any claimed effects (*e.g.* cholesterol lowering or inhibition of platelet aggregation) have required substantial intakes.

4.4 Other ageing-related disorders

There is increasing evidence that plant-derived bioactive compounds may be protective against a number of other chronic age-related disorders. These include specific disorders such as cataract formation and macular degeneration and less specific age-related changes, such as the relative immune deficit seen in elderly people. Further discussion of these potential roles can be found in Chapter 3.

4.4.1 Age-related macular degeneration and cataract

The macula lutea is a pigmented region of the retina which includes the fovea, responsible for the highest visual acuity and which contains the highest density of cone photoreceptors. The human macular pigment is composed primarily of the carotenoids lutein and zeaxanthin (see Section 3.5.2). The macular pigment filters blue light, which is particularly damaging to photoreceptors and to the retinal pigment epithelium. There is increasing interest about whether carotenoids can reduce age-related macular degeneration. The high level of carotenoids may protect the retina by limiting the oxidative stress that results from metabolic processes and from exposure to light. One of the ways in which light can damage the retina is by generating free radicals that lead to the peroxidation of membrane lipids. Lutein and zeaxanthin are powerful antioxidants and so may help protect against free radical damage (Greenway & Pratt, 2001).

4.5 Summary

Our understanding of the pathogenic processes underlying cancers and CVD is developing rapidly and is leading to improved pharmacological means of preventing and treating these disorders.

In parallel with these developments, it has become apparent that there is a very large range of bioactive compounds present in plant-derived foods and drinks that may have protective effects against these disorders. The potential of these compounds to be beneficial to human health appears significant, but many mechanisms of action are likely to be involved. In order to provide clear dietary guidelines aimed at maximising these potential protective effects (see Chapter 13), it will be necessary to understand more clearly the importance and relevance of the different protective pathways and the efficacy of the different compounds in regulating these pathways.

4.6 Research recommendations

- Much more information is required on the effects of plant constituents, *in vivo* and *in vitro*, at concentrations relevant to their normal levels in foodstuffs.
- Novel approaches are required to develop appropriate and relevant models of cancer pathogenesis and CVD in which food constituents can be studied over a realistic timespan.
- Intervention studies to examine the effect of specific plant constituents should utilise 'hard' endpoints in the light of uncertainties about the relevance of surrogate biomarkers to the pathogenetic process (*e.g.* oxidation markers).

4.7 Key points

- Our understanding of the pathogenic processes underlying cancers and CVD is developing rapidly and is leading to improved pharmacological means of preventing and treating these disorders.
- In parallel with these developments, it has become apparent that there is a very large range of bioactive compounds present in plant-derived foods and drinks that may have protective effects against these disorders.
- The potential of these compounds to be beneficial to human health appears significant, but many mechanisms of action are likely to be involved.
- In order to provide clear dietary guidelines aimed at maximising these potential protective effects, it will be necessary more clearly to understand the importance and relevance of the different protective pathways and the efficacy of the different compounds in modulating these pathways.
- Epidemiological data are consistent with the possibility that constituents of fruit and vegetables may play specific roles in prevention of the pathogenesis of certain cancers and CVD.
- The pathophysiological processes involved in the formation of tumours and in CVD are becoming increasingly well understood.
- *In vitro* and cell culture studies have indicated multiple potential steps in the pathophysiological processes at which various plant constituents might act to prevent the formation of tumours or occurrence of CVD.
- Little evidence has been presented demonstrating that any such effects occur *in vivo* and many of the studies have used experimental conditions that do not approximate to nutritional intake levels.

5
Influence of the Gut Microflora

5.1 Introduction

With its stable temperature, high moisture content and abundant nutrients, the interior of the alimentary tract provides an ideal environment for colonisation by micro-organisms. Bacteria utilise a huge variety of organic materials as sources of energy and have evolved an equally diverse array of enzymes to achieve this. The exploitation of bacterial enzymes to augment the digestive capabilities of the host is a common strategy amongst multicellular organisms. In humans, the stomach and small intestine are relatively sterile and the bulk of the gut microflora reside in the large intestine, downstream from the main sites of digestion and absorption. Thus, human colonic bacteria receive undigested dietary residues, together with mucus and digestive juices.

The main functions of the human large intestine are to salvage water, energy and micronutrients from the faecal stream, and to dehydrate and store the faecal material between bowel movements. However, human beings and their intestinal micro-organisms have become adapted to one another over an immense period of evolutionary time and it would be surprising if the relationship did not involve subtle biological interactions that influence the health of the host. This possibility has aroused much popular and commercial interest in recent years. Various functional food products have been designed to increase the levels of supposedly beneficial bacteria in the colon, either by oral supplementation with live bacterial cultures (probiotics), or by provision of fermentable substrates which selec-

tively favour the growth of bacteria already present (prebiotics).

This chapter is not directly concerned with practical measures to manipulate colonic micro-organisms, but will deal instead with the evidence that gut bacteria can influence human health through the formation or metabolism of protective factors which are not traditionally classified as nutrients. The chapter begins with an introductory account of the human colon, its structure and its microflora, and a short discussion of colonic diseases in which protective factors may play a role. The role of the microflora as a source of various substances, including short-chain fatty acids, which may act as protective factors against colorectal disease, is then discussed. Some examples of bacterial metabolism of food-borne plant secondary metabolites that act either directly on the colonic mucosa or on more distant target tissues after absorption are also given.

5.2 The human colon

5.2.1 Anatomy

The size and gross morphology of the large bowel vary between species in ways that reflect their dietary adaptation. Typically, the colon is thick-walled and muscular, often with a separate blind-ending sac, the caecum, opening close to the junction with the small intestine. At 1.5 m in length, the human colon is relatively large, but morphologically it is little more than a simple tube with a minor bulbous enlargement into which the small intestine empties via a sphincter. Although small in volume, the caecum receives a regular supply of unabsorbed water, mucus and digestive residues which ensures that it provides a relatively dilute, nutrient-rich environment, ideal for fermentation. Post-mortem studies have shown that the proximal colon contains around 200 g of semiliquid material (Cummings *et al.*, 1990), over half of which is bacterial cells (Stephen & Cummings, 1980). At intervals, faecal material is transferred from the right colon into the transverse and distal segments, where it undergoes partial dehydration and storage. The total transit time varies considerably between individuals, and the length of time that material spends in transit through the caecum and right colon influences both the extent of fermentation and the faecal bulk (Stephen *et al.*, 1987). Usually, in Western societies, individuals pass semi-solid stools with a frequency varying from once or twice a day to once every 2–3 days.

5.2.2 Mucosal cells

Unlike the small intestine, in which the mucosa is provided with a dense and elaborate array of leaf- or finger-like villi, the mucosal lining of the colon is flat. The surface is composed of mature columnar epithelial cells that are constantly shed into the intestinal lumen, and replaced by new cells formed near the base of the crypts. These closed, tubular structures are amongst the most rapidly proliferating tissues in the body. In addition to the immature colonocytes migrating toward the mucosal surface, the crypts also contain goblet cells that secrete a steady supply of mucus, and endocrine cells that secrete gastrointestinal hormones into the circulation.

The main function of the colonic epithelial cells is to absorb water and solutes from the faecal material in the gut lumen, but they must also protect the underlying tissues and the circulation from toxic materials and infectious agents in the intestinal lumen. Apart from providing a tight physical barrier, the epithelial cells express a battery of enzymes that can metabolise biologically active molecules, including plant secondary metabolites (Peters *et al.*, 1992), toxins and drugs. Thus, like the liver, the colon can be regarded as a metabolic organ (McDonnell *et al.*, 1996),

that can detoxify substances derived from the environment.

Detoxifying enzymes are classified broadly into two classes, Phase I enzymes, including the cytochrome P450 group, which produce hydrophilic but often reactive oxides, and Phase II enzymes, such as glutathione-S-transferase (GST) and UDP-glucuronyltransferase (see Section 4.2.3). Phase II enzymes often combine the products of Phase I metabolism with chemical groups such as glutathione, glucuronic acid or sulphates. These conjugates are relatively inactive, water-soluble products that can be exported easily from the cell and ultimately excreted in urine.

The Phase I and Phase II enzymes of the colonic mucosa differ from those of the liver, and their activities also vary markedly between individuals because of genetic polymorphisms (Sivaraman *et al.*, 1994). Moreover, because these enzymes are inducible, their activities are regulated in response to exposure to substances in the diet or to metabolites derived from colonic bacteria (Rosenberg, 1991). This provides the mechanistic basis for an important commensal relationship between the intestinal micro-organisms and their human host, whereby the metabolic activities of the former modulate biochemical defences of the latter (Treptow van Lishaut *et al.*, 1999).

5.2.3 Microflora

The colon is a highly anaerobic environment, containing both obligate and facultative anaerobes. The typical adult human colonic microflora has been estimated to contain as many as 400 different bacterial species, but the detailed composition is surprisingly poorly characterised, mainly because a large proportion of the species present cannot be cultured *in vitro*. In general, the largest single groups present are Gram-negative anaerobes of the genus bacteroides, and Gram-positive organisms comprising a number of different genera including bifidobacteria, eubacteria, lactobacilli and clostridia (Moore & Holdeman, 1974). Unlike many other mammalian species, spirochaetes are absent.

The fetal intestine is of course sterile, but bacteria are acquired at birth by cross-contamination from the mother, and then more gradually from the environment during infancy (Bullen *et al.*, 1976). The full microbiological complexity is not achieved until after weaning, when individuals tend to acquire and retain a characteristic microbial pattern. An individual's flora remains fairly stable in response to short-term alterations in diet (Bornside, 1978), but over longer periods of time, large variations in the contribution of individual bacterial species have been observed.

5.2.4 Substrates for fermentation

The colonic microflora derive their energy from two sources, undigested food, most of which is starch or cell wall polysaccharides, and endogenous secretions, particularly digestive enzymes and mucus from the small bowel. Most of the bacteria of the human colon utilise carbohydrate as a source of energy, although not all can degrade polysaccharides directly. Many other species of bacteria are also ultimately dependent upon dietary carbohydrate residues for energy, but they utilise the initial degradation products of the polysaccharide utilisers, rather than the polymers themselves. Around 30 g of bacteria are produced for every 100 g of carbohydrate fermented (Cummings, 1987).

It has been estimated that somewhere between 20 and 80 g of carbohydrate enter the human colon every day, of which about half is undigested starch. In the unprocessed storage organs of plants such as tubers (*e.g.* potatoes) and seeds, starch is localised in granules. The glucose polysaccharides of starch occur in two forms, straight chains of amylose and branching chains of amylopectin, which in their native state have a semicrystalline structure, highly resistant to digestive enzymes. Heating the granules in the presence of water causes the polysaccharides to become hydrated and dispersed. Although this gelatinised starch is readily accessible to hydrolytic enzymes, it can still escape digestion if the degraded granules remain enclosed within intact cell walls, as is common in the cooked legume seeds (Wursch *et al.*, 1986) (see Chapter 8). Cooked starch can also become less susceptible to human digestive enzymes if it is cooled and allowed to undergo

retrogradation to a semicrystalline state (Ring *et al.*, 1988) (see Chapter 12). Most types of resistant starch can be broken down by bacterial enzymes but intact starch is excreted in animals fed retrograded amylase (Gee *et al.*, 1991).

The other main sources of food-borne carbohydrate entering the large bowel are the structural polysaccharides that form plant cell walls (dietary fibre), non-digestible sugars, sugar alcohols and oligosaccharides. Fructooligosaccharides and galactooligosaccharides occur only sparingly in plant foods but they are of commercial interest because they can be used as prebiotics to selectively manipulate the numbers of bifidobacteria in the human colon (Gibson *et al.*, 1995). It is widely assumed that this is of some benefit to health, although the evidence for this is somewhat limited. Some studies on bacterial metabolism *in vitro* suggest that under certain circumstances manipulation of the colonic microflora with either pre- or probiotics could lead to increased synthesis of genotoxic products, although the significance of this is not clear (McBain & Macfarlane, 1997).

Apart from digestive residues, a number of endogenous substrates are available for bacterial fermentation. Mucus is an aqueous dispersion of mucins, a complex group of glycoproteins containing oligosaccharide side-chains which account for most of their molecular mass, and provide a major source of nutrients for the colonic microflora. It is known that mucin carbohydrates are utilised as substrates by many colonic bacteria, and even when the colon is surgically isolated and has no access to exogenous substrates it still supports a complex microflora (Miller *et al.*, 1984). The intestinal mucosa is also a major site of epithelial cell proliferation and loss, and degraded cellular proteins and lipids are substrates for bacterial metabolism. In total, endogenous carbohydrate is thought to contribute 2–3 g of fermentable substrate per day to the faecal flora, and endogenous proteins may contribute as much as 4–6 g. The bacterial metabolism of amino acids derived from intraluminal protein leads to the formation of a complex variety of products, many of which are potentially harmful to the host. For example, ammonia is thought to be a potential promoter of neoplasia, as are many amines (Matsui *et al.*, 1995). Increased dietary protein intake leads to a corresponding increase in faecal ammonia and amines in human volunteers (Geypens *et al.*, 1997).

5.3 Colorectal diseases

The large intestine is subject to a range of functional, structural and infectious diseases that are largely outside the scope of this chapter. In the context of food-borne protective factors, the most important classes of colorectal diseases are the inflammatory conditions of unknown cause, Crohn's disease and ulcerative colitis, and colorectal carcinoma, which is the second most common cause of death from cancer in many industrialised societies.

The progressive, multistage model for the development of cancer described in Section 4.2.1 is well illustrated by the natural history of colorectal carcinomas, most of which are thought to arise from adenomatous polyps via the adenoma–carcinoma sequence (Hill *et al.*, 1978). The gradual transition from a normal crypt to a precancerous lesion, and finally to a malignant tumour, is associated with the appearance of mutations in specific genes which are known to be associated with the control of cell proliferation and differentiation (Vogelstein *et al.*, 1988). The mutagenic substances responsible for the induction of DNA damage have not been positively identified. One possibility is that nitrosamines, formed from nitrates derived by bacterial metabolism of residual dietary protein, are important (Bingham *et al.*, 1996). Another possibility is that the heterocyclic aromatic amines formed directly in meat during cooking can act as faecal carcinogens (Sinha *et al.*, 1999). However, in both cases the concentrations present in the human faecal stream are much lower than those needed to induce cancer in animal models.

The influence of diet on the adenoma–carcinoma sequence remains poorly understood. It seems unlikely that the human food chain is a major source of carcinogens, and it is more probable that dietary practices can, in the long term, alter the susceptibility of the epithelial crypts to the initiation and promotion of neoplasia. One hypothesis is that diet causes a form of chronic irritation to the mucosa which may induce a prolonged state of tissue regeneration in which mitosis is relatively high, and programmed cell death (apoptosis) is suppressed to facilitate net cellular growth (Kinzler & Vogelstein, 1996). Rapidly dividing cells are more vulnerable to genetic damage than quiescent cells (Ames, 1989). Furthermore, there is increasing evidence that apoptosis in the dividing cell population at the base of the crypt provides a defence mechanism against the survival of stem cells carrying tumorigenic mutations (Johnson, 2001). The speed at which an established tumour grows depends upon the relative rates of mitosis and apoptosis amongst its constituent cells (Tomlinson & Bodmer, 1995). Mutations that cause a loss of apoptosis appear to be important at every stage of the development of colorectal cancer (Bodmer, 1999).

5.4 Protective factors, intraluminal metabolism and health

Although the metabolic activities of the human colonic bacteria are immensely complicated and still poorly understood, it is possible to identify some general mechanisms by which they may provide the body with biologically active substances that can function as protective factors. Broadly, it is useful to distinguish between the global metabolic effects of the mixed microflora and other mechanisms that depend on the properties of specific classes or strains of bacteria, or the effects of particular metabolites derived from defined substrates. The concepts of *probiotics*, which are live microbial supplements consumed in order to modify the microbial balance, and *prebiotics*, which are non-digestible food ingredients that affect the host by selectively stimulating the growth of beneficial bacteria already present in the microflora, are largely beyond the scope of this review. However, these approaches are mentioned briefly in the following examples, and the interested reader is referred to other recent reviews for a more detailed discussion (Gibson & Fuller, 2000; Rolfe, 2000).

5.4.1 Lactic acid bacteria

The lactic acid bacteria have long been considered beneficial to health. Yoghurt is produced by fermentation of milk by lactic acid bacteria, and so functions both as a source of viable bacteria and of potentially protective bacterial metabolites. Although the epidemiological evidence for the benefits of yoghurt is not strong (World Cancer Research Fund, 1997), there is some experimental evidence to show that it has antimutagenic activity in *in vitro* assays (Bakalinsky *et al.*, 1996), and that this property is associated with bacterial metabolites, including palmitic acid (Nadathur *et al.*, 1996). A number of different strains of lactobacillus have also been shown to inhibit chemically induced DNA damage in the rat colon (Pool-Zobel *et al.*, 1996). It is not firmly established if lactobacilli exert such effects *in vivo* under the mixed culture conditions of the colon, or whether manipulating the levels of such bacteria in the colon by the use of probiotic or prebiotic preparations is of potential benefit to human health. However, it has been shown that, for example, consumption of fermented products containing lactobacilli reduces the level of urinary mutagens after fried meat consumption in humans (Lidbeck *et al.*, 1992; Hayatsu & Hayatsu, 1993). The general principle of manipulating the balance of the colonic microflora by dietary intervention is an area that requires further intensive study (Sanders, 2000).

5.4.2 Short-chain fatty acids

The major fermentation pathway for colonic bacteria is the formation of pyruvate from hexose sugars, yielding ATP in the process. Pyruvate then serves as an intermediate substrate for a variety of other pathways leading to the formation of the short-chain fatty acids acetate, propionate and butyrate (Bernalier *et al.*, 1999). A number of bacterial species, including lactobacilli, bifidobacteria and clostridia, form ethanol in pure culture, but ethanol is rarely found as a major product in the human colon, perhaps because other species utilise it as a substrate. The faeces of some subjects also contain methane, and this has been shown to be due to the presence of two methanogenic bacterial species, *Methanobrevibacter smithii and Methanosphaera stadtmaniae* (Miller & Wolin, 1986).

The colonic epithelial cells are adapted to utilise butyrate preferentially as a source of energy (Clausen & Mortensen, 1994), and butyrate is also known to stimulate the proliferation of normal colonocytes (Marsman & McBurney, 1996) and suppress the proliferation of cancer cells *in vitro* (Gamet *et al.*, 1992). Butyrate also induces apoptosis in tumour cell lines established from human adenomas and carcinomas, at concentrations close to those which occur in the human colon (Hague *et al.*, 1993, 1996). Interestingly, the carcinoma lines were less responsive to butyrate, so the abnormal cells that survive and evolve into malignant tumours may have acquired an adaptive resistance to induction of apoptosis by butyrate. It may be valid to regard butyrate as a protective factor, which can be manipulated by dietary intervention.

It is not yet clear to what extent variations in butyrate supply or metabolism are involved in human disease, but Roediger (1980a) has proposed that a failure of butyrate metabolism may be the underlying metabolic disorder in the inflammatory condition ulcerative colitis (Roediger, 1980b). This remains a matter of controversy (Clausen & Mortensen, 1995), but it is well established that butyrate, and to a lesser extent the other short-chain fatty acids, support the proliferation of normal mucosal cells obtained from human subjects (Scheppach *et al.*, 1992a). Moreover, when solutions of butyrate are given as enemas to patients suffering from ulcerative colitis, there is a significant reduction in the level of inflammation (Scheppach *et al.*, 1992b).

These and other findings have prompted interest in the development of functional food products containing readily fermentable substrates such as resistant starch that could augment the supply of butyrate to the colonic epithelium, over and above that provided by unabsorbed carbohydrates in the normal diet. Care is needed in the selection of such substrates. Lignified plant cell walls and resistant starches are fermented relatively slowly and are therefore probably most suitable for the delivery of butyrate to the more distal regions of the large intestine. Rapidly fermentable substrates such as fructooligosaccharides are increasingly being considered for use as prebiotics because they favour the growth of such potentially beneficial micro-organisms as *Bifidobacterium* sp. (Gibson & Fuller, 2000). However, they may be metabolised too rapidly after entering the right colon to provide an adequate supply of butyrate to the distal bowel. It has been suggested that an over-supply of readily fermented substrates from functional foods could accelerate crypt cell mitosis to a point at which the dividing cells could become vulnerable to induction of DNA damage (Wasan & Goodlad, 1996). No conclusive evidence for or against this suggestion exists, but further research is required to determine the ideal level of butyrate production in the human colon, to discover how and why it varies between individuals, and to determine how best to achieve optimal butyrate yield through manipulation of the diet.

5.4.3 Glucosinolates

The Brassica vegetables (see Section 7.4.3) provide one of the best documented examples of human enzyme induction by plant secondary metabolites in food, and at least part of their effect appears to be due to colonic bacterial metabolism. The order *Cruciferae* includes many familiar varieties of vegetables such as cabbage, broccoli, cauliflower and Brussels sprouts, and also other species used as condiments, including mustard and horseradish. The distinctive, hot or bitter flavours of these foods are caused by various breakdown products of the glucosinolates (Fenwick *et al.*, 1982), a complex group of sulphur-containing compounds peculiar to *Cruciferae* (Fenwick *et al.*, 1983; Mithen *et al.*, 2000). Amongst the most important of the breakdown products are the 'mustard oils' or isothiocyanates (see Sections 2.6.2 and 7.4.3). Glucosinolates remain relatively inert within plant cells until the tissue is damaged by food preparation (see Section 12.7.1) or by chewing. This triggers the release of the endogenous enzyme myrosinase, (thioglucoside glycohydrolase, EC 3.2.3.1), which releases glu-

cose from the glucosinolate, causing the aglycone to undergo further reactions to form a variety of products including isothiocyanates.

In addition to providing flavour and aroma, isothiocyanates have been shown to interact with human liver and intestinal epithelial cells. They can act as 'blocking agents' that modify the activities of Phase I and Phase II enzymes to detoxify carcinogenic substances before they cause DNA damage (Tawfiq *et al.*, 1995) (see Section 4.2.3). They can also induce apoptosis in previously initiated cells (see Section 5.3), thus preventing their further progression to cancer (Smith *et al.*, 1998). With the exception of the work by Nijhoff *et al.* (see below), these are *in vitro* experiments and have not used physiological amounts of isothiocyanates. There have been relatively few studies in humans as yet, but consumption of Brassica vegetables under experimental conditions has been reported to induce increased levels of the α- and π-isozymes of glutathione-S-transferase (GST) in human rectal mucosa (Nijhoff *et al.*, 1995). Recent work on the molecular epidemiology of lung cancer suggests that a high consumption of brassica vegetables can reduce the risk of lung cancer in smokers, but the effect depends critically upon genetic polymorphisms affecting the expression of the GSTs (London *et al.*, 2000). Hence the metabolic effects of glucosinolate breakdown products might account for the strong epidemiological evidence (see Chapter 3) that a high consumption of Brassica vegetables is associated with a relatively low risk of cancers of the large intestine and lung (Verhoeven *et al.*, 1997).

Brassica vegetables may be cooked or processed in a variety of ways before they are eaten, each of which will modify the way in which glucosinolates are presented to the alimentary tract (see Section 12.7.1). If lightly chopped and eaten raw (see Section 12.7.1), the plant tissue will contain a mixture of intact glucosinolates and active myrosinase, and most of the glucosinolate breakdown products will appear in the food or the upper part of the alimentary tract (Verkerk *et al.*, 1997). However, cooking (see Section 12.7.1) will inactivate myrosinase and, although some glucosinolates may be broken down by the heat or lost in cooking water, a substantial quantity will pass through the small intestine to the large bowel (Dekker *et al.*, 2000). Further release of isothiocyanates will take place in the colon because human colonic bacteria are known to exert myrosinase-like activity, liberating glucose for fermentation, and thereby releasing isothiocyanates into the bowel lumen (Michaelsen *et al.*, 1994).

Indirect evidence that colonic micro-organisms from the human gut can liberate biologically active metabolites from glucosinolates was first obtained in animal studies. Germ-free rats showed no signs of any adverse effects due to toxic isothiocyanates from rapeseed, whereas animals inoculated with a human colonic microflora did (Rabot *et al.*, 1993). Rabot and colleagues have since isolated a number of bacterial species from various different genera, including *Bacteroides, Peptostreptococcus, Enterococcus, Escherichia* and *Proteus*, all of which are able to carry out the degradation of the biologically active glucosinolates progoitrin and sinigrin *in vitro* (Rabot *et al.*, 1995).

More direct evidence for the activity of bacterial myrosinase in the human gut is provided by studies in which consumption of raw broccoli gave rise to substantial excretion of isothiocyanate breakdown products such as dithiocarbamates in the urine of human volunteers (Shapiro *et al.*, 1998). In the study of Shapiro *et al.*, the quantity excreted was reduced in subjects who ate broccoli in which myrosinase had been heat-inactivated, and it fell to zero in subjects given antibiotics to reduce the activity of their colonic microflora. These and similar human studies using watercress (Getahun & Chung, 1999) and broccoli (Conaway *et al.*, 2000), are consistent with the hypothesis that at least some food-borne glucosinolates are degraded in the colon, so that their breakdown products are available for interactions with colonic epithelial cells, and for uptake into the circulation via the colonic mucosa. Thus, the glucosinolates provide an interesting example of a mechanism by which the human colonic microflora can influence the exposure of the gut and its circulation to biologically active compounds in food, and thereby regulate potentially important aspects of the host's metabolism.

5.4.4 Phenolic substances

The human diet contains a rich variety of both simple and complex phenolics that originate from plant-derived foods and drinks. Amongst the most important phenolics are the flavonoids, a large and complex group comprising flavonols, flavones and flavan-3-ols (see Section 2.2). The flavonols and flavones are generally present in the form of water-soluble but relatively inactive glycosides, containing a variety of different sugars. Some of the flavonol glycosides are absorbed intact in the small intestine or hydrolysed by mucosal enzymes and absorbed as aglycones (Gee *et al.*, 2000a), but those that pass through the small intestine unabsorbed, or re-enter the gut in the bile, become available for bacterial metabolism in the colon. Collectively, the human colorectal microflora possess all the enzymes necessary to degrade the various phenolic glycosides, and also other conjugates such as glucuronides, formed from flavonoids that have been absorbed and re-secreted into the bile (Scheline, 1973). Further degradation of phenolic rings also occurs in the colon, and the breakdown products are absorbed, metabolised further and secreted in the urine (Hollman & Arts, 2000; Gonthier *et al.*, 2003). The physiological effects, if any, of the bacterial metabolites of flavonoids in humans are unknown (see Section 6.3.3).

The isoflavones are diphenolic compounds (see Section 2.2.1*vi*) derived from plant foods and which bear a structural similarity to mammalian oestrogen (Price & Fenwick, 1985). The glycosides genistin and daidzin, and their respective methylated derivatives biochanin A and formononetin, are found principally in soya products. The parent species are broken down by the intestinal microflora to yield the aglycones genistein and daidzein (see Section 8.6.2), which can be transported across the intestinal mucosa into the circulation. In some individuals, another bacterial product, the isoflavan equol, is produced (Axelson *et al.*, 1982). The inter-individual variations in equol production appear to reflect differences in the composition and metabolic capabilities of their intestinal microflora, rather than those of the human host. A second important group of diphenolic phytoestrogens, the lignan precursors matairesinol and secoisolariciresinol, occur in cereal seeds and vegetables and particularly in flax seeds (see Section 8.6.3). As with the isoflavones, these compounds are degraded by colonic bacteria to yield the active lignans enterolactone and enterodiol, which can be taken up by mucosal epithelial cells and transferred to the circulation (Setchell *et al.*, 1981). In human volunteers given flax seed as a dietary supplement the level of lignans detectable in plasma rose after about 9 h, and there was a dose-related increase in the urinary excretion of lignan (Nesbitt *et al.*, 1999).

Much of the importance of phytoestrogens lies in their ability to exert weak hormone-like activity (see Section 8.6.1). They are thought to bind to oestrogen receptors *in vivo*, thereby effectively blocking the more potent activity of endogenous oestrogens and hence modifying oestrogen mediated processes (Setchell & Cassidy, 1998). Genistein may also exert direct effects on the epithelial cells of the colon because it is a potent inhibitor of protein kinases involved in the regulation of mitosis (Akiyama *et al.*, 1987). In principle, genistein might suppress epithelial cell proliferation, and possibly induce apoptosis in crypt cells carrying DNA damage. These effects on cytokinetics have been observed in intestinal tumour cell lines *in vitro*, but not apparently in animals fed dietary supplements of genistein (Booth *et al.*, 1999a,b). Apart from its effects on protein kinases, genistein is an inhibitor of topoisomerase II, an enzyme that helps to maintain the structure of DNA during mitosis. Both synthetic topoisomerase poisons and genistein are known to be mutagenic *in vitro* (Kaufmann 1998), and genistein supplementation appears to augment the induction of DNA damage in intestinal mucosa when fed in conjunction with a chemical carcinogen (Gee *et al.*, 2000b). There is no epidemiological evidence to suggest any adverse effect of soya products in humans, but caution is obviously necessary when considering the incorporation of such biologically active compounds into functional foods (see Sections 8.6.2, 12.6.1 and 13.6).

5.5 Research recommendations

- Much remains to be discovered about the biochemistry and ecology of the colon, and about the physiological responses of the colon epithelial cells to their environment.
- In view of the current interest in the development of functional food products containing poorly absorbed but readily fermentable substrates, further research is needed to assess the true biological role of butyrate, both as a stimulant to mucosal cell proliferation and as an inducer of potentially beneficial programmed cell death in colorectal epithelial cells.
- The glucosinolates (found in Brassica vegetables such as cabbage, broccoli, Brussels sprouts), and the polyphenols (derived from many other fruits, vegetables and beverages) provide promising evidence of potentially anticarcinogenic defence mechanisms. At least part of their effect appears to be due to colonic bacterial metabolism, but the significance of inter-individual variation in bacterial flora remains unknown. Studies on the effects of the human gut flora need to be integrated into future research on protective factors derived from plant foods.

5.6 Key points

- The mucosal surfaces of the alimentary tract are unique in their direct exposure to food constituents at levels that are often far in excess of those achieved at systemic sites. In the colon, this exposure is extended to include a complex variety of bacterial metabolites, which include both harmful and potentially protective factors.

- The interior of the human alimentary tract provides an ideal environment for colonisation by micro-organisms. Although the stomach and small intestine are relatively sterile, the large intestine contains a rich commensal microflora, strategically located, downstream from the main sites of digestion and absorption. The microflora is an important source of substances derived from undigested plant components, which may act as protective factors against colorectal and systemic disease.

- The colonic microflora derive their energy from two sources, undigested food and endogenous secretions. Most of the bacteria of the human colon utilise carbohydrate as a source of energy, although not all can degrade polysaccharides directly. Around 30 g of bacteria are produced for every 100 g of carbohydrate fermented, and it has been estimated that somewhere between 20 and 80 g of undigested carbohydrate enter the human colon every day.

- The large intestine is subject to a range of functional, structural and infectious diseases, the most important of which are the inflammatory conditions of unknown cause, Crohn's disease and ulcerative colitis, and colorectal carcinoma, which is the second most common cause of death from cancer in many industrialised societies.

- The lactic acid bacteria have long been considered beneficial to health. Evidence for the subtle biological effects of such bacteria is accumulating but, in general, the importance of these for the prevention of disease remains to be established. Some plant foods, *e.g.* artichokes, onions, garlic and chicory, contain prebiotic substances. These cannot be digested by human enzymes, but can be broken down and utilised by some colonic microflora, therefore modifying the profile of gut bacteria. The general principle of manipulating the balance of the colonic microflora by dietary intervention is an area that requires further intensive study.

- The major carbohydrate fermentation pathway for colonic bacteria leads to the formation of the short-chain fatty acids acetate, propionate and butyrate. The colonic epithelial cells are adapted to utilise butyrate preferentially as a source of energy, and butyrate stimulates the growth of normal colon cells and suppresses proliferation of cancer cells *in vitro*. Butyrate also induces apoptosis (programmed cell death) in tumour cells. These and other findings have prompted interest in the development of functional food products containing readily fermentable substrates, such as resistant starch, that could augment the supply of butyrate to the colonic epithelium.

- The Brassica vegetables (cabbage, broccoli, Brussels sprouts) provide some of the best-documented examples of induction of potentially anticarcinogenic defence mechanisms by plant secondary metabolites in food. At least part of their effect appears to be due to colonic bacterial metabolism. Some food-borne glucosinolates remain intact in cooked vegetables, and pass to the colon where they are degraded. Their biologically active breakdown products (isothiocyanates) then become available for interactions with colonic epithelial cells, and for uptake into the circulation via the colonic mucosa.

- The human diet contains a rich variety of phenolic substances that originate from plant-derived foods and drinks, amongst the most important of which are the flavonoids. These are generally present in the form of water-soluble but relatively inactive glycosides, some of which are efficiently absorbed in the upper part of the alimentary tract. A proportion of the unabsorbed flavonoids pass through the small intestine unabsorbed and become available for bacterial metabolism in the colon but the physiological effects of the bacterial metabolites of flavonoids in humans are unknown.

- The isoflavones are diphenolic compounds found principally in soya products, that bear a structural similarity to mammalian oestrogen. The parent species are broken down by the intestinal microflora to yield the aglycones genistein and daidzein, which can be transported across the intestinal mucosa into the circulation. In some individuals, another bacterial product, the isoflavan equol, is produced. A second important group of diphenolic phytoestrogens, the lignan precursors matairesinol and secoisolariciresinol, occur in cereal seeds and vegetables. As with the isoflavones, these compounds are degraded by colonic bacteria to yield the active lignans enterolactone and enterodiol, which can be taken up by mucosal epithelial cells and transferred to the circulation. Much of the importance of phytoestrogens lies in their ability to exert weak hormone-like activity. They may also exert potentially beneficial direct effects on the epithelial cells of the colon through suppression of protein kinases and cyclooxygenases. Further research is needed to assess these effects.

- A great deal remains to be discovered about the biochemistry and ecology of the colon, and about the physiological response of the colon epithelial cells to their environment. Biologically active substances derived from plant foods are an important part of that environment. There may be much to gain through the manipulation of this complex system by dietary intervention.

6
Dietary Intake and Bioavailability of Plant Bioactive Compounds

6.1 Introduction

Knowledge of the chemical form, physico-chemical nature and concentration of bioactive compounds in the diet at their potential sites of action is essential. Many *in vitro* studies have pointed to isolated dietary compounds as bioactive but few of these studies have been undertaken using physiologically relevant concentrations or knowing anything about the metabolic form of the substance in cells.

In terms of whether any potential effects are limited to the gastrointestinal system or can be expected to occur systemically, it is important to know how much of the compound remains intact, is degraded by gut micro-organisms, re-enters the system or re-enters the colon after systemic metabolism.

In order to assess the bioavailability of any food component, it is necessary to have information about the amount that enters the blood circulation following consumption of the food, *i.e.* following its digestion, possible metabolism and passage across the gut wall (*e.g.* in the small intestine or the colon). It is also important to have an understanding of the following:

- whether (and how) the substance is metabolised as it passes through the liver and kidneys
- how quickly it is excreted, by which means (*e.g.* bile and/or kidneys) and in which form
- whether it is stored in body tissues, particularly those that might be of relevance to any specific functions that may be of interest (*e.g.* protection against cancers in particular organs). See Fig. 6.1.

Until recently, there was very little published information about the food sources or bioavailability of plant bioactive compounds, such as flavonoids and phytoestrogens. Before considering the available information on bioavailability, it is worth noting the information now available on dietary sources of a variety of bioactive substances.

6.1.1 Food composition databases

Most studies providing analytical data have been focused on the main dietary sources rather than undertaking the almost impossible task of measuring thousands of substances in thousands of foods. However, many of the databases are now becoming sufficiently comprehensive to provide reasonable estimates of likely total intake.

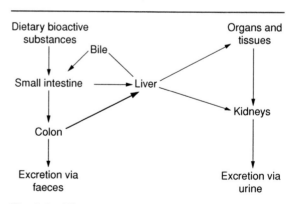

Fig. 6.1 Diagrammatic representation of the major compartments of the body involved in metabolism of dietary bioactive substances.

There are now a number of published values for the flavonoid content of foods (see Section 6.3.1) in a range of populations. Work is under way in the USA to establish a comprehensive database for the polyphenol composition of foods consumed in North America. The USDA has already established databases for carotenoids (members of the terpenoid family, see Chapter 2), isoflavones and flavonoids (available for download at www.nal.usda.gov/fnic/foodcomp). These are based on foods available in the USA, but they will also be of use for estimating intakes in other countries, although their value will be limited by the variations in composition of the dietary components in one country compared with another. An EU-derived carotenoids database was published in 2001 (O'Neill *et al.*, 2001), together with information about current intakes of the major carotenoids across Europe (see Section 6.5.1).

General limitations of this approach to assessing intake include the likelihood that data do not exist for all foods consumed and that, within any food type, there are likely to be fluctuations in concentration which cannot be taken into account, *e.g.* variations between types of apple in their quercetin level and changes in concentration brought about by different types of processing or by cooking (see Chapters 7 and 12).

6.1.2 Total diet study

This approach involves constructing a model diet based on knowledge of the nature of the diets eaten by individuals in a sample population, and then analysing samples of this complete model diet to estimate directly the content of the compounds of interest. This approach has been used in the UK, using the National Food Survey (NFS) data to construct a national, average, domestic diet containing 119 categories of food and drink assigned to 20 food groups to assess content of quercetin, kaempferol, apigenin and luteolin (see Section 6.2.1). Six food groups assessed as most likely to contain significant levels of flavonoids were selected for study; these comprised various categories of vegetables, fruit and fruit products, and beverages (which included samples of red and white wine). Esti-

mated total intake of these four flavonoids was 30 mg/day, with quercetin contributing 64% of the total.

6.2 Methodological aspects in the assessment of bioavailability

In the absence of functional markers for biological activity of carotenoids and other bioactive substances in intact organisms, 'bioavailability' has largely been taken to mean 'assimilation efficiency', or the ability to accumulate carotenoids in some defined body pool (Parker *et al.*, 1999). Such pools may be highly dynamic, such as plasma chylomicrons following a carotenoid-rich meal, total plasma or plasma lipoproteins following subchronic or chronic dietary supplementation or more static pools such as adipose tissue or the macular pigment of the eye. The xanthophylls lutein and zeaxanthin together largely comprise the macular pigment of the human retina, implicating these carotenoids in macular function and prevention of macular degeneration (see Section 3.5.2). Thus, macular pigment density, which can be assessed non-invasively by physical methods to study its relationship with carotenoid intake (Hammond *et al.*, 1997), may emerge as a near-functional indicator of bioavailability of lutein or zeaxanthin.

6.2.1 Absolute bioavailability

Experimentally, absolute bioavailability and utilisation can be determined by administering the substance of interest and studying its kinetics. For example, a flavonoid may be given both intravenously and orally, and then the ratio of plasma levels with time calculated (from the areas under the curve of plasma concentration versus time). These curves reflect the fate of a substance in the body as a result of absorption from the gut, distribution within body fluids and tissues, metabolism in the liver, gut wall and kidneys and excretion. Given the vast number of substances of interest and the relative complexity of this technique, it is not surprising that this has generally not been performed. Most of the studies in humans have used only the oral route. Hence they can only provide information about the relative bioavailability of one food compared with another, again by comparing the areas under the curve of plasma concentration against time for the substance of interest, in response to each of a number of foods (Hollman *et al.*, 1997a–c).

6.2.2 Measurement in biological fluids

Determination of bioavailability is dependent on measurement of the substance of interest in biological fluids, and there are a number of limitations with the available methods (Hollman, 2000). Research has been focused on urinary and biliary excretion, with some attention paid to blood, plasma and tissue concentrations following oral ingestion of substances of interest (*e.g.* specific flavonoids and carotenoids) by humans. However, there is an absence of suitable and sufficiently sensitive and selective methods, which are needed before real progress can be made on the kinetics of such substances.

6.2.3 Methods used to assess bioavailability

The methods discussed below have been used to estimate the bioavailability of carotenoids, but have general applicability for other classes of plant bioactive compound (Parker *et al.*, 1999; van den Berg *et al.*, 2000).

(i) Metabolic balance techniques

Much of the data on absorption from foods and isolates are based on either acute or chronic faecal mass balance methods and show great variability.

(ii) Ileostomy mass balance

In individuals who have undergone an ileostomy, the colon has been surgically removed and the terminal ileum brought to a stoma on the abdominal wall. Ingested food passes through the stomach and ileum in around 6 h, as it would in the intact gut. The ileal effluent can be recovered at regular intervals (*e.g.* 2-hourly) and all the residue from a test meal can be recovered in 12 h if the subsequent meals given to the volunteers are free of the test substance(s). The model has the added advantage that an excretion profile can be obtained, which gives a time span for the absorption, which can in turn be compared with changes in plasma concentration over the 12 h test period. Using this approach, absorption of isolated crystalline β-carotene, given dispersed in milk shake containing a known amount of fat, was found to be around 90% (van den Berg *et al.*, 2000).

(iii) Gastrointestinal lavage technique

In this technique, the entire gastrointestinal tract is washed out by the subject consuming a large volume (4.5 L) of Colyte, containing polyethylene glycol and electrolyte salts. Washout is complete with the production of clear rectal effluent (2.5–3.5 h). Difficulties associated with the method are that it is relatively time consuming, can only be applied to healthy individuals and may give an underestimation if absorption is compromised or normal transit time is reduced owing to the use of Colyte. In addition, as with the faecal mass balance, the method depends upon there being no degradation or loss of the unabsorbed substances of interest. On the other hand, it has the advantage of standardising the residence time in the gastrointestinal tract.

(iv) Plasma and plasma fraction concentration methods

Measurements of absorption are usually carried out by calculating changes in plasma concentration following the administration of an acute or chronic dose of, for example, isolated carotenoid or carotenoid-containing food (van den Berg *et al.*, 2000). This is known as the 'area under the plasma curve' (AUC) approach.

With this method, it is possible to compare different doses and foods and to derive information about the relative absorption by comparison to a standard dose (normally the isolated substance). A crossover design, with an adequate period of washout between treatments, is the most suitable approach so that each individual can act as their own control.

The AUC approach is not appropriate for the calculation of absolute absorption, because the kinetics of absorption, disposal and re-export are not known. For example, with carotenoids, peak plasma concentration occurs at between 6 and 48 h depending on the dose and the frequency of making the measurements. Yet it is known that the dose passes through the ileum in about 6 h. The most likely explanation is that the first peak in plasma concentration is due to the carotenoid present in the newly absorbed chylomicrons and the second peak, or prolonged duration of the first peak, results from hepatically re-exported carotenoid in VLDL and LDL (van den Berg *et al.*, 2000). The transfer of carotenoids from the short-lived chylomicrons to the longer-lived LDL and HDL (which appear to carry most of the carotenoid in fasting subjects) also explains why the plasma concentration remains elevated for up to and beyond 10 days post-dose.

Newly absorbed carotenoids are initially present in plasma chylomicrons before they are sequestered by body tissues and re-exported in, or transferred to, other lipoprotein fractions. Thus, measurement of carotenoids in this fraction, and knowledge of the rate of clearance of the chylomicrons, allow the calculation of rates of absorption, disposal and overall absorption based on AUC measurement. This method has the advantage that few chylomicrons are present in fasting plasma and they are usually devoid of carotenoids (van den Berg *et al.*, 2000), although there are also disadvantages. Another option is to measure the clearance rate of carotenoids from the triglyceride-rich lipoprotein (TRL) fraction.

In chronic studies with supplements or foods, dosing needs to be carried out until the plasma concentration reaches a plateau. Again using carotenoids as an example, this normally takes a period of weeks when supplementing with dietary-achievable amounts (*e.g.* 15 mg/day of carotenoids) and may increase the plasma concentration of β-carotene up to 10-fold, with other common carotenoids showing smaller increases. Again, absolute absorption cannot be measured, but the data may allow comparisons between isolated compounds and foods and between different foods. Decay curves of falling plasma con-

centration of carotenoids, when supplementation is discontinued, may also provide some data on the half-life of the body carotenoid pool.

(v) Isotope methods

There are now ethical constraints against the use of radioactive tracers in human volunteers to determine kinetics. The use of stable isotopes is more ethically acceptable. Studies with β-[^{13}C]carotene, for example, have suggested that about 64% of the ^{13}C entered the plasma as retinyl esters, 21% as retinol and 14% as β-[^{13}C]carotene. The very high level of conversion of the β-[^{13}C]carotene is in line with the data from two earlier studies with radiolabelled β-carotene (van den Berg *et al.*, 2000).

In another study, which tracked β-carotene and retinol (labelled with a stable isotope) in human volunteers for up to 24 days after an oral dose, 22% of the carotenoid dose was absorbed, 17.8% as carotenoid and 4.2% as retinoid. This result is close to the 11% absorption of β-carotene found by van Vliet *et al.* (1995) but indicates a much lower percentage conversion to retinol than that found using very small oral doses of β-[^{13}C]carotene.

Newer methods using stable isotopes offer the potential to measure absolute absorption and subsequent metabolism in human subjects in the presence of both dietary exogenous and endogenous supplies of the substances of interest. Ideally, the use of stable isotope-labelled food materials coupled with the measurement of the isotopomers of the native compounds in plasma fractions should provide the best possible measure of bioavailability.

(vi) Conclusions

With regard to carotenoids, van den Berg and colleagues concluded that plasma AUC may not be an appropriate method for measuring bioavailability because of the probable re-export of hepatically absorbed carotenoid into the plasma in VLDL while absorption from the gut is still active (van den Berg *et al.*, 2000). For mass balance methods, the gastrointestinal lavage technique and ileostomy models offer a direct measurement of absorption. For the plasma response to hydrocarbon carotenoids, the use of the TRL fraction offers the best prospect of assessing absorption, especially if the chylomicron fraction can be isolated and the conversion to retinol is taken into account. For the more polar carotenoids (xanthophylls), the TRL fraction may not be appropriate, especially if they are not exclusively carried by the chylomicrons when freshly absorbed.

Much of the published work has been focused on isolates of bioactive substances. However, it has to be acknowledged that, once in a food matrix, the substance may act differently, and that the bioavailability is likely to vary from one food matrix to another. Cooking and processing of the food are also likely to affect the bioavailability of constituents (see Chapter 12). For example, *cis/trans* isomerisation occurs on heat processing.

6.3 Current intakes and bioavailability of flavonoids

6.3.1 Estimations of dietary intakes

Flavonols, flavones and flavan-3-ols constitute the three major sub-classes of flavonoids (see Chapter 2). The flavan-3-ol sub-group includes

the substances referred to as catechins and the proanthocyanidins. Also in the flavonoids group are flavanones (*e.g.* naringen and hesperidin) [a review is available (Tomás-Barberán & Clifford, 2000a)], anthocyanidins and isoflavones. These are described in more detail in Chapters 2, 7 and 9. The main dietary sources of these flavonoids are shown in Table 6.1. A substantial amount of information about the content of selected flavonoids, from these three major sub-classes (flavonols, flavones and flavan-3-ols), in fruits and vegetables available in The Netherlands has now been published using state-of-the-art HPLC techniques [see below and the literature for a summary of the data (Hollman & Arts, 2000)]. A USDA database is also now available (see Section 6.1.1).

Historically, one of the first important sources of information on dietary intakes of flavonoids was the Zutphen Elderly Study (Hertog *et al.*, 1993a,b; Keli *et al.*, 1996). Mean baseline flavonoid intake was estimated to be 25.9 mg, the major sources being tea (61%), onions (13%) and apples (10%). The average intake of a particular flavonoid, the flavonol quercetin, was 16 mg/day, provided mostly in tea (48%), onions (29%) and apples (7%) (Hertog *et al.*, 1993b). A study among over 4000 free-living Dutch adults had previously

Table 6.1 Principal dietary sources of flavonoid sub-classes.

Flavonoid	Examples of major food sources
Flavonols, *e.g.* quercetin, kaempferol, apigenin, luteolin, myricetin	Onions, kale, broccoli, apples, cherries and berries, tea and red wine
Flavones,	Parsley, thyme and celery
Flavan-3-ols, *e.g.* (+)-catechin, (–)-epicatechin and proanthrocyanidins	Catechins: tea, apples, apricots and cherries. Proanthrocyanidins: apples, chocolate and red wine
Flavanones, *e.g.* hesperidin and naringin	Citrus fruit
Anthocyanidins, *e.g.* cyanidin, delphinidin, malvidin, pelargonidin and peonidin, and petunidin	Grapes and cherries
Chalcones and dihydrochalcones	Heavily hopped beer, tomatoes (with skins), apple juice and cider
Isoflavones, *e.g.* daidzein and genistein	Soya beans, soya products and legumes

Source: information derived from Hollman (1997), Scalbert & Williamson (2000) and Tomás-Barberán & Clifford (2000a). See also Chapters 2, 7, 8 and 9.

indicated that average intake of flavonols and flavones in the Netherlands was 23 mg/day, of which the flavonol quercetin contributed 16 mg/day, kaempferol 3.9 mg/day and myricetin 1.4 mg/day; thus flavones provided only a minor fraction, about 7% (Hertog *et al.*, 1993b). Tea was the major source of these flavonols in this population) (48% of intake), followed by onions (29%) and apples (7%). In a cohort of nearly 35 000 male professionals in the USA aged 40–75 years, the contribution from tea was proportionately less, but the overall intake was similar to that for the Dutch cohorts at about 20 mg/day (Rimm *et al.*, 1996b). A small study in Welsh middle-aged men found an average intake of 26 mg/day (Hertog *et al.*, 1997).

Although these figures are widely quoted as *total flavonoid* intake, taking the Zutphen study as an example, the values apply not to flavonoids in general, but are restricted to three flavonols (quercetin, kaempferol and isorhamnetin) and two flavones (luteolin and apiginin), and the calculation is based on aglycones rather than conjugates. It is, therefore, almost certainly a serious underestimate of flavonoid ingestion. At the other end of the scale, Kühnau proposed an intake of over 1000 mg/day in the USA (Kühnau, 1976). This figure is based on all phenols being glycosides (*i.e.* conjugates), and is likely to be an overestimate of flavonoid consumption.

It is to be expected that the relationships between the predominant flavonoids and their sources will vary between populations, and that there will be wide inter- and intra-individual variations in intakes of individual compounds, because of the substantial differences that occur in dietary patterns around the world. Hence it is not surprising that an analysis of data from the Seven Countries study, pertaining to the diets consumed in Japan, the Netherlands, the former Yugoslavia, the USA, Finland, Italy and Greece in the early 1960s, found that red wine was the main source of the flavonol quercetin for the Italians, tea the dominant source in Japan and the Netherlands, and onions in Greece, the former Yugoslavia and the USA (Hertog *et al.*, 1995). Flavonol intake was highest in Japan (64 mg/day) and lowest in Finland (6 mg/day).

(i) Flavonols and flavones

Flavonols and flavones are usually present in the diet as glycosides, *i.e.* bound to sugar molecules. With regard to flavonols and flavones, quercetin has been shown to be present in a wide range of fruits and vegetables (Hollman & Arts, 2000). Levels have been shown to be generally below 10 mg/kg in vegetables, except for onions (280–490 mg/kg), kale (110 mg/kg), broccoli (30 mg/kg) and green beans (445–60 mg/kg). In most fruits, the quercetin content averaged about 15 mg/kg, except for apples (20–70 mg/kg), apricots (25 mg/kg) and blackcurrants (37 mg/kg). Kaempferol could only be detected in kale (210–470 mg/kg), endive (15–90 mg/kg), broccoli (670 mg/kg) and leek (10–60 mg/kg). The contents of myricetin, luteolin and apigenin generally were below the level of detection (about 1 mg/kg), except for beans (30 mg/kg myricetin), sweet red pepper (15–39 mg/kg luteolin) and celery stalks (5–20 mg/kg luteolin, 15–60 mg/kg apigenin). Quercetin levels in red wine were 5–15 mg/L and levels in fruit juice were generally below 5 mg/L. Various black tea infusions contained 15–25 mg/L of quercetin, 7–17 mg/L of kaempferol and 2–5 mg/L of myricetin. No luteolin or apigenin was detected in any of the beverages. It should be noted that seasonal variation was large in leafy vegetables such as lettuce, endive and leek, with the flavonol contents of these being 3–5 times higher in summer than in other seasons. Some forms of cooking and processing are also recognised to affect the concentrations present. For example, Crozier *et al.* reported that the quercetin content of tomatoes and onions is affected to varying degrees by cooking: boiling reduced the content by 80%, microwave cooking by 65% and frying by 30% (Crozier *et al.*, 1997). See Chapter 12 for a detailed discussion of the effects of cooking and processing on the polyphenol content of foods.

In the UK, a study focusing on four specific flavonoids (the flavonols quercetin, kaempferol, apigenin and luteolin) estimated the total intake of these to be 30 mg/day, with quercetin contributing 64% of the total (Wearne, 2000) (see Fig. 6.2). Beverages contributed 82% of the total

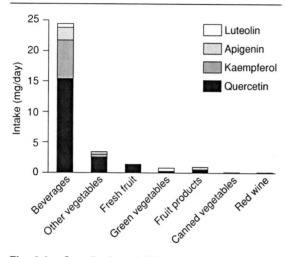

Fig. 6.2 Contribution of different food groups to average UK intakes of four flavonoids. Source: From Wearne (2002) with kind permission of the Royal Society of Medicine.

intake of these flavonoids, and this was mainly attributed to tea, as wine provided very little of the particular flavonoids studied.

In a study comparing total flavonol plus flavone consumption in free-living subjects from 14 countries, de Vries *et al.* found that the contribution of quercetin was 68–73% of the total intake (average total flavonoid intake was 27.6 mg/day) and the major sources were tea (37%), onions (26%), vegetables (14%), fruit (22%) and red wine (1%) (de Vries *et al.*, 1997a).

(ii) Flavan-3-ols

Flavan-3-ols, sometimes referred to as flavanols (see Section 2.3.3), are widespread in plant foods, including tea, fruits and legumes (Hollman & Arts, 2000), with tea being the most important source in many countries because the amount present is relatively large and tea is often drunk in substantial amounts (see Chapter 9). Tea contains substantial amounts of flavan-3-ols, including epicatechin, epigallocatechin and epigallocatechin gallate (Hollman *et al.*, 1997a). These constitute about 30% of the dry weight of green tea and 9% of the dry weight of black tea, in which condensa-

tion products (large multi-unit molecules) predominate (see below) (Arts *et al.*, 2001b). Wine, particularly red wine, is also a contributor to intake of catechin and epicatechin. Depending on the type of grape used, levels in red wines of the flavan-3-ols, (+)-catechin and (−)-epicatechin are typically in the range 8-60 mg/L (see Chapter 9, Table 9.14).

Arts and co-workers have published a detailed survey of flavan-3-ol intake in the Dutch population, based on 2-day dietary records from a national survey of 6200 males and females aged 1–97 years (Arts *et al.*, 2001b). They found that the average intake (in the total population) was 50 mg/day (ranging from 0 to 958 mg/day), with intake increasing with age. Average intake was higher in women (60 mg/day) than in men (40 mg/day). Only 7% of the population had an intake of 140 mg/day or more.

In the Dutch study, tea was the main source in all age groups. The second largest source was chocolate among the children (83% of children ate chocolate on at least one survey day). In adults, apples and pears were closely followed by chocolate as the second most important sources, and in the older people, pears and apples were the second source. Wine, other fruits (*e.g.* cherries, strawberries and peaches) and legumes (*e.g.* kidney beans) contributed only marginally to total intake (Table 6.2). Flavan-3-ol intake was lower in smokers than in non-smokers, and increased with socio-economic group. A high intake was weakly associated with a high intake of fibre, vitamin C and β-carotene, after adjustment for total energy intake. The specific flavan-3-ols that contributed to this total can be found in Table 6.3.

A similar average intake has been published for the Danish population (Dragsted *et al.*, 1997) which used the Danish Household Consumption Survey to arrive at an estimate of 20–50 mg/day. These figures bring into question the published estimate for the USA of 220 mg/day (Künhau, 1976), particularly as tea consumption tends to be much lower in the USA.

The manufacture of black tea results in the enzymatic oxidation of green tea flavan-3-ols and the subsequent production of condensation (multi-unit) products: theaflavins, thearubigens, epitheaflavic acids and bisflavanols (Hollman *et al.*, 1997a). See also Chapter 9.

(iii) Other flavonoids

Proanthocyanidins, also within the flavan-3-ol categorisation, are found in apples, dark chocolate and red wine (Scalbert & Williamson, 2000). According to a review by Santos-Buelga and Scalbert, very few studies have been focused on the bioavailability of proanthocyanidins in ani-

mals and none have been conducted in humans (Santos-Buelga & Scalbert, 2000).

To date, little attention has been paid to the dietary burden of flavanones, chalcones and dihydrochalcones in European diets, although there is a small amount of data from studies in Japan. However, intakes may be considerable in those who consume oranges and orange juice regularly: 250 mL of orange juice will provide 25–60 mg of flavanones (aglycone equivalents) and consumption of the flesh of an orange could provide 125–375 mg. The main sources of dihydrochalcones are apple juice and cider, with 250 mL supplying 1–5 mg of phloretin (dessert apples would supply 1 mg). Heavily hopped beers can be a source of chalcones but the only significant source will be tomatoes eaten with their skin, with 100 mg supplying up to 0.7 mg. It is thought that the absorption of at least some of these substances requires the intervention of the gut microflora to cleave the sugar moiety from the aglycone (Tomás-Barberán & Clifford, 2000a).

Table 6.2 Percentage contribution from different food sources to flavan-3-ol intake.

	Children (1–18 years) $n = 1539$	Adults (19–64 years) $n = 3954$	Older people (>65 years) $n = 707$
Tea	65.2	83.3	87.3
Chocolate	20.1	5.7	2.6
Apples and pears	12.0	5.9	5.3
Other fruits	1.5	1.4	2.1
Wine	0.1	2.8	1.5
Legumes	0.2	0.3	0.7
Other foods	0.9	0.7	0.6
All foods (mg/day)	25.5 ± 27.2	55.6 ± 60.2	75.1 ± 63.4

Source: derived from Arts *et al.* (2001b).

6.3.2 Absorption of flavonoids

Relatively little information is available on the absorption and subsequent distribution, metabolism and excretion of flavonoids in humans, although a considerable amount of work has been conducted in animals. All flavonoids except flavan-3-ols (catechins) are present in plants bound to sugars as glycosides. Free flavonoids, without

Table 6.3 Average intakes of a range of flavan-3-ols in Dutch people.

	Mean ± s.d. flavan-3-ol intake (mg/day)	
	Males ($n = 2885$)	Females ($n = 3315$)
Total flavanols	39.5 ± 46.4	59.4 ± 62.5
(+)-Catechin	3.5 ± 3.6	4.4 ± 4.1
(−)-Epicatechin	10.2 ± 9.0	12.8 ± 10.1
(+)-Gallocatechin	1.8 ± 2.6	3.0 ± 3.6
(−)-Epigallocatechin	2.8 ± 4.1	4.6 ± 5.6
(−)-Epicatechin gallate	12.1 ± 17.8	20.1 ± 24.4
(−)-Epigallocatechin gallate	9.0 ± 13.2	14.9 ± 18.1

Source: derived from Arts *et al.* (2001b).

their attached sugar molecules, are known as aglycones. Sugar molecules, can bind at various positions to the flavonoid and more than 80 different sugars have been found bound to flavonoids in plants. This serves to emphasise the diversity and heterogeneity of these compounds, *e.g.* 1779 different glycosides of quercetin alone have been described in nature (Hollman & Arts, 2000). With the exception of the cells lining the gastrointestinal tract, Depeint *et al.* suggest that all other cells in the body are only exposed to the flavonoid metabolites and degradation products (Depeint *et al.*, 2002).

(i) Flavonols

The absorption of flavonols (*e.g.* quercetin) from the diet was long considered to be negligible because they are present in plants as glycosides. Whilst it was thought that aglycones in the diet (free flavonoids without a sugar molecule), *e.g.* flavan-3-ols such as (+)-catechin, might be available for absorption, in experiments with rats, the enzymes necessary for liberating the aglycone were not thought to be present in the intestinal wall or secreted in the gut (Hollman & Arts, 2000). Hydrolysis of the bond that attaches the sugar molecule to the flavonoid was known to take place in the colon by a process that is mediated by the gut bacteria, which possess a diverse range of enzymes (see Section 6.3.3). However, it was recognised that this process also extensively degraded the flavonoid molecule, and the capacity for absorption in the colon was much lower than in the small intestine.

However, opinions changed following some experiments in ileostomy patients (chosen to circumvent the possibility of microbial degradation, see Section 6.2.3), in whom it was demonstrated that absorption of quercetin glycosides from onions was in fact superior to absorption of the pure aglycone (52% compared with 24%). These experiments also demonstrated that the extent of absorption would appear to be dependent on the nature of the sugar moiety of the molecule (although matrix effects of the food cannot be ruled out). Pure rutin, a major quercetin glycoside in tea, which has a rhamnose molecule as its

sugar moiety, was relatively poorly absorbed (17%) compared with other glycosides. The mechanism by which the glycosides are absorbed intact is still not clearly understood (Hollman & Arts, 2000). However, there is evidence that the glycosides interact both with the brush border glucose transporter, and with the brush border enzyme, lactose-phlorizin hydrolase (Gee *et al.*, 2000a). For quercetin in particular there is now evidence that absorption does occur. There is also evidence that it accumulates in the blood and that it is present there for some time (half-life of elimination is 24 h). This alone, of course is not evidence of bioavailability. The presence of quercetin glycosides (including rutin) in the plasma of unsupplemented individuals has been reported (Paganga & Rice-Evans, 1997), but more recent evidence suggests that only quercetin conjugates are present in human plasma, principally glucuronides derived from intestinal and hepatic metabolism of quercetin aglycone (Day *et al.*, 2001). It has been suggested that quercetin may be able to contribute to reduction of risk of cardiovascular disease, perhaps by enhancing antioxidant capacity. To support this, the Zutphen Elderly Study revealed an inverse association between high flavonol intake and the risk of death from coronary heart disease and stroke (Hertog *et al.*, 1993a; Keli *et al.*, 1996); a similar association was not found with cancer (Hertog *et al.*, 1994). However, so far, supportive data are lacking on the tissue distribution of quercetin. Work by Hollman and colleagues on other aspects of bioavailability, namely distribution of quercetin within the body and elimination, suggests that this is a gradual process, with 5% of the initial plasma level still being present 48 h after the peak plasma level was recorded, which occurred almost 3 h after the oral dose was given (Hollman *et al.*, 1996).

(ii) Flavan-3-ols

Flavan-3-ols are present in the diet in the aglycone form, *i.e.* not attached to sugar molecules. With regard to flavan-3-ols, most of the published work has been conducted with tea, and this suggests that absorption occurs and is rapid, as is elimination from the plasma (Hollman & Arts, 2000). Details can be found in Hollman *et al.* (1997a). Knowledge about the bioavailability of catechin condensation products (*e.g.* thearubigins) is scarce but there are some indications that they are absorbed, possibly following microbial degradation or metabolism in the colon (Hollman *et al.*, 1997a; Hollman, 2000). See Chapter 7.

Tea flavonoids have a strong affinity for transition metals and form insoluble complexes with iron ions, making both partners less available for absorption (Hollman *et al.*, 1997a). There is evidence from acute feeding studies of reduced iron uptake following consumption of tea (Hallberg & Hulthen, 2000; Zijp *et al.*, 2000).

(iii) Other flavonoid subclasses

The extent of absorption of other flavonoid sub-classes, such as anthocyanidins, has not been studied in humans, and only a small amount of animal work has been reported (Hollman, 1997). Because of their high molecular weight, proanthrocyanidin polymers are unlikely to be efficiently absorbed in the small intestine and published evidence for absorption is scarce (Santos-Buelga & Scalbert, 2000). Very little is known about the fate of orally ingested flavanones, although they appear to be absorbed (Hollman, 1997).

6.3.3 Metabolism

Two body compartments are of importance in any consideration of the metabolism of flavonoids: the colon (and its resident gut flora) and the tissues in which biotransformation enzymes are located, in particular the liver, but also the kidneys and the small intestine. Flavonols and flavan-3-ols are metabolised primarily in the colon and liver. The colon contains 10^{12} micro-organisms/cm^3 and has enormous catalytic and hydrolytic potential.

The bacteria produce enzymes capable of stripping flavonoid conjugates of their sugar moieties, enabling free aglycone to be absorbed. Unlike the enzymes in human tissues, the enzymes produced by gut bacteria can break down the polyphenols

to simple compounds. Hence a variety of derivatives can be produced through the actions of gut bacteria, some of which have antioxidant properties (see Chapter 5). The hydroxylation pattern of the flavonoids determines their susceptibility to microbial degradation and the type of fission products formed (Hollman, 1997).

Similarly, these flavonoids can be transformed in the liver (and to some extent in the intestinal wall) to a variety of products, in particular via glucuronidation and sulphation of the phenolic hydroxyl groups and *O*-methylation of the catechol groups (Hollman & Arts, 2000). The pathways are common to those that are utilised in the metabolism of drugs and foreign compounds, to facilitate their excretion from the body, and are described in some detail in a review (Scalbert & Williamson, 2000). There is evidence from a number of studies that metabolism is extensive in humans; in studies only 0.2–2% of ingested quercetin was excreted unchanged in urine as quercetin or its conjugates (Hollman & Arts, 2000). Similarly, extensive metabolism of flavan-3-ols has been reported. However, with the exception of the conjugates mentioned above, virtually no metabolites have been characterised in humans.

Future research requirements include the need for a better understanding of the bioavailability of flavonols, flavones and flavan-3-ols, in particular the identification and quantification of metabolites in body fluids and tissues.

Scalbert and Williamson reported that plasma concentrations of the intact parent polyphenol are often low and do not account for reported increases in the antioxidant capacity of plasma following consumption (Scalbert & Williamson, 2000). It is thought that metabolites contribute to these increases. Absorbed microbial metabolites might be particularly important in this respect, as has been shown with equol (see Section 6.4.1).

To gauge the impact of various flavonoid-providing foods on the total antioxidant capacity of plasma, comparisons have been made with ascorbic acid, the other main water-soluble dietary antioxidant. For example, consumption of 300 mL of red wine (providing 500 mg of polyphenols) has been reported to induce an increase in plasma antioxidant capacity similar to that of 1 g of ascorbic acid (Scalbert & Williamson, 2000). The average intake of ascorbic acid in the UK in 1999 was 62 mg/day (MAFF, 2000b). It has been calculated by several researchers, including Duthie *et al.*, that 500 mg of ingested polyphenols might be expected to result in a plasma concentration of total polyphenols of about 50 μm, which is about 10 times higher than the expected peak concentration of the parent polyphenols originally present in the diet (Duthie *et al.*, 1998). This suggests that metabolites formed in body tissues and via the colonic microflora contribute significantly to the total levels reaching the plasma and, hence, potentially antioxidant capacity (Scalbert & Williamson, 2000). Currently, little is known about these metabolites or their potential, and better knowledge of the consumption and bioavailability of dietary polyphenols will be essential in the future to evaluate their potential role in health and disease prevention.

6.4 Current intakes and bioavailability of phytoestrogens

This group of compounds comprises isoflavones (categorised as flavonoids) (see Section 2.2.7), lignans and stilbenes (see Section 2.3.3). Information on food sources of these can be found in Chapter 8, which shows that although phytoestrogens are present in a range of foods, the major sources quantitatively are soya beans and soya products.

Two databases of the isoflavone content of foods have been developed. The first is a collaborative effort between US institutions (http://www.nal.usda.gov/fnic/foodcomp). The second was compiled by European researchers involved in an EC Concerted Action project termed VENUS (Vegetal Estrogens in Nutrition and Skeleton; http://www.venus-ca.org). It includes the content of isoflavones, lignans, coumestrol and indols of foods commonly consumed in Europe.

Isoflavones are present either as the aglycone (genistein or daidzein), *e.g.* in fermented soya products such as miso and tempeh, or as various glycoside conjugates (the usual form), *e.g.* genistin and daidzin. These conjugates can be metabolised in the gut, after ingestion, either in the stomach via acid hydrolysis or in the large bowel by the resident bacteria, releasing the aglycone. The aglycones can also be released as a result of food processing (see Chapters 8 and 12).

Although lignans are present in most fibre-rich foods and hence are potentially a ubiquitous source of phytoestrogens, the levels present are low for most foods that have currently been analysed (Section 8.6.3). Stilbenes (Section 2.3*iii*) are also widely distributed in the plant kingdom, with *trans*-resveratrol (present in peanuts, grapes and wine) being the main focus of research in this area. Stilbenes are synthesised from cinnamic acid derivatives (see Section 6.6), *e.g.* resveratrol is derived from 4-coumaric acid (Cassidy *et al.*, 2000).

It has long been recognised that the gut bacteria play a role in the metabolism of phytoestrogens, as reviewed by Setchell & Cassidy (Setchell & Cassidy, 1999); however, understanding of the factors that influence the bioavailability and pharmokinetics of phytoestrogens remains limited (see Section 8.6). For example, lignans as they occur in plants, are not active plant oestrogens; this is only achieved following metabolism in the gut by bacteria (Setchell *et al.*, 1981).

6.4.1 Absorption and metabolism of phytoestrogens

Absorption is facilitated by removal of the sugar moiety, whether by β-glucosidases of human intestinal bacteria, gastric hydrochloric acid or β-glucosidases in food. Recent rat studies on the pharmacokinetics of genistein confirm that, in common with endogenous oestrogens, isoflavones undergo an enterohepatic circulation and biliary secretion. Infused genistein rapidly appears in bile and, after secretion via bile back into the small intestine, conjugated isoflavones and lignans may again be deconjugated by the intestinal bacteria. In common with steroid hormone metabolism, the liver probably plays a key role in the further metabolism of phytoestrogens. Evidence suggests that the aglycones are conjugated predominantly as glucuronides and to a lesser extent as mono- and disulphates. Although little is definitively known about the metabolism of the isoflavone precursor daidzein in humans, even less information is available on the metabolic fate of the isoflavone precursor genistein.

The ability to absorb isoflavones such as equol (formed from dietary isoflavone precursors by the action of gut bacteria) was recognised when it was observed that the addition of soya protein to rat and human diets caused a dramatic increase in urinary equol levels (Cassidy *et al.*, 2000).

To date, only a few studies have addressed the pharmacokinetics of these compounds. Studies conducted in premenopausal women focused on the apparent bioavailabilities, determined from the plasma appearance/disappearance curves following a single-bolus oral dose of 50 mg of the pure isoflavones (genistein and daidzein) or their glycosides (genistin and daidzin). They revealed that plasma genistein concentrations are consistently higher than daidzein concentrations when equal amounts of the two isoflavones are administered (Setchell *et al.*, 2001). The systemic bioavailability of genistein was much greater than that of daidzein, and bioavailability of both of these isoflavones was greater when ingested as the glycosides (daidzin and genistin) rather than as the aglycones.

Lignan absorption and utilisation also require a series of deconjugation and conjugation steps, but few quantitative data are available from human studies. Comparatively few studies have been carried out to examine the metabolism of natural stilbenes.

6.4.2 Metabolic response

There is considerable individual variability in metabolic response to a dose of isoflavone-rich food. Plasma concentrations of isoflavones in the range from 50 to 800 ng/mL have been reported in adults after consumption of 50 mg of isoflavones per day (Cassidy *et al.*, 2000). These values are similar to the plasma concentrations of the Japanese consuming their traditional diet. When soya is consumed on a regular basis, plasma isoflavone levels typically far exceed normal plasma oestradiol levels, which generally range between 40 and 80 pg/mL. However, the rapidly changing eating habits in Japan and China now make it difficult to generalise accurately about the intake of isoflavones in these countries. Recent estimates indicate intakes of 20–50 mg/day, but this may vary between urban and rural areas and with other lifestyle factors. In Western populations, the average daily dietary intake of isoflavones is typically negligible (<1 mg/day).

Under controlled conditions, Cassidy *et al.* showed that a daily challenge of 45 mg/day of conjugated isoflavones, fed as 60 g/day of TVP over a 1-month period, resulted in a 1000-fold increase in isoflavone metabolite excretion (Cassidy *et al.*, 1994). Total urinary isoflavone excretion levels ranged from 1 to 17 µg/day during the period when the control diet was consumed, while levels increased to between 0.4 and 8 mg/day on the TVP diet. Urinary equol excretion varied between individuals (Cassidy *et al.*, 1994): only two of the six subjects excreted substantial levels of equol, while the other four subjects predominantly excreted the aglycones, daidzein and genistein. Similar findings have been reported by Setchell *et al.* (1984). This inability of some individuals to produce equol following a soya challenge may be due to the absence from the gut flora of the bacterial enzymes responsible for the conversion of isoflavone precursors to equol, or to transit time variations, with rapid transit effectively preventing such metabolism (Cassidy *et al.*, 2000). These results also imply individual variability in metabolic capacity and/or differentially active metabolic pathways, as suggested by Kelly *et al.* (1993). These studies in premenopausal women indicate that the biological effects observed when isoflavones are consumed are not dependent on the conversion of the aglycones to equol and suggest that the aglycones or other unidentified metabolites are also biologically important *in vivo*.

Dietary fibre, or other components of a high-fibre diet, may also influence isoflavone excretion/absorption, by promoting the growth and/or activity of bacteria responsible for equol production in the colon in women (Lampe *et al.*, 1998).

This study adds further weight to the *in vitro* findings, which showed that a high-carbohydrate environment enhanced the conversion of the lignan or isoflavone precursors to their respective metabolites (Cassidy *et al.*, 2000).

The links between intake, metabolism, absorption and potential biological effects remain an area of active research. Studies are also under way to address the effects of age, gender, food matrix and food composition on the absorption and metabolism of this class of phytoestrogens.

In summary, more extensive data are required on the absorption and endogenous metabolism of these phytoestrogens in humans, and clarification of the biological activity of the metabolites. It is also necessary to identify the key gut microorganisms responsible for the conversion of the plant constituents to the biologically active derivatives, and the factors that determine their occurrence in the gastrointestinal tract. The interactions of phytoestrogens with each other and with endogenous steroids should also be further investigated.

6.5 Current intakes and bioavailability of carotenoids

6.5.1 Dietary sources of carotenoids

The five most commonly occurring carotenoids (categorised as terpenoids, see Section 2.4*vi*) in blood are β-carotene, lycopene, lutein, β-cryptoxanthin and α-carotene. A new EU-funded survey indicates that the main sources of these in the UK are carrots, tomatoes/tomato products, peas, citrus fruit and carrots, respectively (O'Neill *et al.*, 2001). The main sources in populations of European countries (France, Republic of Ireland, UK, the Netherlands, Spain) are shown in Table 6.4. For more details see the paper by O'Neill *et al.* Median intake of total carotenoids in the UK is 14.4 mg/day in adults (range: 11.77–19.1), with the largest contributions coming from β-carotene (5.6 mg/day) and lycopene (5.0 mg/day). The related ranges and median intakes in other European counties are shown in Table 6.5. Median β-carotene intakes ranged from 2.96 mg/day in Spain to 5.84 mg/day in France. Median lutein (and zeax-

Table 6.4 Major contributors to carotenoid intake in adults.

Carotenoids	Major contributors to intake in Europe
β-Carotene	Carrots, spinach, tomato products
Lutein	Spinach, peas, broccoli, lettuce
Lycopene	Tomatoes and tomato products (including pizza)
α-Carotene	Carrots, oranges, tangerines
β-Cryptoxanthin	Oranges and orange juice, tangerines

Source: derived from O'Neill *et al.* (2001).

Table 6.5 Comparison of carotenoid intakes (mg/day) in adults from five European countries.

Country	Total carotenoid* intake	
	Median	Interquartile range
Spain	9.54	7.16–14.46
France	16.06	10.3–22.1
UK	14.38	11.77–19.1
Republic of Ireland	14.53	10.37–18.9
The Netherlands	13.71	9.98–17.7

Source: adapted from O'Neill *et al.* (2001).
*In this context, total carotenoids comprises β-carotene, lutein, lycopene, α-carotene and β-cryptoxanthin. Determined by food frequency questionnaire during the winter months.

anthin) ranged from 1.56 mg/day in the Republic of Ireland to 32.5 mg/day in Spain. Median lycopene intakes ranged from 1.64 mg/day in Spain to 5.0 mg/day in the UK. Median α-carotene intakes ranged from 0.29 mg/day in Spain to 1.23 mg/day in the Republic of Ireland. Median β-cryptoxanthin intakes ranged from 0.45 mg/day in France to 1.3 mg/day in Spain. These data were collected in winter but there was generally little evidence of seasonal variation (O'Neill *et al.*, 2001). O'Neill *et al.* noted that these findings, obtained using a food frequency questionnaire, have provided higher estimates of intake than previous studies that used other methods, such as weighed records. However, information on contributions from different foods to the overall carotenoid intake is quantitatively similar to that of studies using other methods, and the findings are very similar to those of studies using a similar food frequency questionnaire methodology. Several explanations may be pertinent. Firstly, there can be a tendency with food frequency questionnaires for people to overestimate their consumption of certain foods with a positive image, such as vegetables, particularly when they are presented with a long list of choices. Another reason may be related to characteristics of the various populations studied, which affected their carotenoid intake to different extents.

Carotenoid intake varies with age (Carroll *et al.*, 1999) and other lifestyle factors, especially smoking (Margetts & Jackson, 1996); β-carotene and lycopene intakes were 36% and 58% lower, respectively, in the older population.

6.5.2 Absorption of carotenoids

Compared with the flavonoids, far more is known about the absorption and transport of carotenoids. These are passively absorbed from mixed micelles at the brush border along with dietary lipids, lipid hydrolysis products, sterols and bile salts. The absorbed carotenoids are transported through the cells lining the gut wall (enterocytes), where they are packaged in chylomicrons and transported via the lymphatic system through the thoracic duct into the circulating blood.

About 80% of β-carotene and lycopene (hydrocarbon carotenoids) found in fasting plasma is carried by LDL (low-density lipoproteins). It is not known how much of the carotenoid is distributed to the tissues by lipoproteins (and how quickly), but uptake of LDL particles by adipose tissues is likely to be a major carotenoid 'sink' (van den Berg *et al.*, 2000).

The hydroxycarotenoids (lutein, zeaxanthin) are almost equally distributed between the LDL and the high-density lipoproteins (HDL) in fasting subjects. The reason for this is unclear.

Carotenoids from oil solutions appear to be more bioavailable than those from food matrices, although very few foods have been examined. The increased bioavailability of lycopene from tomatoes and β-carotene from carrots are important examples (see Chapter 12). Heating foods appears to increase carotenoid bioavailability, although important variables such as severity of heat or commodity-specific effects remain largely unknown (see Chapter 12 for more details). Progress in this area has been hampered by the lack of methods suitable for the reliable measurement of carotenoid bioavailability or vitamin A yield.

Currently, relative bioavailability of carotenoids is more readily assessed than absolute bioavailability (see Section 6.2.3). The most commonly applied methods include measuring the increase in plasma carotenoid concentration following supplementation over a period of time, and the use of postprandial chylomicron (PPC) carotenoid or retinyl ester response following a single dose of carotenoid. The advantages and limitations of these approaches, together with examples of each, are discussed elsewhere (Parker *et al.*, 1999; van den Berg *et al.*, 2000) and are summarised in Section 6.2.3.

6.5.3 Interactions between carotenoids

There is no evidence to suggest that retinol-replete individuals absorb β-carotene or the other carotenoids less efficiently. However, individual carotenoids can interact. For example, lutein and β-carotene can interact to reduce the apparent absorption of lutein as measured by the AUC method (see Section 6.2.3*iv*), and in some instances lutein has been shown to reduce the AUC for β-carotene. Short-term supplementation of volunteers with β-carotene, either as a pure compound or as the major constituent of a natural β-carotene source, has also been found to reduce the plasma concentration of lutein. However, in a long-term study (4 years) of β-carotene supplementation, although there was a trend, the reduction in plasma lutein was not significant (van den Berg *et al.*, 2000). Currently it is unclear at what stage of absorption (mass transfer from food, dissolution in the lumenal lipid structures, absorption from the micelle, transport within the enterocyte or incorporation into chylomicrons) the interactions occur.

Alcohol intake has been shown to increase the plasma concentration of β-carotene and α-carotene and to reduce the concentrations of lutein and zeaxanthin, but it is notable that in alcoholic men, serum carotenoids were found to be lower than in controls (van den Berg *et al.*, 2000).

6.6 Hydroxycinnamates

The interest in hydroxycinnamates (see Section 2.3*ii*) as bioactive components of the diet has grown rapidly in the last 5–10 years, and progress has been reviewed (Kroon & Williamson 1999; Clifford 2000b). These compounds are phenolic acids and their conjugates possess potent antioxidant properties *in vitro*. The main dietary hydroxycinnamates are ferulic acid and caffeic acid, the latter being found in high levels in coffee, but at more modest levels in other foods. Heavy coffee drinkers may consume as much as 2000 mg/day of chlorogenic acid (the ester of caffeic acid). Ferulic acid, for example, is thought to play an important role in the lignification of plants and is abundant in cereal bran. The group also includes 4-coumaric acid and sinapic acid. Consumers of large quantities of cereals may achieve intakes of >100 mg/day of ferulic acid. Clifford's review indicates that the most important dietary sources are as follows:

- caffeic acid: coffee, blueberries, apples, cider
- 4-coumaric acid: spinach, cereal brans
- ferulic acid: coffee, citrus juices, cereal brans
- sinapic acid: broccoli, kale, other leafy brassicas, citrus juices.

Clifford also provides information on the sources of the major classes of cinnamate conjugates (Clifford 2000b). As yet, little is known about the uptake and metabolism of hydroxycinnamates in humans or their effect on biomarkers of human health (Clifford 2000b). However, a recent study with ileostomy volunteers indicated that 30% of ingested chlorogenic acid and almost all caffeic acid are absorbed in the small intestine (Olthof

et al., 2001). There is also a need for a more detailed understanding of typical intakes in the UK and elsewhere.

Meanwhile, there is considerable interest in the function of hydroxycinnamates within the plant, and their metabolism (Rechner *et al.*, 2001). Work is also under way to improve the understanding of the potential to use these substances in food processing and as functional food ingredients (Kroon & Williamson, 1999).

6.7 Plant sterols

The principal sources of plant sterols (see Section 2.5.5) in the diet are vegetable oils, with levels ranging from 1 to 5 g/kg. Cereals are the next most important source, with levels ranging from 0.5 to 1.8 g/kg. Nuts are also a good source (0.3–2.2 g/kg) (see Chapters 8 and 10). Typical intakes in the diet as a whole are 140–400 mg/day and might be as high as 1000 mg/day in those with a high intake of vegetable oils (see Chapter 10 for details). Recently, spreads enriched with plant sterols and stanols have become available (see Chapter 10), which could make a substantial contribution to intake in those who consume such products.

Plant sterols are very poorly absorbed, and it is this property that has caused plant sterol and stanol esters to gain prominence as ingredients within products designed to help reduce blood cholesterol levels (see Chapter 10). The US Food and Drug Agency (FDA) granted health claim approval for spreads containing plant sterols and the related derivatives, stanols, in September 2000 (Jones & Raeini-Sarjaz, 2001). The mechanism of action is suppression of cholesterol absorption. Cholesterol is present in the gut via the diet and also as a result of secretion of cholesterol via the bile; the absorption of dietary cholesterol and the reabsorption of the bile-secreted cholesterol are both suppressed by the presence of plant sterols (and plant stanols) in the diet.

Hydrolysis of conjugated plant sterols in the human intestine has been incompletely studied, especially regarding the glucosides. However, there is evidence that esterified plant sterols and stanols are hydrolysed effectively in the upper intestine and transferred to a micellar phase. Thus, about half of the esterified sterols and stanols are hydrolysed during passage of the first 0.5 m of the upper small intestine. Free and less esterified sterols are transferred to the micellar phase. The higher the free sterol/stanol content in the micellar phase, the more cholesterol remains in the oil phase, retarding its absorption. This appears to be the mechanism for the inhibition of cholesterol absorption by plant stanols and sterols (Piironen *et al.*, 2000). Unabsorbed sterols can be detected in faeces, as can their bacterial conversion products (see Chapter 10).

Although these plant substances are generally viewed as safe for long-term use for almost all sectors of the population (Jones & Raeini-Sarjaz, 2001), there are still some concerns about the impact of consumption of plant sterols on other lipid soluble nutrients, especially fat-soluble vitamins (Weststrate & Meijer, 1998; Hallikainen *et al.*, 2000). However, others in the field remain unconcerned (Gylling & Miettinen, 1999a).

6.8 Glucosinolates

Glucosinolates are sulphur-containing compounds found in Brassica vegetables (see Section 2.5*i*). The structural diversity and chemical reactivity of glucosinolate breakdown products, and the complexities of the matrix from which they have to be isolated, have long inhibited progress in understanding how these compounds are handled in the body. However, improvements in analytical methods for detecting and quantifying isothiocyanates and their excretory metabolites are now transforming this situation. This topic has recently been reviewed (Mithen *et al.*, 2000) and is also addressed in Chapter 5.

When the Brassica plant tissue is disrupted, *e.g.* by chopping, fermentation, cooking or chewing, the glucosinolates present are brought into contact with, and hydrolysed by, the endogenous plant enzyme myrosinase. This releases a range of breakdown products including the bitter tasting isothiocyanates commonly termed 'mustard oils', which are often volatile and have an acrid smell (see Chapters 2, 5, 7 and 12). Cooking reduces glucosinolate levels by about 30–60% and, after

prolonged cooking, breakdown products are barely detectable (see Chapter 12). There is growing interest in these breakdown products because of evidence from animal studies that certain isothiocyanates and their conjugates can inhibit the cytochrome P450 enzymes that activate nitrosamines to alkylating carcinogens (Mithen *et al.*, 2000) (see Chapter 5), and can induce Phase II enzymes, which detoxify carcinogens (Zhang *et al.*, 1992) (see Chapter 4).

Generally, each food source contains up to four different glucosinolates in significant amounts (Mithen *et al.*, 2000). Table 6.6 provides information derived from one study but published values show considerable variation, which may result from the use of different varieties, growing conditions and analytical methods. Although over 100 different glucosinolates have been identified, they fall into three principal groups: the aliphatic group (*e.g.* sinigrin and progoitrin), the aromatic group (*e.g.* gluconasturtiin) and the indolyl group (*e.g.* glucobrassicin and neoglucobrassicin) (see also Chapter 2). Current evidence suggests that when plant myrosinase is active in the ingested Brassica vegetables, glucosinolates are rapidly hydrolysed, and isothiocyanates are absorbed in

Table 6.6 Glucosinolate levels of freeze-dried Brassica vegetables (µmol/g dry weight).

	Total aliphatic/ aromatic glucosinolates	Indolyl glucosinolates
Cauliflower	0.7	1.1
Brussels sprouts	28.3	6.6
Savoy cabbage	10.0	4.7
Broccoli	13.5	3.2
Red cabbage	6.2	4.2
Green cabbage	17.9	8.1
White cabbage	11.5	3.9
Kohl rabi	0.5	2.0
Chinese cabbage	0.5	2.9
Swede	6.4	2.3
Radish	6.0	1.0
Horseradish	10.2	0.7

Source: derived from Mithen *et al.* (2000).

the proximal gut (Conaway *et al.*, 2000). If myrosinase is deactivated, *e.g.* by prolonged cooking of the vegetables before consumption, the ionised nature of glucosinolates may be expected to enable them to reach the large bowel where they could be metabolised by bacterial enzymes. This hypothesis was first tested and confirmed by studies in which antibiotic treatments were used to reduce the number of large bowel microflora. More direct evidence was eventually obtained from experiments in which the introduction of a whole faecal flora from rats or humans into initially germ-free rats resulted in the disappearance of intact glucosinolates in the caecal and colonic content, coupled with evidence of glucosinolate hydrolysis. It appears that the ability to degrade glucosinolates is widely distributed among intestinal bacteria.

Little is known of the structure of microbial glucosinolate derivatives, although the contribution of the digestive microflora to the production of isothiocyanates *in vivo*, in the large bowel, has been recently demonstrated using gnotobiotic rats harbouring a human digestive strain of *Bacteroides* (Elfoul *et al.*, 2001).

Glucosinolate degradation in the upper digestive tract is probably entirely a result of plant myrosinase activity because no endogenous activity has ever been found in gut tissues. Intact glucosinolates may also be partly absorbed, as indicated by reports of small amounts of intact glucosinolates in the blood and urine of poultry fed rapeseed meal, by experiments with hamster tissues (Michaelsen *et al.*, 1994) and studies with germ-free rats (Elfoul *et al.*, 2001).

Following rapid absorption from the upper gastrointestinal tract, the major route of isothiocyanate metabolism in humans is via conversion to *N*-acetylcysteine derivatives. This proceeds by initial conjugation with glutathione, promoted by glutathione-S-transferases, followed by hydrolysis of the resulting conjugates to the cysteine derivatives and final N-acetylation (Mithen *et al.*, 2000). Studies in human subjects have found evidence of metabolism and excretion of isothiocyanates, the effect being dependent upon the contributions of plant and microbial myrosinases. The post-absorptive fate of glucosinolate derivatives other than isothiocyanates has received comparatively little attention.

Although *in vitro* studies can contribute valuable information about the mechanisms of interaction between glucosinolate breakdown products and their target tissues, the major priority for future research must be *in vivo* studies with human volunteers. Mithen *et al.* recommend that such studies should preferably be conducted with chemically defined *Brassica* vegetables, and employ protocols which enable the dose–response relationship for both beneficial and adverse effects to be properly quantified (Mithen *et al.*, 2000). As with other classes of plant bioactive compounds, the major technical challenge will be the development of biomarkers to provide a comprehensive picture of the individual subject's physiological response to dietary glucosinolates. It is now well known that glutathione-S-transferase isoenzymes vary considerably in their specificities for isothiocyanates, as genes coding for these enzymes are polymorphic in humans. Consequently, the overall metabolism of isothiocyanates in individuals may ultimately depend on an individual's genotype (London *et al.*, 2000).

It is becoming clear that the fate of glucosinolates in fresh vegetables during food production is extremely complex since it depends on several mechanisms of degradation and biosynthesis, which seem to occur simultaneously (Verkerk *et al.*, 2001). The development of a robust predictive model to quantify the effects of these phenomena, and the integration with it of models describing the bioavailability and biological activity of those glucosinolates considered to be the most important for humans, should be the ultimate goal for future research in this area (Dekker *et al.*, 2000).

6.9 Hydroxybenzoic acid derivatives

This group (also known as phenolic acids, see Section 2.3*i*) includes benzoic acid and derivatives such as salicylic acid. Benzoic acid may be obtained from the diet either as a natural constituent, as for example in cranberries, or as an antimicrobial additive. Benzoic acid may also be formed endogenously from β-oxidation of

3-phenylpropionic acid, a gut flora metabolite of tyrosine in humans and of some flavonoids, at least in animals. Another source is from the aromatisation of dietary quinic acid in the liver.

Metabolic transformations include conjugation with sulphate, glucuronate and glycine. Methylation may also occur, as may demethylation, dehydroxylation and decarboxylation. In humans, benzoic acid is excreted mainly as hippuric acid (glycine being the rate-limiting factor) with a much smaller amount as the glucuronide, except at very high intakes when the glucuronide becomes more important.

Salicylic acid is excreted largely unchanged, but also as ester and ethereal conjugates with glucuronic acid, and as the glycine conjugate (salicyluric acid). However, the levels of salicylic acid in food are generally low and hence may have no biological significance in humans. Furthermore, some individuals are intolerant of dietary salicylic acid.

The intake of this group of compounds has been estimated for a Bavarian population using 7-day dietary records and data from the literature for food composition (Radtke *et al.*, 1998). The estimates obtained for daily intake of eight hydroxybenzoates were as follows: 4-hydroxybenzoic acid up to 1.69 mg; protocatechuic acid up to 4.17 mg; vanillic acid 0.03–4.09 mg in men and 0.24–2.03 mg in women; salicylic acid 0.11–10.27 mg; gentisic acid up to 2.20 mg; and syringic acid up to 4.48 mg. The equivalent data for gallic acid and ellagic acid (up to 17.83 and 91.80 mg, respectively) are included here for ease of comparison but are more fully discussed by Clifford and Scalbert, who pointed out that the ellagic acid contents of wine and grape juice used by Radtke *et al.* in the calculations (24 and 15 mg/L, respectively) may be higher than commonly encountered (Clifford & Scalbert, 2000).

It is clear from these data that total HBA burden, at least in one area of Germany, is very variable (from <1 up to ~ 95 mg/day) and dominated by ellagic acid. However, these data do not fully consider all conjugated forms of hydroxybenzoates, especially gallic acid, the formation of various HBAs by the gut microflora, the exposure to salicylates through medication or the burden of hydroxybenzoates or gallates added to foods as preservatives or antioxidants, respectively. The average daily burden in the UK has been estimated as 48.9 mg for benzoic acid and its salts (E210–E213), 0.1 mg for methyl, ethyl and propyl esters of benzoic acid (E214–E219) and virtually zero for propyl, octyl and dodecyl gallates (E310–E213).

On the basis of very limited data for the composition of black tea leaf and beverage, and the known consumption in the UK of a daily average of 3.4 cups, it seems likely that for many people this will be the major source of gallic acid. For others it would be wine, particularly red wine. It seems very likely, therefore, that in the UK and Ireland (heavy consumers of tea) and southern Europe (heavy consumers of red wine) the Bavarian gallic acid burden of approximately 18 mg/day could be exceeded by an appreciable margin. Heavy consumers of potato might also exceed the Bavarian burden of protocatechuic acid, since a 100 g serving might supply between 5 and 20 mg (compared with a maximum of 4.71 mg). Rosaceous fruits, although probably consumed less regularly, and certain herbs and spices generally consumed in small quantities, could also make significant contributions of certain HBAs.

Even heavy and regular consumers of tea, red wine, potato and herbs/spices would be unlikely to achieve the levels that have been used in *in vitro* or animal studies (generally above 10 mg/kg body weight), suggesting that the biological effects associated with dietary sources, if any, are likely to be weak. However, any attempts to increase the content of HBAs in foods should have regard to their sensory properties that could limit acceptability.

In view of the considerable potential that commodities such as tea, potato, red wine and rosaceous fruits might make to the consumption of hydroxybenzoates, there is a need for more representative analytical data. There is also a need for a better understanding of the role of the gut microflora in determining the burden of hydroxybenzoates. This should encompass not only the extent to which the flora deconjugates the hydroxybenzoates (particularly gallic and ellagic acids), but also the extent to which degradation of other classes of phenols (*e.g.* cinnamates and flavonoids) contributes to the burden of hydroxy-benzoates. These issues have been reviewed (Tomás-Barberán & Clifford, 2000b).

6.10 Enhancement of bioavailability

There is currently considerable interest in the potential to enhance the bioavailability of polyphenols in plants, via conventional breeding techniques and also by genetic modification technology (Farnham *et al.*, 1999; Kochian & Garvin, 1999). Studies are needed to evaluate whether modification of a plant's bioactive compound content will affect other attributes such as yield, post-harvest stability and storage, taste or processing qualities (Grusak *et al.*, 1999). It will also be important to know whether enhancement of one compound reduces the bioavailability of another, perhaps more critical substance.

Many of the substances referred to in this chapter are plant defence compounds and are present in wild-type forms of plants. It is likely that classical plant breeding will have reduced the amounts present in currently available food crops because they confer bitterness or other undesirable characteristics to the consumer or processor. However, because of their role in the plant, the consequence of reducing levels might be to increase the dependence on chemical treatments.

There is good evidence that some processing techniques can increase bioavailability (see Chapter 12).

Whether such changes are, on balance, of benefit from the perspectives of human and animal health and the environment remains to be established. Currently there are insufficient data to enable such a judgement to be made.

6.11 Research recommendations

More information is needed about the bioavailability of bioactive substances in plant foods in order to help establish whether the effects reported *in vitro* are relevant *in vivo*

- Assessment of the biological effects of specific plant components is currently confounded by numerous technical barriers. Particularly important among these is the need to develop practical and feasible tests for measurement of biological effects, which take account of the need for high sensitivity measurement of small changes in endpoint. More ^{13}C-labelled compounds are required for human metabolic studies.
- There is a need for comprehensive food composition databases for bioactive plant substances in order to assess the range of likely intakes of individual compounds in a diversity of populations.

- The basic mechanisms of action of these substances need to be worked out, along with an understanding of how the activity of these compounds in isolation differs from their activity when delivered in their natural (plant) milieu, and how this activity can be modified by the effects of other plant substances and by food processing and preparation methods.
- Some compounds may have important effects in the gastrointestinal tract and may not need to be systemically absorbed to be protective. This requires investigation.
- It is important to understand the synergies and interactions of plant bioactive substances from various sources, including spices and herbs.
- More information is required about the compositional changes in plants as a consequence of modern plant breeding methods and the range of levels that are found in commercial varieties.

6.12 Key points

- In order to assess the bioavailability of a food component, it is necessary to have information about the amount that enters the blood circulation intact following consumption of the food, *i.e.* following digestion and absorption. This knowledge is essential in order to understand the potential role of dietary components in the prevention of disease.

- There remains a need for a comprehensive and thorough survey of the occurrence in food and progress through the body of the various types of bioactive compounds (*e.g.* flavonoids and allied compounds, terpenoids, alkaloids, nitrogen-containing alkaloids and sulphur-containing compounds) using selective, sensitive and well-standardised methods, which are applicable to blood, plasma, urine and tissues.

- Although intestinal absorption can be high, there is evidence of extensive metabolism of absorbed flavonoids, as changes in plasma antioxidant capacity generally considerably exceed changes in levels of the parent flavonoid in plasma. Absorption from the colon, following the action of colonic bacteria on ingested flavonoids and related compounds, is thought to be important in contributing to antioxidant capacity in plasma but little is known about the precise role of the microflora in the bioavailability of such substances and, apart from a limited understanding of why flavonol glycosides are better absorbed than their aglycones, little is known about the influence of other structural parameters.

- For the flavonoids and carotenoids in particular, research is beginning to provide information on the amounts of selected compounds in foods, and typical intakes in a number of populations world wide. However, compared with the flavonoids, much more is known about the absorption and transport of carotenoids. Assessment of relative bioavailability is also receiving considerable research attention. Functional markers for carotenoids

are required, however, to enable research into potential health benefits to progress.

- Flavonoids (*e.g.* flavonols, flavones, flavan-3-ols, flavanones and isoflavones) account for about two-thirds of the dietary phenols, with phenolic acids accounting for the remainder. The main sources are fruit, beverages (fruit juice, wine, tea, coffee, cocoa and beer) and chocolate. Vegetables, dry legumes and cereals also contribute. The total intake of phenols is estimated to be about 1 g/day.

- The potential beneficial effects of flavonoids justify a thorough understanding of the bioavailability in humans of these abundant dietary constituents. The limited data available suggest that dietary concentrations are potentially high enough to give biological effects.

- The five most commonly occurring carotenoids in blood are β-carotene, lycopene, lutein, β-cryptoxanthin and α-carotene. The main dietary sources of these are, respectively, carrots, tomatoes/tomato products, peas, citrus fruit and carrots. Average intake of total carotenoids in UK adults is 14.4 mg/day, with the largest contributions coming from β-carotene and lycopene.

- A beneficial role for plant sterol and stanol esters, in relation to reducing plasma cholesterol, has been established. Their action hinges on their very low absorption rates and their structural similarity to cholesterol and hence their competition in the micellar phase with dietary and endogenous cholesterol, reducing uptake of the latter.

- More data are required on the absorption and endogenous metabolism of phytoestrogens in humans, and clarification is also needed of the biological activity of the metabolites. It is necessary to identify the key gut microorganisms responsible for the conversion of the plant constituents to the biologically active derivatives, and the factors that determine their occurrence in the gastrointestinal tract. The interactions of phytoestrogens with each other and with endogenous steroids should also be investigated further.

- Glucosinolates are sulphur-containing compounds found in Brassica vegetables. Disruption of the plant tissue (*e.g.* by chopping or cooking) releases myrosinase which converts the glucosinolates to a number of substances including isothiocyanates. There is also evidence that conversion to isothiocyanates can occur in the colon; ability to degrade glucosinolates is widespread among bacteria. There is growing interest in these breakdown products and animal evidence that they may have anti-cancer effects.

- Interest is growing in the hydroxycinnamates (*e.g.* caffeic and ferulic acids) and hydroxybenzoates (ellagic acid). Although there is some information about the uptake and metabolism of hydroxybenzoates in humans, further research in this area is required.

7
Fruit and Vegetables

7.1 Introduction

Current advice is that for optimum health, people should consume on a daily basis at least five portions of fruit and vegetables (World Cancer Research Fund, 1997; Department of Health, 1998b), each weighing at least 80 g (see Section 13.2) (Williams, 1995). The epidemiological evidence for the benefit of consuming diets that are high in fruit and vegetables is quite compelling (see Chapter 3). The evidence for specific vegetables, and indeed specific compounds, is less convincing, although epidemiological studies of cancer suggest that it is mainly the highly coloured green or yellow vegetables that are associated with reduced incidence and mortality rates.

The use of the terms 'fruit' and 'vegetable' is a culinary rather than a botanical distinction. In a botanical context, 'vegetables' such as tomatoes, cucumbers, courgettes, peppers (capsicums) and avocado pears are classified as fruits. To avoid confusion, in this chapter foods will be classed according to their common usage. Some vegetables, such as potatoes, cassava and yams, serve as staple foods although they tend to have a high starch content. Such staples are not generally classed as 'vegetables' for the purposes of dietary guidelines (see Chapter 13). Outside the provision of a dietary staple, vegetables are used for dietary variety, colour and taste and can be purchased in a range of processed states (see Chapter 12), including fresh, frozen, canned and dried. In contemporary Western society, fresh vegetables may also be processed to a high degree, including washing and slicing or shredding. The most widely consumed vegetables in the world that are not used as staples are onions and tomatoes. Fruits and vegetables are generally low in fat, may contain significant amounts of dietary fibre (non-starch polysaccharides) and, apart from vitamins and minerals, contain a wide range of compounds called 'phytochemicals' that may have biological activity in humans. Trends in fruit and vegetable consumption and the nutrients provided by fruits and vegetables are discussed in Chapter 1.

Plants may be consumed as leaves, stems, roots, tubers, buds, fruits, seeds and flowers. Usually only one part of a particular plant is considered desirable for consumption.

In this chapter, we identify the bioactive compounds, including those contributing to colour, known to be present in fruits and vegetables which, together with the vitamins and minerals also present, may be the basis for their beneficial effects. Authoritative figures for contents of macronutrients, vitamins and minerals are given in food tables (McCance & Widdowson, 1991) and these will not be repeated in this chapter. Similarly, vegetables in general are a source of fibre and the levels will not be identified for each individual species. These figures are also available in food tables.

In addition to the references cited throughout this chapter, other information about the historical context of fruit and vegetables can be found in a number of books (Simpson & Conner-Ogorzaly, 1986; Tannahill, 1988; Readers Digest Association Ltd, 1996; Mason & Brown, 1999; Pavoro, 1999; Whiteman, 1999).

7.2 Bioactive compounds found in fruits and vegetables

There are four principal classes of bioactive compounds: terpenoids, phenolics and polyphenolics, nitrogen-containing alkaloids and sulphur compounds (see Chapter 2) the members of which have been suggested to have positive effects on human health. It is a truism that the effect produced depends on the amount consumed. For example, within the class of glucosinolates, progoitrin can be converted to goitrin (Fig. 7.1) which is a potent goitrogen. Glucobrassicin (Fig. 7.1) is mutagenic at high doses. However, in the levels found in the normal diet, both progoitrin and glucobrassicin may be protective (Rhodes & Price, 1998).

In the growing plant, bioactive compounds have roles in metabolism and in the interaction of the plant with the environment. The occurrence of the bioactive compounds of interest varies throughout the plant kingdom from the widespread carotenoids, to the glucosinolates that are found only in the Cruciferae and a few members of some other families of dicotyledonous angiosperms (Fenwick *et al.*, 1983). Carotenoids are ubiquitous in leaves and stems because they are an essential part of the photosynthetic process, involved in light harvesting and protecting against photo-oxidative damage (van den Berg *et al.*,

2000). Sterols generally control membrane fluidity and permeability, while some have further specific roles (Piironen *et al.*, 2000). Phenolic compounds, on the other hand, appear to be mainly associated with the defence of the plant against a range of attacks, from browsing animals through insects, bacteria and fungi to inhibiting the growth of competing plants. Flavonols in epidermal cells of leaves and the skins of fruit provide protection against the damaging effects of UVB irradiation. They also are involved in fertilisation by promoting the growth of pollen tubes in the style of flowers. Polyphenols and carotenoids provide colour to stems, leaves, flowers and fruits. The carotenoids provide yellows with some orange and red, whereas the polyphenolics, most notably the anthocyanins, are more numerous and provide a greater range of colours from orange to blue.

Glucosinolates have been shown to affect insect predation; some act as feeding deterrents to certain species of insect, but other insects such as the large white butterfly larvae are attracted by specific glucosinolates. There is also evidence that glucosinolates have antifungal and antibacterial activities and their presence in the plant may contribute to resistance to infection by mildew and other fungi.

Members of the terpenoid family are diverse in structure, and have an extremely wide range of actions. For example, the complex limonoid azadirachtin (Fig. 7.2) from the neem (*Azadirachta indica*) tree is a powerful insect antifeedant, whereas the monoterpene linalool (Fig. 7.2) is an attractant bringing insects to fertilise flowers. Others terpenoids are the active ingredients in

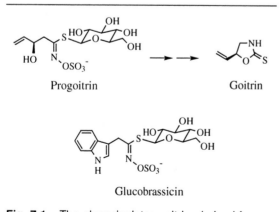

Fig. 7.1 The glucosinolates goitrin, derived from progoitrin, and glucobrassicin can have either adverse or positive effects on health depending upon the amount consumed.

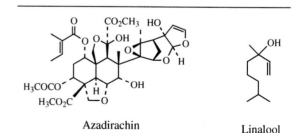

Fig. 7.2 An example of the diverse structures of terpenoids.

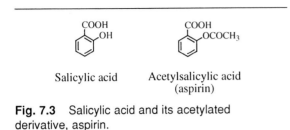

Fig. 7.3   Salicylic acid and its acetylated derivative, aspirin.

essential oils while diterpene resins block insect attack on conifer trees (Croteau *et al.*, 2000). Limonoids are oxygenated triterpenoids that are found in only two plant families. The citrus limonoids are only found in the Citrus genus where in the leaves and young fruit they act as antifeedants (Hasegawa *et al.*, 2000).

Salicylic acid (Fig. 7.3) is produced rapidly in some plants as a signal molecule that initiates defence responses following attack by insects, fungi, bacteria and viruses. Salicylic acid and acetylsalicylic acid (aspirin) levels have been monitored in a range of fruits, vegetables, herbs, spices and beverages (Venema *et al.*, 1996). Acetylsalicylic acid was not detected in any of the samples and with the exception of some herbs and spices, most notably cinnamon (*Cinnamonum verum* syn. *C. zeylandicum*), oregano (*Origanum vulgare*) and rosemary (*Rosmarinus officinalis*), salicylic acid levels were less than 1 mg/kg fresh weight. It is thought that the levels of salicylates present in most diets are too low to have an impact on health (Janssen *et al.*, 1996b).

It is important to be aware of the sheer numbers of plant bioactive compounds. Attention tends to be focused on a few representatives of each class, but 25 000 members of the terpenes have been identified, around 8000 phenolics and there are even 250 different sterols.

7.3   Quantification

7.3.1   Units of measurement

With some significant exceptions, plant bioactive compounds are present in relatively small amounts in fresh fruit and vegetables. While the tea leaf contains in excess of 15% flavan-3-ols by weight (Haslam, 1998), it is more common for levels to be of the order of mg/kg (*i.e.* 0.001%). Quantifications are reported in a variety of units: mg/kg, mg/g, mg/100 g or even mol/g. For consistency, in this chapter all such contents will be given in mg/kg.

7.3.2   Variability within and between plants

Where studies on plant material have been compared, it is not unusual for reported levels to vary by a factor of 20, with the difference in some cases being as much as 100-fold (Price *et al.*, 1987; van den Berg *et al.*, 2000). The levels of plant bioactive compounds recorded have to be considered in context and no single figure can be regarded as representative of a plant species. The content of individual fruits and vegetables is affected by many factors:

- variety
- soil
- climatic conditions
- agricultural methods
- physiological stress under which they are grown
- degree of ripeness, storage conditions and length of storage before consumption.

Not all references have recognised the resultant variability, and results from a single unnamed variety purchased in a supermarket have often been taken as representative of the species (van den Berg *et al.*, 2000). Major cultivated crops in the developed world have been bred so that they are true to type; naming the variety is sufficient to define the plant. This is not necessarily the case where local varieties are still grown. Genotype influences not only the overall content of a class of compound, but also the proportions of individual chemicals. The form in which vegetables are available is also changing. In the past spinach was typically a mature leaf purchased loose from the greengrocer. The product available in a modern supermarket is pre-packed young leaf cut to a prescribed length.

The levels of compounds vary within the plant; within fruits many are concentrated in the skin, and within vegetables in the outer leaves. For

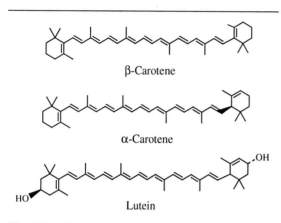

β-Carotene

α-Carotene

Lutein

Fig. 7.4 Carotenoids found in the leaves of Savoy cabbage.

example, the outer leaves of Savoy cabbage contain more than 150 times the level of lutein (Fig. 7.4) and 200 times the level of β-carotene (Fig. 7.4) present in the inner leaves (van den Berg *et al.*, 2000). Glucosinolates are also heterogeneously distributed within the plant, and a study has shown a varying composition even in different parts of a swede root tuber (Adams *et al.*, 1989).

7.3.3 Methodologies used and analysis of data

It is not just the inherent variability discussed above that needs to be considered. The bioactive compound content can be reported in three ways: as individual compounds, cumulatively as groups of compounds and by application. Thus, for example, polyphenols may be measured as pure compounds and total polyphenols by mode of action. Measures of total polyphenol content are prone to overestimation, while measures of specific compounds may not identify all those present in a sample.

As analytical techniques have improved, so have both the identification of individual compounds and the accuracy of the quantitative determination. The validity of earlier results depends to some extent on the compound of interest and on the method used. For example, many results on individual polyphenols obtained in the 1960s stand up today, whereas some determinations of

glucosinolates would now be regarded as rather high.

The nutritional implications of polyphenols have often been determined simply in terms of antioxidant capacity. Many methods of estimation of antioxidant capacity have been developed which are based on *in vitro* tests. They give different results and are not all equally valid. Furthermore, results cannot be extrapolated to the *in vivo* situation.

7.4 Vegetables

In the following sections each vegetable will be discussed briefly. Particular compounds will be highlighted, but this should not be taken as an indication that these are the only ones associated with the foodstuff as it is evident that the contents of some dietary fruits and vegetables have been investigated in detail whereas others have received very little, if any, attention.

7.4.1 Root crops (*e.g.* carrots, turnips, swedes, parsnips)

Root crops include carrot (*Daucus carota*), turnip (*Brassica campestris*), swede (*Brassica napus*) (also known as rutabaga), parsnip (*Pastinaca sativa*) and Jerusalem artichoke (*Helianthus tuberosus*). These were important dietary items during the 19th and early 20th centuries; turnip and swede were more common at the beginning of the 20th century, but carrot is now the most popular root vegetable after the potato. Changes in dietary habits have also seen a decrease in consumption of the leaves of root crops as vegetables. Originally, leaves were the only part of the beetroot that was consumed, and carrot leaves were eaten until the middle of the 19th century in the UK (Anon, 1897). Young turnip leaves are still considered an early season delicacy in some countries, and beetroot leaves are still eaten in the UK. Interestingly, in comparison, the leaves of leaf beet are eaten as spinach and the root discarded.

The carrot was introduced into Europe from Arabia in the 14th century. The original carrots were purple and yellow, and the orange carrots

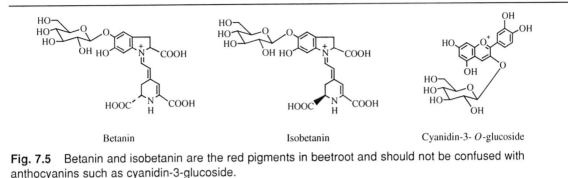

Betanin   Isobetanin   Cyanidin-3-*O*-glucoside

Fig. 7.5 Betanin and isobetanin are the red pigments in beetroot and should not be confused with anthocyanins such as cyanidin-3-glucoside.

that we use today originate from selective breeding in the Netherlands in the 17th century. Nowadays, different varieties of carrot are grown both for immediate consumption and for storage (see Section 12.4). The principal compounds of interest in carrots are α-carotene and β-carotene (Fig. 7.4) and carrots are a rich source, containing up to 650 mg/kg (van den Berg *et al*., 2000). Carrots also contain polyphenols (Lister & Podivinsky, 1998) and sterols (Piironen *et al*., 2000).

Beetroot contains β-carotene in the leaves while red pigmentation in the roots is due to betanin and isobetanin (Fig. 7.5), which are betalains. Betalains were long thought to be related to anthocyanins, even though they contain nitrogen and are structurally quite distinct (Fig. 7.5). Betalains are restricted to 10 plant families, all of which are members of the order Caryophyllales which lack anthocyanins. Beetroot extract is used as a food colouring (E162).

Swedes and turnips are both Brassicas in which the principal compounds of interest are glucosinolates, found throughout the plant but particularly in the root. Parsnip is a member of the Umbelliferae family and like many members of this family, including celery (*Apicum graveollens*), contains psoralen (Fig. 7.6), which in sensitive people can cause blistering on exposure to light (see Section 7.5.4*ii*).

7.4.2 Onions and garlic

Members of the family Alliaceae have been an important part of the human diet for thousands of

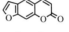

Psoralen

Fig. 7.6 Some people are very sensitive to psoralen, which occurs in Umbelliferous plants and causes blistering of the skin on exposure to sunlight.

years; even in ancient times they were used extensively throughout the northern hemisphere. Onions (*Allium cepa*), leeks (*Allium porrum*) and garlic (*Allium sativum*) were important in the diet of the Romans, who probably introduced them to the UK. Now a considerable array of varieties, red, white, yellow and silver skin onions, spring onions (scallions), shallots, leeks, chives (*Allium schoenoprasum*) and garlic, are available throughout Europe and other varieties are eaten on other continents. It is believed that all members of the genus *Allium* are edible. World onion production is estimated to be in excess of 30 billion kg per annum. Garlic is reputed to have benefits for protection against cardiovascular diseases, cancer, microbial infections, asthma, diabetes and vampires! Although there is some evidence for the first two effects, the rest of the list is largely speculation or folklore. Garlic has been commercially exploited and is available as essential oil of garlic, garlic pearls and other extracts in the form of tablets or capsules.

S-Alkylcysteine sulphoxides are found in all members of the *Allium* genus (Fig. 7.7). All

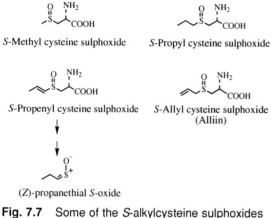

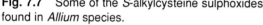

S-Methyl cysteine sulphoxide   *S*-Propyl cysteine sulphoxide

S-Propenyl cysteine sulphoxide   *S*-Allyl cysteine sulphoxide
                                        (Alliin)

(*Z*)-propanethial *S*-oxide

Fig. 7.7 Some of the *S*-alkylcysteine sulphoxides found in *Allium* species.

species contain *S*-methylcysteine sulphoxide but *S*-propylcysteine sulphoxide is the major component in chives, and the *S*-1-propenyl derivative predominates in onions and *S*-allylcysteine sulphoxide (alliin) in garlic. When cutting onions, conversion of *S*-propenylcysteine sulphoxide to (*Z*)-propanethial *S*-oxide (Fig. 7.7) results in the well known phenomenon of onion-induced kitchen tears as (*Z*)-propanethial S-oxide is a lachrymatory factor.

Fresh garlic has little smell and can be eaten raw but tissue damage by cutting, crushing or biting results in alliin being cleaved by the enzyme alliinase, resulting in the formation of diallyl thiosuphinate (allicin) (Fig. 7.7). Allicin gives crushed garlic its characteristic aroma. Alliin and alliinase are both stable when dry so dried garlic retains the potential to release allicin when moistened and crushed. Nonetheless, the composition of dried garlic and assorted garlic powders and oils is very variable, with reported values for the alliin content differing by 10-fold.

Allicin is very unstable to heat, so cooking garlic results in its degradation to a number of compounds including diallyl sulphides and ajoenes (Fig. 7.8). Bad breath which follows the ingestion of garlic products is due to a range of sulphide compounds, including diallyl disulphide and diallyl trisulphide (Fig. 7.8).

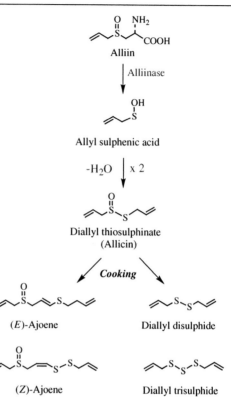

Alliin

Alliinase

Allyl sulphenic acid

$-H_2O$ x 2

Diallyl thiosulphinate
(Allicin)

Cooking

(*E*)-Ajoene   Diallyl disulphide

(*Z*)-Ajoene   Diallyl trisulphide

Fig. 7.8 The characteristic aroma of garlic is due to allicin, which is formed from alliin when the cloves are cut or crushed. When garlic is cooked, allicin breaks down to a number of products including diallyl sulphoxides, which are responsible for bad breath after eating garlic-flavoured foods.

Most studies on the potentially protective effects of garlic have used extracts or preparations rather than cooked garlic. There have been very few investigations using raw garlic, arguably because the flavours and smells are so strong that double-blinded, placebo-controlled trials are not possible. There is epidemiological evidence (see Chapter 3) associating reduced risk of colonic cancer (Steinmetz *et al.*, 1994) and CHD (Keys, 1980) with regular consumption of garlic. Five of six intervention studies using fresh garlic or freshly prepared extracts demonstrated a lowering of serum cholesterol, increased fibrinolytic activity and inhibition of platelet aggregation (Kleijnen

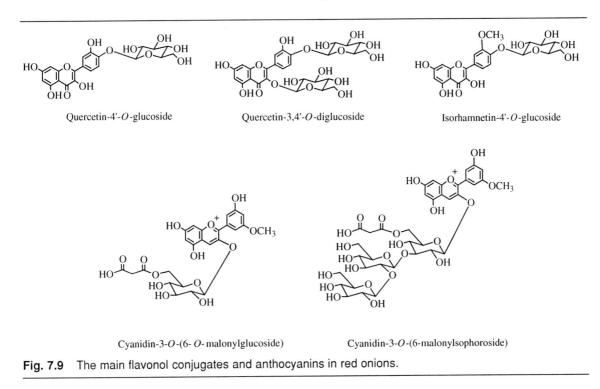

Quercetin-4'-*O*-glucoside   Quercetin-3,4'-*O*-diglucoside   Isorhamnetin-4'-*O*-glucoside

Cyanidin-3-*O*-(6-*O*-malonylglucoside)   Cyanidin-3-*O*-(6-malonylsophoroside)

Fig. 7.9   The main flavonol conjugates and anthocyanins in red onions.

et al., 1989). Another study also showed significant reductions in systolic blood pressure (Steiner *et al.*, 1996). However, these effects were generally achieved at very high levels of intake, the equivalent of between 7 and 28 cloves per day, and this produces side effects that are unacceptable to many people, including body odour, bad breath and flatulence. There are claims that allicin and ajoene are the bioactive agents in garlic, but there is limited evidence to substantiate this view.

The main flavonols in onions are glycosylated derivatives, principally quercetin-4'-glucoside and quercetin-3,4'-diglucoside with smaller amounts of isorhamnetin-4'-glucoside (Fig. 7.9) and other quercetin conjugates (Tsushida & Suzuki, 1995). Yellow onions form one of the main sources of flavonols in the Northern European diet, the edible flesh containing between 280 and 490 mg/kg (Hollman & Arts, 2000). Even higher concentrations are found in the dry outer scales (Chu *et al.*, 2000). By contrast, leeks have been found to have only 10–60 mg/kg of kaempferol and no quercetin. The flavonols in onions appear to be particularly well absorbed from the gut with a recovery of only about 15% in ileostomy effluent. White onions are all but devoid of flavonols. Red onions, like their yellow counterparts, are rich in flavonols and also contain up to 250 mg/kg of anthocyanins (Clifford, 2000a), the main components being cyanidin-3-(6-malonylglucoside) and cyanidin-3-(6-malonylsophoroside) (Fig. 7.9).

7.4.3 Cabbage family and greens (*e.g.* Brussels sprouts, broccoli, cabbage)

Members of the genus *Brassica* (in the family Cruciferae) have been cultivated for thousands of years, although the main use in ancient times was probably for medicine. Carbonised seed of brown mustard has been found at a site in China dating to around 4000 BC (Fenwick *et al.*, 1983). The Romans cultivated a number of members of the genus, including mustard, cabbage, kale and possibly broccoli and kohl rabi, and introduced the crop to the UK. Cauliflower is mentioned in the 12th century and the most recent member

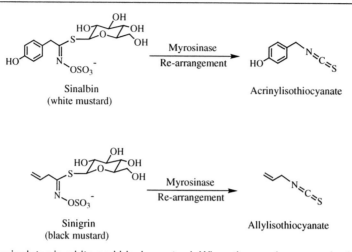

Fig. 7.10 Glucosinolates in white and black mustard. When the seeds are crushed and moistened, sinalbin is converted to acrinyl isothiocyanate and sinigrin to allyl isothiocyanate.

of the family to be discovered was Brussels sprouts in around 1750. Varieties of only one species, *Brassica oleracea*, are the most commonly consumed vegetables in the UK and include broccoli, Brussels sprouts, cabbage, calabrese, cauliflower, kale and kohl rabi.

Within the Brassica, all parts of the plant are consumed, roots (turnip, swede, kohl rabi), leaves (cabbage, kale), apical buds (Brussels sprouts), flower heads (broccoli and cauliflower) and seeds (mustard). In addition to being consumed fresh, worldwide considerable tonnages of these crops are processed, mainly into sauerkraut, coleslaw and pickles. Fermented Brassica crops are important constituents of Asia–Pacific diets.

All members of the genus contain glucosinolates. These break down on chewing as the enzyme myrosinase is released (see below) and yields compounds that are responsible for the spicy/hot flavour of mustard and a number of other cruciferous plants which are not Brassicas, including radish (*Raphanus sativus*), horseradish (*Armoracia rusticana*), watercress (*Nasturtium officinale*) and rocket (*Eruca sativa*).

The glucosinolate sinalbin accumulates in white mustard (*Sinapis alba* syn. *Brassica hirta*) seed and when moistened and crushed the glucose moiety is cleaved by myrosinase and a

sulphonated intermediate that is formed undergoes rearrangement forming acrinylisothiocyanate (Fig. 7.10) which is responsible for the hot, pungent taste of the condiment. Black mustard (*Brassica nigra*) seeds contain sinigrin which is similarly hydrolysed to allylthiocyanate (Fig. 7.10), which is considerably more volatile than acrinyl isothiocyanate which gives black mustard powder a pungent aroma and a hot spicy taste.

While glucosinolates are desired for their intense flavour, as in mustard, their presence in leaf crops such as Brussels sprouts can make these foods less attractive to consumers, particularly the young. Glucosinolates are not biologically active of themselves but once the glucose moiety has been removed by myrosinase, the resulting aglycone is unstable and rearranges, forming active compounds including isothiocyanates, thiocyanates, nitriles and indole derivatives. In the plant, myrosinase is a membrane-associated enzyme, but when the plant is chewed or processed, cellular compartmentation is disrupted and myrosinase comes into contact with glucosinolates that are localised in the cell vacuoles. Much of the myrosinase will be inactivated by cooking (see Section 12.7.1), which means that in most foodstuffs both intact glucosinolates and

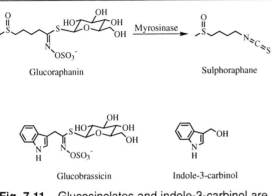

Fig. 7.11 Glucosinolates and indole-3-carbinol are found in *Brassica* species.

breakdown products will be ingested (see Section 5.4.3).

There have been reports of cabbage having a goitrogenic effect in animals fed on a diet low in iodine, and thyroid, liver and kidney enlargement in rats fed a diet rich in rapeseed. There is no evidence that direct consumption of Brassicas causes goitre, but it has been suggested that endemic goitre in certain regions of Europe could be caused by the consumption of milk containing the goitrin precursor progoitrin (see Fig. 7.1) from the ingestion by cattle of cruciferous forage or weeds, together with marginal or deficient iodine status. This question has not yet been resolved unequivocally.

Some glucosinolate derivatives, including sulforaphane, are potent, selective inducers of Phase II enzymes. The sprouting seedlings of some cultivars of broccoli and cauliflower contain 10–100 times the level of glucoraphanin, the glucosinolate precursor of sulforaphane (Fig. 7.11), than mature plants (Fahey *et al.*, 1997). Furthermore, these immature plants do not contain significant levels of the indole glucosinolates, such as glucobrassicin, and related indoles including indole-3-carbinol (Fig. 7.11) that can enhance tumorigenesis, although protective effects have also been reported. Broccoli sprouts, very similar to mustard and cress, are available commercially as a 'health food', and their consumption may provide scope for significantly increasing glucosinolate intake without large increases in the consumption of Brassica vegetables. These products may be more palatable to those who dislike the taste of the mature form.

In addition to glucosinolates, broccoli florets contain quercetin-3-sophoroside (65 mg/kg) kaempferol-3-sophoroside (166 mg/kg) and conjugates of the hydroxycinnamate sinapic acid (336 mg/kg) (Fig. 7.12) (Plumb *et al.*, 1997).

Other members of this genus are consumed as roots (turnip and swede) and as salad leaves [Chinese cabbage (*Brassica pekinensis*), rocket and watercress]. Other leaves are consumed cooked as greens. These include spinach (*Spinaceae oleraceae*), the closely related spinach beet and Swiss chard (*Beta vulgaris*). Swiss chard has a high flavonoid content estimated at 2700 mg/kg, compared to spinach with 1000 mg/kg and red onion with 900 mg/kg (Gil *et al.*, 1999). Spinach contains

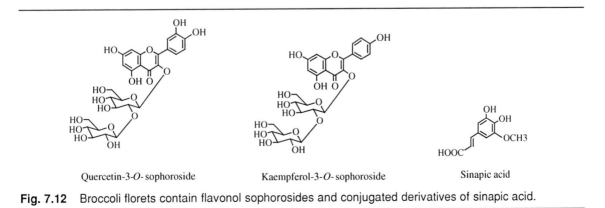

Quercetin-3-*O*-sophoroside   Kaempferol-3-*O*-sophoroside   Sinapic acid

Fig. 7.12 Broccoli florets contain flavonol sophorosides and conjugated derivatives of sinapic acid.

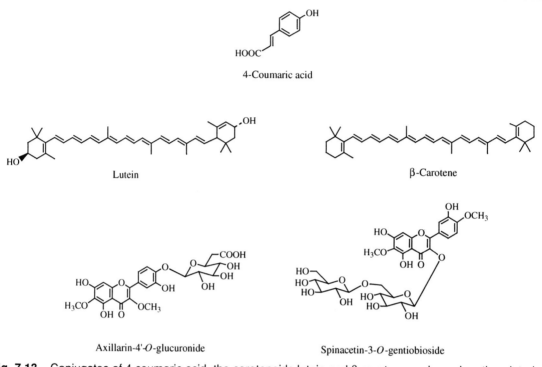

Fig. 7.13 Conjugates of 4-coumaric acid, the carotenoids lutein and β-carotene and novel methoxylated flavonols occur in spinach.

conjugates of 4-coumaric acid (Fig. 7.13) and high levels of carotenoids; lutein contents have been determined ranging from 20 to 203 mg/kg and β-carotene from 8 to 240 mg/kg (van den Berg *et al.*, 2000). Spinach is devoid of the common flavonols conjugated quercetin and kaempferol but contains axillarin-4'-glucoside and spinacetin-3-gentobioside (Fig. 7.13) (Kidmose *et al.*, 2001), and other novel methoxyflavonol derivatives (Zane & Wender, 1961), some of which have antimutagenic properties (Edenhardener, 2001).

7.4.4 Salad vegetables

Salad vegetables are taken from a wide range of botanical families. Lettuce (*Latuca sativa*) was consumed by the Romans and Egyptians, the latter possibly as early as 4500 BC.

(i) Lettuce

Lettuce is a source of carotenoids, containing both lutein and β-carotene, although the concentrations determined have varied by a factor of 60, the highest being 45.3 mg/kg for lutein (van den Berg *et al.*, 2000). The red-leafed lettuce Lollo Rosso contains the anthocyanin cyanidin-3-(6-malonylglucoside) and several flavonols including the major component quercetin-3-(6-malonylglucoside), and the hydroxycinnamate derivatives caffeoyltartaric acid, dicaffeoyltartaric acid, 5-*O*-caffeoylquinic acid (chlorogenic acid) and 3,5,-*O*-dicaffeoylquinic acid (isochlorogenic acid) (Fig. 7.14) (Ferreres *et al.*, 1997). The levels of flavonols, measured as quercetin released by acid hydrolysis, is 911 ± 27 mg/kg fresh weight in the outer leaves and around half this amount in the inner leaves of Lollo Rosso. Other varieties have much lower flavonol levels with Round lettuce

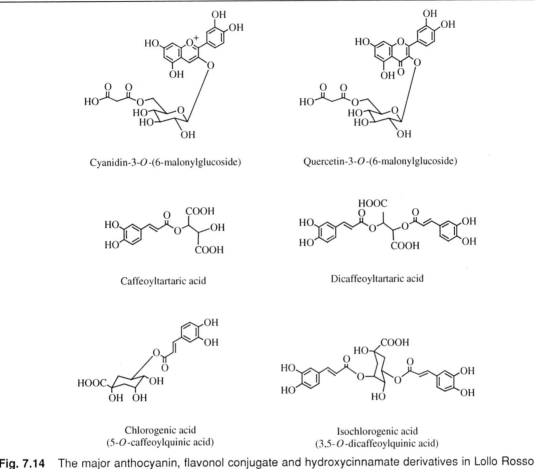

Cyanidin-3-*O*-(6-malonylglucoside)

Quercetin-3-*O*-(6-malonylglucoside)

Caffeoyltartaric acid

Dicaffeoyltartaric acid

Chlorogenic acid
(5-*O*-caffeoylquinic acid)

Isochlorogenic acid
(3,5-*O*-dicaffeoylquinic acid)

Fig. 7.14 The major anthocyanin, flavonol conjugate and hydroxycinnamate derivatives in Lollo Rosso lettuce.

containing only 11 mg/kg and Iceberg, which is used widely in commercial salads and sandwiches, a mere 2 mg/kg (Crozier *et al.*, 1997, 2000).

(ii) Celery

Celery was cultivated as a medicine by the ancients and was not used as a food until 1623. Celery contains conjugates of the flavones luteolin and apigenin (Fig. 7.15) although the amounts can be variable (Crozier *et al.*, 1997). Fungal infection of celery results in the accumulation of psoralen and other furocoumarins such as the methoxylated derivatives xanthotoxin and bergapten (Fig. 7.15). People harvesting infected plants by hand can become very sensitive to the UVA component of ultraviolet light and develop a sunburn-type rash (phytophotodermatitis). The level of psoralen is considerably reduced by cooking, especially boiling. Psoralen is now used in the treatment of skin disorders such as psoriasis. Celeriac (*Apicum graveollens* var. *rapaceum*) has a similar flavour to celery but the root rather than the stem is eaten, either peeled and parboiled in salads or as a cooked vegetable.

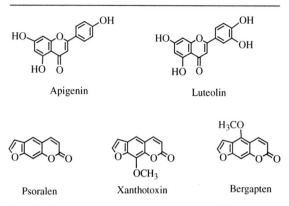

Fig. 7.15 Celery contains conjugates of the flavones apigenin and luteolin. Following fungal infection, furocoumarins, including psoralen, xanthotoxin and bergapten, accumulate.

(iii) Asparagus

Asparagus (*Asparagus officinalis*) is native to the Mediterranean. It was cultivated by the Romans as both food and medicine and has been cultivated in Northern Europe since the beginning of the first millennium. Asparagus contains β-carotene, the level varying with the colour of the spear.

(iv) Avocados

Avocados (*Persea americana*) are found in archeological deposits in Mexico, which date to 7000 BC. There are three cultivated varieties with differing oil content in the pulp. The West Indian variety, which can weigh up to 1 kg, has only 8–10% oil, whereas the Mexican variety, which is smaller, contains about 30% oil. It thus has the highest energy content of any fruit pulp (with the possible exception of olives). Avocado is becoming increasingly popular, being used in salads, sandwich fillings, dips and spreads. The flesh contains vitamins B, C and E, carotenes and chlorophyll.

(v) Cucumber

Cucumber (*Cucumis sativus*) is considered one of the first vegetables to be cultivated, being men-

tioned in the Bible (Numbers 11:5). It is a member of the squash family (Cucurbitaceae).

7.4.5 Tomato and related plants (tomatoes, peppers, aubergines)

The tomato *Lycopersicon esculentum* (Family Solanaceae), was introduced into Europe in the 16th century from South America but took nearly three centuries to become widely accepted as a foodstuff. The original tomato was yellow, which is reflected in the Italian – pomodoro – pomo d'oro, golden fruit.

(i) Tomatoes

Many different types of tomatoes are now available, ranging from the very small, cherry, through plum tomatoes to the giant beefsteak type that can weigh several pounds each. Colours range from yellow through green to purple. Together with onions, tomatoes are the most widely consumed non-staple food.

In the UK, tomatoes are eaten as an important component of salads, soups and sauces, while tomatoes play a central role is what is seen to be the traditional diet of Mediterranean countries. In the USA the consumption of tomato and tomato products is second only to that of potatoes.

Green tomatoes contain the steroidal alkaloid tomatine, which disappears as the fruit ripens. All tomatoes contain the carotenoids lycopene, β-carotene and lutein (Fig. 7.16), which are produced in the flesh as the fruit ripens (see Section 6.5). Lycopene is quantitatively the most important carotenoid and extensive research has identified the cultural conditions to optimise levels. The content is affected by nitrogen, calcium and potassium in fertilisers, by light, temperature and irrigation, being reduced by excessive light and by temperatures over 32°C. Lycopene levels as high as 600 mg/kg have been reported in the literature (van den Berg *et al.*, 2000), but other references consider 200 mg/kg to be exceptionally high (Grolier *et al.*, 2001). Tomatoes also contain flavonols, mainly as quercetin-3-rutinoside (rutin), which accumulates in the skin, and, because of their high skin:volume ratio, cherry tomatoes are

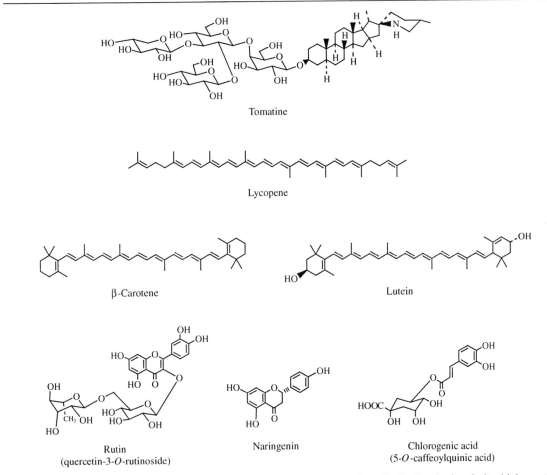

Fig. 7.16 Green tomatoes contain the steroidal alkaloid tomatine. Levels decline in ripe fruit which contain the carotenoids β-carotene and lutein and also lycopene, which is responsible for the red colour. Rutin, naringenin and chlorogenic acid are also present.

an especially rich source (Stewart *et al.*, 2000). In addition, the flavanone naringenin and chlorogenic acid (Fig. 7.16) have also been detected in tomato (Paganga *et al.*, 1999).

(ii) Peppers and aubergines

Peppers (*Capsicum annuum*) and aubergines (*Solanum melongena*) are also fruits of members of the Solanaceae family. Peppers are native to Mexico and were introduced to Europe from the West Indies by Columbus. There are two main types: bell peppers, which tend to be large and

sweet and are available in a range of colours from green through yellow to orange, red and purple, and chilli peppers, of which there are many varieties, which are smaller and much hotter. Capsaicin (Fig. 7.17) has been identified as the chemical that gives the heat to chilli peppers. Bell peppers are often eaten raw in salads and are used in many Mediterranean dishes. They contain a number of carotenoids, the main components being lutein and β-carotene. However, the overall level of carotenoids in bell peppers is typically only one tenth of the total carotenoid content of tomatoes. Special varieties have been bred with vastly

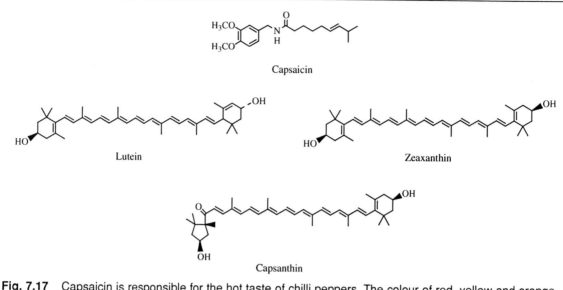

Fig. 7.17 Capsaicin is responsible for the hot taste of chilli peppers. The colour of red, yellow and orange bell peppers is due to the accumulation of lutein, zeaxanthin and capsanthin, respectively.

increased levels of different carotenoids, which result in different colours. Yellow bell peppers accumulate lutein, zeaxanthin is the major component in orange peppers and capsanthin (Fig. 7.17) predominates in red varieties (see Fig. 2.21).

Aubergines (*Solanum melongena*) are native to South East Asia and have been used as a vegetable in China for over 2000 years but only comparatively recently in Europe. They are low in energy but can absorb a great deal of fat during cooking. They contain anthocyanins in the form of delphinidin conjugates in the skin and other phenolics including chlorogenic acid in the flesh.

7.4.6 Other vegetables

(i) Squashes

Marrow, pumpkin, squash and courgette (zucchini) are all *Cucurbita* species and members of the Cucurbitaceae, as are melons (*Cucumis melo*). Squashes were very important to early inhabitants of Southern and Central America, as important as corn and beans. Fossilised remains of squashes in Peru have been dated to 4000 BC. Originally the

flowers, seeds and flesh were eaten. The seeds provided a source of sulphur-containing amino acids. Wild members of the family are thin-skinned and bitter. There are few data available on the bioactive compounds in the flesh of squashes. Butternut squash has been found to contain 350 mg/kg of total phenolics (Lister & Podivinsky, 1998).

(ii) Sprouted seeds

A wide range of sprouted seeds are eaten both raw and stir-fried. The seeds include grains and lentils (*Lens culinaris*), aduki (*Phaseolus angularis*) and mung beans (*Phaseolus aureus*), fenugreek (*Trigonella foenum-graecum*), alfalfa (*Medicago sativa*), mustard (*Brassica juncea*) and cress (*Lepidium sativum*). During the process of germination the seed produces a range of enzymes and vitamins.

(iii) Mushrooms and fungi

Mushrooms are the fruit bodies of fungi. There are very many species; unfortunately, some are poisonous. Since medieval times the mushroom

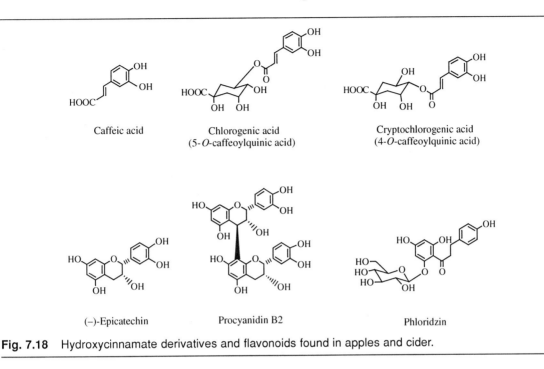

Fig. 7.18 Hydroxycinnamate derivatives and flavonoids found in apples and cider.

has been regarded with suspicion in the UK whereas in continental Europe it has always been a useful part of the diet, and the truffle, the fruit body of *Tuber aestivum*, is considered a gastronomic delicacy. While many species are still collected from the wild, commercial production can be traced back to the 18th century. *Fusarium graminearum* is now being grown commercially in fermenters for processing into Quorn®, a high-protein food.

(iv) Sea vegetables (algae, e.g. laver bread)

Seaweed has been consumed in the UK for centuries. In Wales, Devon and Scotland the fronds of *Porphyra umbilicalis* are washed, stewed and eaten as laver bread. Other varieties of seaweed are eaten as green or purple laver. Other seaweeds are used worldwide in the production of alginates (E400–405), agar (E406), carageenan (E407) and processed eucheuma seaweed (E407a). Seaweed consumption is more significant in Asia where it is used in sushi. These sea-weeds have been shown to contain a number of flavonoids (Yoshie & Suzuki, 2000).

7.5 Fruits

As in the sections on vegetables, in the following sections each fruit will be discussed briefly. Particular compounds will be highlighted but this should not be taken as an indication that these are the only compounds associated with the foodstuff.

7.5.1 Tree fruits

(i) Apples and pears

Small, bitter, crab apples are very widely distributed throughout the world and have been eaten since prehistoric times. However, the first apples resembling modern apples (*Malus* × *domestica*) probably grew on the slopes of the Tien Shan between China and Kazakhstan. The Romans first cultivated the fruit, grew at least a dozen

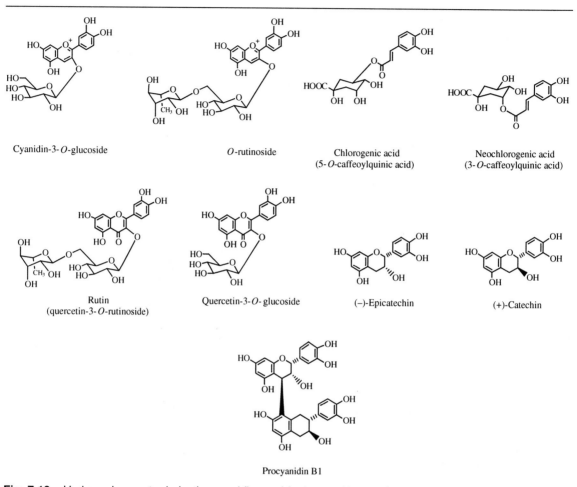

Cyanidin-3-*O*-glucoside | *O*-rutinoside | Chlorogenic acid (5-*O*-caffeoylquinic acid) | Neochlorogenic acid (3-*O*-caffeoylquinic acid)

Rutin (quercetin-3-*O*-rutinoside) | Quercetin-3-*O*-glucoside | (−)-Epicatechin | (+)-Catechin

Procyanidin B1

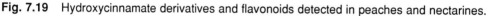

Fig. 7.19   Hydroxycinnamate derivatives and flavonoids detected in peaches and nectarines.

varieties and are believed to have introduced it to Northern Europe including Britain. The Pilgrim fathers took pips to America. Cox's Orange Pippin was first grown in England in 1826 and later that century Granny Smith was grown in Australia. More than 7000 named varieties are now known worldwide.

Apples are a good source of flavonoids (Podsedek *et al.*, 1998). Between 2310 and 4880 mg/kg have been determined in macerated apple including chlorogenic acid, caffeic acid, phloridzin, (−)-epicatechin (Fig. 7.18) and its oligomers. The oligomers have been shown to have an average degree of polymerisation of

between 3.1 and 8.5 (Sanoner *et al.*, 1998). These compounds have a major influence on taste: too much, as in the wild apple, and the fruit is inedible; too little, and it is insipid (Haslam, 1998). The main contributors to the antioxidant capacity of apples are chlorogenic acid, caffeic acid and (−)-epicatechin (Bandoniene & Murkovic, 2000). The flavan-3-ols are important components in the flavour and body of cider, which contains phloridzen, procyanidin B2, chlorogenic acid and its isomer 4-*O*-caffeoylquinic acid (crytochlorogenic acid) (Fig. 7.18).

Pears (*Prunus communis*) were cultivated by the Phoenicians and later by the Romans. There are now in excess of 500 named varieties world-wide. Apples and pears are among the main sources of proanthocyanins in the diet (Santos-Buelga & Scalbert, 2000).

(ii) Apricots and peaches

The apricot (*Prunus armeniaca*) was introduced into Europe from China by silk merchants and arrived in England during the reign of Henry VIII.

Peaches (*Prunus persica*) originate from mountainous regions of Tibet and western China. The fruit was cultivated by the Chinese as early as 2000 BC and reached Greece around 300 BC. It was grown by the Romans in the first century. Peaches were taken along the silk route to Persia and from there were introduced to Greece and Rome. They were introduced to Mexico by the Spaniards in the 1500s. Peaches are now cultivated commercially in many countries, with the fruit being consumed fresh, canned, frozen, dried and processed into jelly, jam and juices. There is increasing usage of nectarines (*P. persica* var. *nectarina*), a smooth-skinned variety of peach. Peaches and nectarines contain cyanidin-3-glucoside, cyanidin-3-rutinoside, quercetin-3-glucoside, rutin, chlorogenic acid, 3-*O*-caffeoylquinic acid (neochlorogenic acid), (+)-catechin, (–)-epicatechin and procyanidin B1 (Fig. 7.19).

Apricots and peaches both contain carotenoids principally in the form of β-carotene. Enzymic browning during processing lowers the carotenoid content.

(iii) Cherries

Sweet cherries were known to the Egyptians and Chinese. Sour cherries were cultivated by the Greeks. Modern varieties are either pure-bred sweet (*Prunus avium*) or sour (*Prunus cerasus*) or hybrids of the two. Both contain anthocyanins, mainly cyanidin-3-(2^G-*O*-glucosylrutinoside), with lower levels of other anthocyanins, including cyanidin-3-*O*-sophoroside (Fig. 7.20), the amounts being reflected in the colour (Wang *et al.*, 1997). Like peaches, they also contain non-anthocyanin phenolic compounds, including (–)-epicatechin and chlorogenic acid (Friedrich & Lee, 1998).

(iv) Plums

Plums were first cultivated by the Assyrians and were extensively hybridised by the Romans. They were introduced to Northern Europe by the crusaders. Prunes are plums that have been dried without being allowed to ferment. Numerous varieties of plums, mainly *Prunus domestica*, are cultivated world wide and they are a rich source of anthocyanins in the form of cyanidin-3-glucoside and cyanidin-3-rutinoside, which are also found in peaches (Fig. 7.19). They also contain significant quantities of chlorogenic acid, neochlorogenic acid and procyanidin dimers and trimers (Tomás-Barberán *et al.*, 2001). Dried plums lack anthocyanins but chlorogenic acid and neochlorogenic acid are present together with the non-phenolic compounds 5-(hydroxymethyl)-2-furaldehyde and sorbic acid (Fig. 7.21).

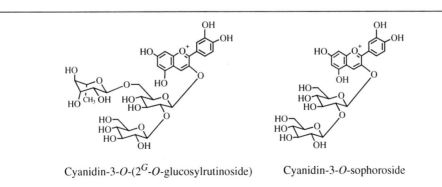

Cyanidin-3-*O*-(2^G-*O*-glucosylrutinoside)   Cyanidin-3-*O*-sophoroside

Fig. 7.20 The main anthocyanins in cherries.

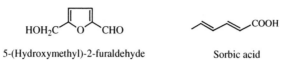

5-(Hydroxymethyl)-2-furaldehyde   Sorbic acid

Fig. 7.21   In addition to a range of phenolic compounds, plums contain sizable amounts of 5-(hydroxymethyl)-2-furaldehyde and sorbic acid.

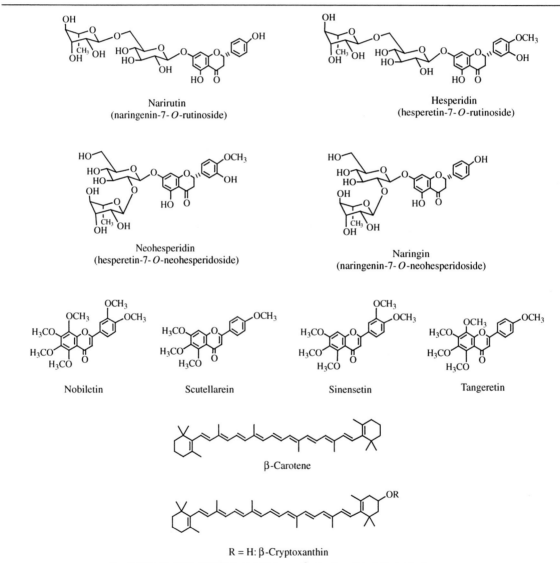

Narirutin
(naringenin-7-*O*-rutinoside)

Hesperidin
(hesperetin-7-*O*-rutinoside)

Neohesperidin
(hesperetin-7-*O*-neohesperidoside)

Naringin
(naringenin-7-*O*-neohesperidoside)

Nobiletin   Scutellarein   Sinensetin   Tangeretin

β-Carotene

R = H: β-Cryptoxanthin
R = laurate, myrisate, palmitate, stearate: β-cryptoxanthin fatty acid esters

Fig. 7.22   Flavanone conjugates, polymethoxylated flavones, β-carotene, β-cryptoxanthin and its fatty acid esters are found in citrus fruit.

(v) Citrus fruits

With the exception of the grapefruit (*Citrus paradisi*), citrus fruits originate from Asia. Orange (*Citrus sinensis*) and tangerine (*Citrus reticulata*) originated in China and were brought to Rome by Arab traders. The Romans and Greeks only knew of the bitter orange (*Citrus aurantium*). Sweet oranges were brought to Europe from India in the 17th century. Lemons (*Citrus limon*) originated in Malaysia or India. They were introduced into Assyria where they were discovered by the soldiers of Alexander the Great who took them back to Greece. The crusaders introduced them into Europe. Limes (*Citrus aurantifolia*) originated in India and were introduced as a crop into the West Indies. The original grapefruit was discovered in Polynesia and introduced to the West Indies where it was developed and brought to Europe in the 17th century.

Citrus fruits are significant sources of flavonoids, principally flavanones, which are present in both the juice and the tissues that are ingested when fruit segments are consumed. The tissues are a particularly rich source but are only consumed as an accidental adjunct to the consumption of the pulp. It is difficult to estimate dietary intake in such cases because it is so heavily dependent on the amount of tissue surrounding the segments after peeling. Citrus peel and to a lesser extent the segments contain the conjugated flavonone naringenin-7-rutinoside (narirutin) and also hesperetin-7-rutinoside (hesperidin) (Fig. 7.22), which is included in dietary supplements and is reputed to prevent capillary bleeding. Naringenin-7-neohesperidoside (naringin) from grapefruit peel and hesperetin-7-neohesperidoside (neohesperidin) from bitter orange are intensely bitter flavanone glycosides. Orange juice contains polymethoxylated flavones such as nobiletin, scullaretin, sinensetin and tangeretin, which are found exclusively in citrus species and the relative levels of these compounds can be used to detect the illegal adulteration of orange juice with juice of tangelo fruit (*Citrus reticulata*). A further distinguishing feature is that β-cryptoxanthin and its fatty acid esters are present in higher amounts relative to β-carotene (Fig. 7.22) in tangelo juice than orange juice (Pan *et al.*, 2002).

Citrus fruits also contain significant amounts of terpenoids. The major constituent of lemon and orange oils is the monoterpene (+)-limonene (Fig. 7.23). Citrus fruits also contain the more complex limonoids, which are modified triterpenoids. The bitterness due to limonoids is an important economic problem in commercial citrus juice production. Among the more than 30 limonoids that have been isolated from citrus species, limonin (Fig. 7.23) is the major cause of limonoid bitterness in citrus juices. Nomilin (Fig. 7.23) is also a bitter limonoid that is present in grapefruit juice and other citrus juices, but its concentration is generally very low so its contribution to limonoid bitterness is minor. As the fruit ripens, the concentration of limonoid aglycones, such as limonoate A-ring lactone (Fig. 7.23), declines and bitterness decreases. This natural debittering process was known for over a century, but the mechanism was not understood until the discovery of limonoid glucosides in citrus fruit in 1989, when it was shown that limonoid aglycones are converted to their respective glucosides in fruit tissues and seeds during the later stages of fruit growth and ripening. In contrast to their aglycones, limonoid glucosides, such as limonin-17-glucoside (Fig. 7.23), are practically tasteless (Hasegawa *et al.*, 2000). *In planta* limonoids appear to act as insect antifeedants; however, they also have a variety of medicinal effects in animals and humans including some anticarcinogenic effects on *in vitro* human cancer cell lines and animal tests. Other limonoid properties include antifungal, bactericidal and antiviral effects.

(vi) Pineapple

Pineapple (*Ananas comosus*) is a member of the family Bromeliacea, cultivated in southern America and was first brought to Europe by Columbus. It is now grown in a number of tropical and subtropical countries and is consumed fresh, canned and processed to give juice. The fruit is notable for the presence of a proteolytic enzyme, bromelain, which is used to prevent a proteinaceous haze in chill-proof beer when refrigerated.

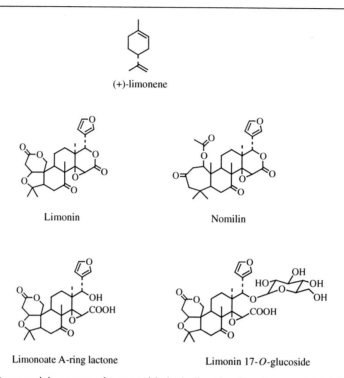

(+)-limonene

Limonin

Nomilin

Limonoate A-ring lactone

Limonin 17-*O*-glucoside

Fig. 7.23 Citrus fruit are a rich source of terpenoids including the C_{10} diterpenoid (+)-limonene and a number of more complex limonoids which are distinctive in that the glucosides are tasteless whereas the aglycones have a bitter taste.

(vii) Dates

Dates (*Phoenix dactylifera*) are probably the oldest cultivated fruit, having been cultivated for over 5000 years. It is a major crop in the Middle East and there are over 2000 cultivars. As with other palms, the sap is tapped for fermentation into 'toddy' which is also distilled. A well-managed tree will produce 400–600 kg of dates per year from the age of 5 years for up to 60 years.

(viii) Mango

Mango (*Mangifera indica*) has been eaten for over 6000 years in India and Malaysia and was introduced to South America and the West Indies in the 18th century. Mango is a good source of β-carotene and vitamin C, and is a major contributor of these nutrients especially in developing countries. The leathery skin of the fruit contains a latex to which some people are sensitive. Extracts of mango stem bark, which contains the xanthone mangiferin (Fig. 7.24) and gallic acid and benzoic acid derivatives as well as (+)-catechin and (–)-epicatechin, are used in Cuba as traditional nutritional supplements to treat a number of conditions including diarrhoea, diabetes and skin infections (Núñez-Sellés *et al.*, 2002).

(ix) Papaya

Papaya (*Carica papaya*) is native to Central America but is now grown widely in the tropics. It fruits all year round. Compared with other fruits it is high in carotenes. The unripe fruit is a source of the enzyme papain, which is used as a meat tenderiser and a beer clarifier.

(x) Fig

The fig is among the oldest known fruit crops, its seeds having been found in early Neolithic sites dating to 7000 BC. It was probably cultivated from about 2700 BC in Egypt and Mesopotamia. The

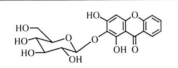

Mangiferin

Fig. 7.24 The xanthone mangiferin is found in mango bark.

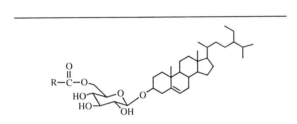

6-*O*-Palmitoyl-β-glucosyl-β-sitosterol (R = palmitate)
6-*O*-Linoleyl-β-glucosyl-β-sitosterol (R = linoleate)

Fig. 7.25 Sitosterol derivatives with potential anti-tumour activity are found in latex released when figs are picked.

genus *Ficus* contains over 1000 species, the most important of which as a commercial fruit crop is *Ficus carica*, which is widely used as a food and as a medicine in the Middle East. The latex released on picking fruits has anti-tumour activity and there is evidence that the bioactive components are 6-*O*-palmitoyl- and 6-*O*-linoleyl-β-glucosylsito-sterol (Fig. 7.25) (Rubnov *et al.*, 2001).

(xi) Olive

The olive tree (*Olea europa*) has been cultivated for thousands of years. The oil is the most important constituent (see Chapter 10), but olives also contain phenolics, including vanillic acid, ferulic acid, the flavones luteolin and apigenin together with substantial amounts of oleuropein glucoside (Fig. 7.26), which is bitter and is commonly neutralised by treatment with caustic soda before the olives can be eaten. Olives contain up to 40% oil of which, typically, three-quarters is a mono-unsaturated fatty acid, oleic acid (C18:1), 14% saturated fatty acids (mainly palmitic acid, C16:0) and 9% polyunsaturated fatty acids. Olive oil is also rich in oleic acid and the main phenol is oleuropein, which is produced by enzymatic degradation. The aglycone contains a hydroxytyrosol group, which is the antioxidant moiety. The oil also contains hydroxytyrosol itself, derived from oleuropein but in smaller amounts than the aglycone (Fig. 7.26). Hydroxytyrosol and

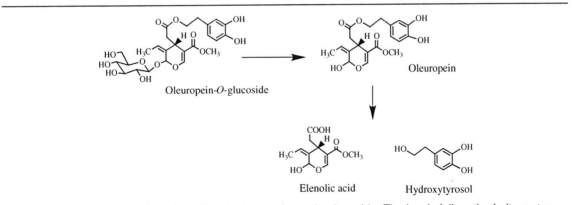

Oleuropein-*O*-glucoside

Oleuropein

Elenolic acid

Hydroxytyrosol

Fig. 7.26 The bitter taste in unripe olives is due to oleurpein glucoside. The levels fall as the fruits mature and the aglycone oleuropein accumulates. Olive oil contains the aglycone and hydroxytyrosol, both of which are strong antioxidants.

oleuuropein are unique phenolic compounds found only in olives and olive oil.

7.5.2 Soft fruits (*e.g.* berries and currants)

This section includes those fruits which in strict botanical terms are berries but which are commonly known as currants, and agglomerates, which perversely are widely referred to as berries. A wide range of berries are consumed. Most are cultivated but some are picked from the wild. The range includes strawberry (*Fragaria × ananassa*), raspberry (*Rubus idaeus*), blackberry (*Rubus* spp.), blueberry (*Vaccinium corymbosum*), elderberry (*Sambucus nigra*), cranberry (*Vaccinium oxycoccus*), gooseberry (*Ribes grossularia*) and black (*Ribes nigrum*), red (*Ribes rubrum*) and white currants. Soft fruits make up only a tiny part of the diet in the UK but are more important in some Nordic countries. They tend to be susceptible to decay and have to be processed to extend the shelf life. Until the introduction of canning in the mid-19th century, preservation was almost impossible but now a range of methods are available, including processing into jam.

The modern strawberry is the descendant of the tiny woodland strawberry that was grown by the Romans. Modern cultivated strawberries derive from a cross between an American and a Chilean variety that occurred around 1750. Raspberries are native to Europe and have been cultivated since the Middle Ages. Cloudberries (*Rubus chamaemorus*) are grown either side of the Arctic Circle and are relatives of the raspberry. Blackberries have been eaten since Neolithic times and the Greeks prized them for the medicinal value of the leaves.

A number of crosses have been made between raspberries and blackberries, including the loganberry (*Rubus loganbaccus*) and the Tayberry. The blueberry is native to North America and is cultivated both there and in Europe. Cranberries grow wild in both northern Europe and northern USA. Native Americans prized them for both their nutritional and medicinal properties and are said to have introduced the first Europeans to cranberries to help them prevent scurvy. Cranberry juice is currently popularly used for preventing

urinary tract infections (Schenker, 2001). The cranberry is *Vaccinium oxycoccus* while *Vaccinium macrocarpon* is the large or American cranberry which is grown commercially in both America and Europe. Gooseberries were popular in Medieval England but were not cultivated until the 16th century. They are little consumed outside the UK.

The currants grow wild throughout northern Europe but were not cultivated until the 16th century. Anthocyanin-deficient whitecurrants are rarely grown now and redcurrants are generally only grown for jelly. The main end products of blackcurrant cultivation are juice drinks and jam. Consumption is therefore relatively low.

The berries contain anthocyanins and a small amount of other flavonoids (Hallikainen *et al.*, 1999). The coloured berries are generally very good sources of anthocyanins and processing techniques are being developed to release more of these from the skin during juice processing. The major berry anthocyanins are illustrated in Fig. 7.27. Raspberry, strawberry and blackberry contain ellagitannins (Clifford & Scalbert, 2000) and raspberries in particular are an especially rich source, the major components being sanguiin H-6, which has a molecular weight of 1870, and to a lesser extent lambertianin C, with a molecular weight of 2806 (Fig. 7.28). Anthocyanins and vitamin C also contribute to the antioxidant capacity of the berries, but vasodilation properties are limited to the two ellagitannins (Mullen *et al.*, 2002).

Berries are reputed to be a rich source of ellagic acid (Fig. 7.28) and are advertised in the USA on this basis. In practice, however, raspberries contain very little ellagic acid and it only appears in high concentrations after extracts of the berries have been subjected to acid treatment, which results in the hydrolysis of sanguiin H-6 and lambertianin C and the release of substantial amounts of ellagic acid (Mullen *et al.*, 2002).

7.5.3 Other fruits

(i) Melons

Melons (*Cucumis melo*) are relatives of cucumbers. The first melons were bitter but they were bred to produce sweeter fruit and introduced into

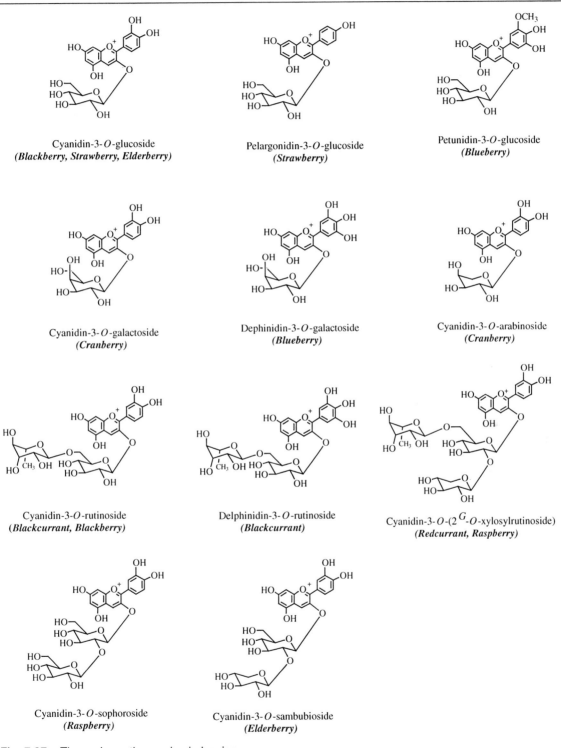

Fig. 7.27 The major anthocyanins in berries.

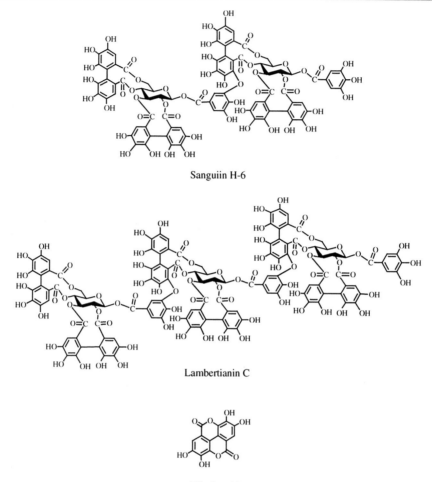

Sanguiin H-6

Lambertianin C

Ellagic acid

Fig. 7.28 Raspberries contain high concentrations of two ellagitannins, sanguiin H-6 and lambertianin C. When extracts are treated with acid the elligitannins are hydrolysed, releasing substantial quantities of ellagic acid.

Europe from Africa by the Moors. They reached France in the 15th century and were taken to the New World by Columbus. Melons and cantaloupes contain high levels of carotenes. Watermelons (*Citrullus lanatus*) are distant relatives of melons, widely spread throughout Africa. They were known to the Egyptians and wild watermelons grow in the Kalahari desert. Watermelons were introduced to Europe in the 15th century. Watermelons can contain high levels of caro-

tenes, particularly lycopene; levels of 23.0–72.0 mg/kg have been reported (van den Berg *et al.*, 2000).

(ii) Grapes

Grapes were among the earliest cultivated crops. The Egyptians, Greeks and Romans all made wine and the Romans bred many new varieties. Concord grapes (*Vitis labrusca*) are characterised

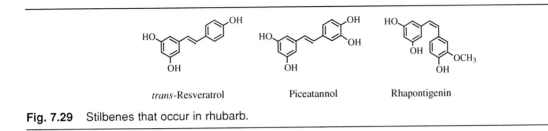

trans-Resveratrol   Piceatannol   Rhapontigenin

Fig. 7.29   Stilbenes that occur in rhubarb.

by a red-coloured flesh and skin. They are grown in America and are a different species from the European grape *Vitis vinifera*. Fresh red *V. vinifera* grapes contain in the region of 4 mg/kg of phenolic material, mainly in the skin and seeds, including gallic acid, caftaric acid, anthocyanins, monomeric flavan-3-ols and oligomeric proanthocyanidins. Some of this phenolic material is carried into the grape juice, which is either sold as such or fermented. However, red wine fermented over skins and seeds tends to have a higher phenolic content as additional phenolics are extracted in the presence of alcohol. A further factor may well be that grapes used to make red wine are generally of better quality than those used to produce juice. White grapes also contain phenolic material in the seeds but care is taken to ensure this is not extracted in the preparation of white wine (Haslam, 1998) (see Section 9.6). Table grapes are picked earlier and do not ripen to the same extent as grapes used to make wines. They are therefore likely to contain much lower levels of polyphenols. Nowadays, red grapes for table use are usually seedless varieties and so will contain much lower levels of flavan-3-ols and their oligomers than grapes used to make red wine.

Raisins are grapes that have been dried in the full sun, whereas sultanas are dried in partial shade and treated with sulphur compounds to prevent darkening. Both raisins and sultanas are generally made from the Thompson seedless grape. Currants are dried, small, black, seedless grapes originally grown in the region of Corinth, from which they derive their name; they were originally known in the UK as raisins of Corinth.

(iii) Rhubarb

Botanically, rhubarb (*Rheum raphonticum*) is a vegetable not a fruit. It was originally cultivated some 2000 years ago in northern Asia as a medicinal and ornamental plant. It is rich in salicylates and contains up to 2000 mg/kg of anthocyanins. The leaf contains oxalic acid, a poison. Several stilbenes have been isolated from rhubarb, including *trans*-resveratrol (see Section 2.3.3), and piceatannol and rhapontigenin (Fig. 7.29).

(iv) Kiwi fruit

Kiwi fruit (*Actinidia deliciosa*) was first grown in China, imported to the UK in the 19th century and seeds from Kew were sent to New Zealand in 1906. Kiwi fruit contain vitamin C and, like avocados are rich in chlorophyll, which is unusual for fruits. Lymphocytes collected from human volunteers after the consumption of a kiwi fruit juice supplement are less susceptible to oxidative DNA damage, as determined by the Comet assay, and this potentially protective effect is not entirely attributable to vitamin C (Collin *et al.*, 2001).

(v) Bananas, plantains

The original banana grew in South East Asia but contained many bitter, black seeds so that the fruit would have been almost inedible. Bananas are recorded in the reports of Alexander the Great in India where they were introduced by 600 BC. Cultivation of bananas (*Musa cavendishii*) commenced in the West Indies in the 17th century. There are both sweet and cooking bananas, the latter sometimes called plantains. Cooking bananas contain more starch and less

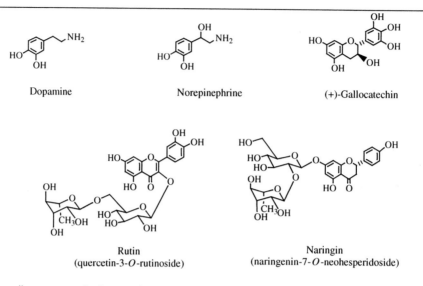

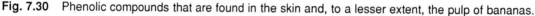

Fig. 7.30   Phenolic compounds that are found in the skin and, to a lesser extent, the pulp of bananas.

sugar than the dessert varieties and are a staple food in East Africa. Bananas are reported to contain lutein, α-carotene and β-carotene (van den Berg *et al.*, 2000) and high concentrations of the catecholamine dopamine, which is a strong antioxidant, together with norepinephrine, gallocatechin, naringin and rutin (Fig. 7.30). Typically, much higher levels of these components are found in the peel than the pulp (Kanazawa & Sakakibara, 2000).

7.6 Research recommendations

- There is a need to establish a system to quantify compounds in plant foods which can be used to formulate quantitative guidelines for specific fruits and vegetables. The available evidence indicates that large differences exist and that certain foods may be especially rich in bioactive compounds.
- There is a need to determine which bioactive compounds in commonly consumed foods contribute to the health effects.
- Once the compounds responsible for the bioactive activity have been identified, there is a need to determine their fate after being eaten:
  (i) Are they metabolised to any extent in the gastrointestinal tract?
  (ii) Do the dietary components and their metabolites provide any benefit during passage through the gastrointestinal tract?

(iii) To what extent are they absorbed, in what form and where: small intestine or large intestine?
(iv) What is the fate of compounds that are absorbed? How long do they survive in the bloodstream? Do they reach and are they deposited in body tissues? Are they deactivated and removed from the blood stream, *e.g.* by excretion in urine? Does consumption of any particular product have a demonstrable benefit in the long term, and what is the mechanism of action?

A key component to the success of such studies is the development of more reliable and specific biomarkers of protective effects, which should be reviewed as more data are collected.

7.7 Key points

- In the growing plant, bioactive compounds have roles in metabolism and in the interaction of the plant with the environment. The occurrence of the compounds of potential nutritional interest varies throughout the plant kingdom from the widespread carotenoids to the glucosinolates (found only in the Cruciferae).
- Polyphenols and carotenoids provide colour to stems, leaves, flowers and fruits. The carotenoids provide yellows with some orange and red while the polyphenolics, most notably the anthocyanins, are more numerous and provide a greater range of colours from orange to blue.
- Some bioactive compounds affect insect predation, some act as feeding deterrents to certain species of insect but to others insect larvae are attracted.
- Some bioactive compounds have antifungal and antibacterial activities and their presence in the plant may contribute to resistance to pathogen attack.
- The role of bioactive compounds in protecting crops poses a dilemma. It is the very compounds that make a crop less palatable that have ensured their survival in different environments. However, levels of some of these compounds tend to be lower in modern plant varieties because they have been deliberately bred out (*e.g.* the bitter-tasting glucosinolates in Brussels sprouts). More attention needs to be given to the changes in plant composition that have occurred given the potential health benefits of these constituents.

- It is important to be aware of the sheer numbers of compounds. Attention tends to be focused on a few representatives of each class, but 25 000 members of the terpene family have been identified, around 8000 phenolics and there are even 250 different sterols.
- The bioactive compound content of individual fruits and vegetables is affected by variety, soil, climatic conditions, agricultural methods, physiological stress under which they are grown, degree of ripeness, storage conditions and period of storage before consumption. Not all references have recognised the resultant variability, and results from a single unnamed variety have often been taken as representative of the species.
- The levels of bioactive compounds also vary within the plant; within fruits many are concentrated in the skin, and within vegetables in the outer leaves. The content determined by analysis will therefore depend on the amount discarded and exactly which part of the plant is analysed.
- Bioactive compounds, including those contributing to colour, are known to be present in fruits and vegetables. Together with the vitamins and minerals, they may be the basis for the beneficial effects of these foods. The fact that particular bioactive compounds are highlighted should not be taken as an indication that these are the only ones associated with the foodstuff.
- The epidemiological evidence for the benefit of consuming diets that are high in fruit and vegetables is quite compelling but the evidence for specific vegetables, and indeed specific compounds, is less convincing.

8
Cereals, Nuts and Pulses

8.1 Introduction

Cereals, nuts and pulses have constituted a substantial proportion of the food eaten by humans for thousands of years. The 'cereal-and-bean' combination is a feature of many cuisines worldwide, in general with the cereal assuming the role of staple, the main source of energy, and the legumes used as accompaniments. For example, the British eat baked beans on toast, the Indians have dhal as an accompaniment to rice and the Asians consume soya products with rice.

Those foods derived from cereals are generally consumed as staple items (*e.g.* cereals, bread, rice, pasta) within the diet. The dietary guidelines in the UK (see Chapters 1 and 13) place a lot of importance on these 'starchy carbohydrates' as a food group. Baked beans (haricot beans) are also classed as a vegetable, and nuts, pulses and legumes are important sources of protein as alternatives to meat and fish. The contribution of all these foods to the nutrient intake in the UK is discussed in Chapter 1.

8.2 Cereals

This category covers all grains eaten as food, *e.g.* barley (*Hordeum vulgare*), maize (corn) (*Zea mays*), millet (*Panicum miliaceum* or *Sorghum bicolor*), oats (*Avena sativa*), rice (*Oryza sativa*), rye (*Secale cereale*) and wheat (*Triticum* sp.). Many cereals, such as rye and barley, also form the basis of other plant-derived foods such as alcoholic beverages (see Chapter 9) and many seeds are used as spices to add flavour and colour to foods (see Chapter 11).

Approximately 50% of the food protein available is derived from cereals, and in developing countries they provide two thirds of energy and protein intake. Cereals are an important source of energy and provide 1400–1600 kJ per 100 g of whole cereal (Table 8.1). They also constitute a rich source of both non-starch polysaccharides (NSP) and starch, which together comprise 70–77% of the weight of the grain (Allman-Farinelli, 1999). The NSP and starch can escape digestion and absorption in the small intestine

Table 8.1 Nutrient content of cereal grains (per 100 g raw grains).

	Protein (g)	Fat (g)	Carbohydrate (g)	Thiamin (mg)	Niacin (mg)	Calcium (mg)	Iron (mg)
Wheat	12.6	2.7	72.4	0.5	6.1	35.0	3.7
Rice (brown)	7.5	1.9	77.4	0.34	4.7	32.0	1.6
Maize	9.0	3.9	72.2	0.37	2.2	22.0	2.1
Millet	10.0	2.9	72.9	0.73	2.3	20.0	6.8
Oats	15.0	7.0	69.0	0.6	1.0	53.0	4.5

Source: Lorenz & Kulp (1991).

and are fermented by micro-organisms in the large intestine to form short-chain fatty acids and gases (see Chapter 5). Much recent research has been focused on the proposed health benefits of the undigested starch and unabsorbable sugars, as they make a significant contribution to colonic fermentation, and therefore may improve the health of the large bowel (see Chapters 3 and 5). There is also the possibility that diets rich in NSP and starch may decrease the bioavailability of minerals such as iron, calcium and zinc, but there is currently little evidence that deficiencies result in practice.

Protein accounts for 6–15% of the weight of cereals; the limiting amino acid is lysine, although maize is also low in tryptophan (Allman-Farinelli, 1999). Gluten is the major protein in wheat and rye, and oryzenin the major protein in rice. Whole grains are a good source of thiamin, their germ is rich in vitamin E and they contain significant amounts of minerals, particularly potassium, phosphorus, magnesium, iron and zinc. The phytate content of cereals may also impart health benefits; however, phytate also binds to some minerals and inhibits their absorption. Unleavened bread, for example, contains high levels of phytate, which may outweigh any benefits of its micronutrient content.

Processing of cereal products not only increases digestibility but also alters the nutritional content. Typically, fibre, vitamins and minerals are concentrated in the outer bran and aleurone layers of the grains and the extent to which these layers are removed determines nutrient content. Starch and protein are concentrated in the endosperm of the grain and as a result are less affected by processing (Allman-Farinelli, 1999) (see Chapter 12).

8.3 Pulses

Pulses, the collective noun for the dried edible seeds of leguminous vegetables, have for centuries been at the heart of European peasant culture and are a practical way of storing vegetables for winter. Pulses include chick peas (*Cicer arietinum*), green and split peas (*e.g. Pisum sativa*), lentils (*Lena cultivare*), kidney, haricot, French and black beans (*Phaseolus vulgaris* cultivars), soya beans (*Glycine max*) and peanuts or groundnuts (*Arachis hypogea*). Legumes were often considered an inferior food, eaten by peasants, and never assumed the importance of a staple food like the cereals wheat, rice, maize and barley. However, they play an important role with staple foods in meeting nutritional requirements. Of all foods, legumes most adequately meet the recommended dietary guidelines for healthy eating. They are high in carbohydrate, and NSP, in general low in fat, supply adequate protein while being a good source of vitamins and minerals. Cooked legumes contain about 6–9% by weight of protein, significantly more than cereal foods, with the exception of soya beans and peanuts that contain 14 and 24%, respectively, when cooked. The limiting amino acids of the legumes are sulphur-containing methionine and cysteine, but since they are rich in lysine, legume proteins are well complemented by cereals (Allman-Farinelli, 1999). Legumes not only provide significant levels of carbohydrate and NSP but also contain oligosaccharides, which escape digestion in the gut and are fermented by bacteria in the colon (see Chapter 5). This is responsible for the abdominal discomfort experienced by some people and is perhaps the factor limiting consumption.

Although in general legumes are low in fat (approximately 2.5%), soya beans and peanuts contain 8 and 47%, respectively (mostly mono- and polyunsaturated fatty acids). Legumes supply vitamins and minerals including thiamin, niacin, iron, zinc, calcium and magnesium (Table 8.2). The substances present in uncooked legumes do inhibit their nutritional quality, but most of these compounds are either inactivated or destroyed by normal cooking or processing. For example, trypsin inhibitors may reduce the effectiveness of the digestive process; phytate binds metals such as iron, decreasing their absorption. However, because most uncooked, dried legumes are virtually indigestible and inedible, processing is essential and improves both the nutritional quality and digestibility (see Chapter 12). Although the leguminous family contains many nuts, most are not important in relation to human consumption,

Table 8.2 Nutrient content of nuts and pulses.

Nutrient	Range in nutrient content per 100 g of cooked beans
Protein (g)	5.4 (baked beans) – 25.6 (peanuts)
Fat (g)	0.4 (lentils) – 7.3 (soya beans)
Carbohydrate (g)	5.1 (soya beans) – 22.5 (aduki beans)
NSP (g)	1.9 (lentils) – 6.7 (kidney beans)
Thiamin (mg)	0.1 (chickpeas) – 0.79 (peanuts)
Riboflavin (mg)	0.05 (kidney beans) – 0.19 (pine nuts)
Niacin (mg)	0.2 (butter beans) – 13.8 (peanuts)
Calcium (mg)	16.0 (lentils) – 83.0 (soya beans)
Iron (mg)	1.4 (mung beans) – 3.0 (soya beans)
Zinc (mg)	0.7 (kidney beans) – 2.3 (aduki beans)

Source: McCance & Widdowson (1991).

except for peanuts. Today peanuts and soya beans account for most of the legume products eaten worldwide. Soya beans are made into a range of products including soya protein isolates, textured products, flour, 'milk' and tofu. Because of their low cost, many soya products are used in the manufacturing of food products, including bread, confectionery, processed meat products, ice creams and low-fat spreads. Peanuts are made into butters and used in confectionery, baked goods and sauces.

8.4 Nuts

Nuts have been valued for their oils as much as a food source since the earliest civilisations. Nuts come from several different plant families: peanuts (*Arachis hypogea*, a member of the Leguminosae family, see above) and tree nuts (one-seeded fruit in a hard shell). Tree nuts include almonds (*Prunus amygdalus dulcis*),

Brazil (*Bertholletia excelsa*), cashew (*Anacardium occidentale*), chestnut (*Castanea sativa*), hazel (*Corylus avellana*), macadamias (*Macadamia ternifolia*), pecan (*Carya illinoensis* or *C. pecan*) and walnut (*Juglans regia*). Nuts (and seeds) are processed for their oil (see Chapter 10), ground into pastes, used as ingredients in baked goods or eaten raw or roasted as snack foods. They contain a number of nutrients that have received attention in relation to potential health effects. They have a high energy content and are a good source of protein, vitamins, essential fatty acids and minerals, overall making them a highly nutritious food. The quantity and type of fat in nuts varies, for example chestnuts contain low levels of fat but other nuts contain 45–74% fat. The majority of nuts contain unsaturated fatty acids, either polyunsaturated (walnuts, high in linoleic and α-linolenic acids) or monounsaturated (macadamia, high in oleic acid). The protein content of nuts ranges between 2 and 25%, and they are good sources of NSP (5–11% by weight), B vitamins, vitamin E, folic acid, iron, zinc magnesium, potassium and calcium. Recent evidence also suggests they are one of the best dietary sources of selenium (Brazil nuts) (Allman-Farinelli, 1999; British Nutrition Foundation, 2001a).

Over the last decade, consumption of nuts has decreased, in part because of the health concerns relating to eating foods rich in fat. However, studies suggest that nut intake only accounts for approximately 2.5% of total fat intake in the USA while Mediterranean countries, whose healthy diets are frequently praised, consume almost double this level of nuts (Dreher *et al.*, 1996). The contribution of nuts to nutrient intake in the UK is discussed in Chapter 1, and fatty acids and vitamin E are discussed in Chapters 1 and 10. The epidemiological studies that have looked at the relationships between nuts and CHD are also discussed in Chapter 3.

8.5 Potentially bioactive substances in cereals, nuts and pulses

Currently, substantial interest is growing in the 'non-nutrient' content of cereals, nuts and pulses.

These food groups constitute one of the most important dietary sources of a range of bioactive compounds that are suggested to be beneficial for human health, including the dietary flavonoids phytoestrogens.

8.5.1 Selenium

In the 1960s, selenium was recognised as being an essential trace element in the diets of both animals and humans. It forms an essential part of a number of enzymes where it is present as the amino acid selenocysteine. The best known examples are the antioxidant glutathione peroxidase enzymes, which prevent free radical damage. Therefore, research interest has been focused on the potential chemopreventative and cardiovascular benefits of selenium-rich diets. However, since selenium also plays an important role in thyroid hormone metabolism and has been shown to be an important component in sperm motility and testosterone metabolism (British Nutrition Foundation, 2001a), the need for adequate dietary intake of selenium is more far reaching than initially considered (Rayman, 2000).

Selenium enters the food chain via plants, which in turn obtain it from the soil in which they grow. Wide international variations in intakes have been observed, in part, because of wide differences in selenium soil content and differences in selenium bioavailability from different foods. Selenium levels are highest in protein-rich foods, but the content is greatly influenced by the growing conditions. Selenium is predominantly obtained from cereals, fish, poultry, meat and bread, in the UK diet (MAFF, 1999). In 1997, 22% of total selenium intake was obtained from cereals and cereal products, and in particular Brazil nuts were identified as the richest source of selenium (levels up to 5300 µg/g) as previously reported (Thorn *et al.*, 1978). However, the selenium content of Brazil nuts varies considerably, depending on the soil conditions in which the tree grows.

Some grain and cereal products do make a significant contribution to the total dietary intake but wide variability in levels has been determined between different samples of a food. Among the cereal grains, rice contains the highest levels

(10–13 µg/100 g) while recent analyses of levels in bread (6–9 µg/100 g) suggest that levels have decreased over the last 20 years, and are significantly lower than levels in US bread samples (32–44 µg/100 g) (MAFF, 2000c). Wheat is a good source of selenium in North America, as the wheat is grown in soils rich in selenium. In Europe, although levels in wheat are lower, bread and cereals make a significant contribution to selenium intake, because they are consumed frequently (22% of total selenium intake in the UK) (Rayman, 2000). In 1997, the average intake for individuals from the household diet was 39 µg/day (see Chapter 1).

The differences in selenium intake between the USA and Europe are reflected in serum and whole blood selenium concentrations. Although a serum value of 100 µg/L is the suggested level required for optimal activity of cytosolic glutathione peroxidase (an indicator of selenium repletion), current levels in the EU appear to be below this level, with mean serum selenium levels in seven European countries calculated as 79 µg/L (Rayman, 1997).

8.5.2 Folate

Recent results from the National Food Survey suggest that cereals and vegetables together provide almost two thirds of the average intake of folic acid (250 µg/day as average intake) (MAFF, 2000b). For the contribution made by cereals and pulses (and their products) to the UK diet, see Table 1.3. Currently, many breads and breakfast cereals are voluntarily fortified with folic acid, and this in part may explain the importance of cereal sources to the folic acid intake for the UK population. The COMA panel (Department of Health, 2000a) endorsed the importance of women consuming extra folic acid preconception and in early pregnancy to reduce the risk of neural tube defects in babies (400 µg/day). However, more recently, the potential role of folic acid intake in cardiovascular disease risk and cancer risk and its effects on cognition have been investigated. Concentrations of homocysteine, a potential predictor of cardiovascular disease, can be lowered by folic acid. However, recent evidence suggests that to lower homocysteine maximally by food alone would be difficult because dietary folates are less bioavailable than the synthetic form, folic acid (Hughes & Buttriss, 2000). Because cereals and breads fortified with folic acid are more bioavailable (Cuskelly *et al.*, 1996) these dietary sources may be the most effective way of ensuring optimal folic acid intake. The relationships between folate and health, and fortification issues, are discussed in more detail in Chapters 1 and 13. Because it is yet to be established if the effects on homocysteine lead to a reduction in risk of cardiovascular disease, COMA suggests that such evidence would be required prior to advocating folic acid supplementation for those at risk of heart disease, but recommended the importance of a folate-rich diet as an integral part of a healthy diet. COMA concluded that fortification of wheat flour with 240 µg of folic acid per 100 g as consumed would have a significant effect in preventing the risk of neural tube defects without leading to unacceptably high intakes in any group of the population (see Chapter 13).

8.6 Phytoestrogens

Although the bioactive compounds in plant-derived foods and drinks discussed in this report are widely distributed within the plant kingdom, to date the richest sources of dietary phytoestrogens are cereals, nuts and pulses. Phytoestrogens encompass a wide range of structurally dissimilar compounds with common characteristics (Chapter 2), which are synthesised in plants from phenylpropanoids and simple phenols (Cassidy *et al.*, 2000). Isoflavones, lignans and stilbenes are intrinsic plant compounds, while the resorcyclic acid lactones are not directly present in plants but occur as products of moulds which flourish in the warm, moist conditions of poorly stored grains and other produce. In plants, phytoestrogens function as anti-fungal agents and levels have been shown to increase as a direct response to microbial or insect attack.

Quantitatively in relation to human health the isoflavones and lignans are considered to be the most important phytoestrogens. However, as the scientific evidence and interest in these compounds grows, novel phytoestrogens may be identified that may be biologically more important than those currently under scrutiny.

8.6.1 What are phytoestrogens?

The phytoestrogens are multifunctional compounds and only one of a series of their potential mechanisms relates to their ability to bind to oestrogen receptors (Setchell & Cassidy, 1999).

Given the similarity in chemical structure between phytoestrogens and the mammalian oestrogen oestradiol (see Fig. 8.1), it is not surprising that these compounds bind to oestrogen receptors (ER). At least two ERs exist, ERβ and the 'classical' ERα subtype. The isoflavone class of phytoestrogens has a stronger binding affinity for ERβ than ERα, suggesting that phytoestrogen-rich diets may exert more potent effects in ERβ-expressing tissues (which include brain, bone, bladder and vascular epithelium).

If dietary phytoestrogens can be shown to exert tissue-selective effects, these compounds would therefore have the potential to act as oestrogen agonists, which may prove beneficial in postmenopausal women with respect to risk factors for heart disease, menopausal symptoms and osteoporosis. Paradoxically, under some conditions dietary phytoestrogens may act as anti-

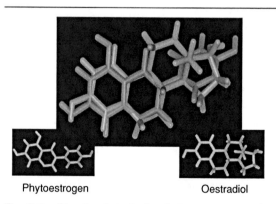

Phytoestrogen   Oestradiol

Fig. 8.1 Structural similarity phytoestrogens and oestrogens.

Table 8.3 Dietary sources of phytoestrogens.

Lignans	mg per typical portion	Isoflavones	mg per typical portion
Linseed	13.5	Soya bean	35–229
Oat bran	0.25	Tofu	10–88
Asparagus	0.46	TVP	28–47
Carrot	0.21	Soya 'milk'	3–18
Broccoli	0.20	Miso	5–16
Lentils	0.72	Soy sauce	Negligible
Pear	0.27	Other legumes	3–6

Adapted from Thompson *et al.* (1991) and Reinli & Block (1996).

oestrogens and this may assist in protecting against the development of breast cancer. However, we still understand little about age-dependent differences in exposure to these classes of compounds. Numerous other biological effects independent of the ER (*e.g.* antioxidant capacity, antiproliferative and antiangiogenic effects) have been ascribed to phytoestrogens and some of these are common to other plant phenolics (Setchell & Cassidy, 1999).

8.6.2 Isoflavones

Although present in several legumes (*e.g.* chick peas, kidney beans), the principal food source of isoflavones in the human diet is soya beans (Table 8.3). Most soya bean proteins and derived foods available for human consumption contain significant levels of isoflavones. However, there is a large variability in concentration and chemical composition among different soya beans or soya protein products as the levels present depend on genetic differences, geographical and environmental conditions and the extent of processing (Barnes *et al.*, 1994) (see also Chapter 12).

Isoflavones are present in plant foods either as the aglycone (genistein or daidzein) (*e.g.* in fermented soya products such as miso or tempeh) or as different types of glycoside conjugates including acetyl- and malonylglycosides, and daidzin and genistin, the β-glucosides of daidzein and genistein (Kudou *et al.*, 1991). The relative proportion of conjugates varies considerably between different soya foods because the malonyl-

and acetylglycosides are susceptible to heat and can be readily converted to the more stable β-glycoside (Barnes *et al.*, 1994). However, recent evidence suggests that the biologically active aglycones are very stable to high temperatures and although the conjugation profile may be influenced by heat, the total isoflavone concentration in the soya protein product remains constant (K. Setchell, personal communication). Isoflavone conjugates are also metabolised after ingestion, either by acid hydrolysis in the stomach or by intestinal bacteria (see Chapter 5). Therefore, irrespective of the relative proportions of the individual isoflavone conjugates in different soya products, the aglycones are ultimately released either by processing, preparation or by intestinal bacterial metabolism (Setchell *et al.*, 1984).

Table 8.3 illustrates the wide range of total isoflavone concentrations in soya protein and soya foods and other legumes. The highest levels are found in soya flours and concentrates. Whilst tofu and soya 'milks' contain significant amounts of isoflavones, the concentrations vary considerably between type and brand (Dwyer *et al.*, 1994; Setchell *et al.*, 2001). In contrast, soya oils contain only trace levels of isoflavones (Coward *et al.*, 1993) because the highly polar glycoside conjugates in soya beans are unable to partition into the lipophilic oil.

There are striking compositional differences between the types of soya protein commonly consumed in Japan and China compared with those incorporated into Western diets (Coward *et al.*,

1993). Many soya foods commonly consumed in the East are produced from fermented soya products (*e.g.* miso, tempeh) and the fermentation processes hydrolyse the glycoside conjugates, resulting in foods that are predominantly aglycone in their phytoestrogen profile (Coward *et al.*, 1993). This compositional difference may well be relevant in relation to the metabolism and bioavailability of these compounds *in vivo* and in relation to the effects of food processing (see Chapters 6 and 12).

8.6.3 Lignans

Lignans are widely distributed as minor constituents of some plants and are defined as compounds possessing a 2,3-dibenzylbutane structure (Cassidy *et al.*, 2000). Several plants contain high concentrations of lignans, *e.g.* linseed (flaxseed) is the richest identified source of the lignan precursor secoisolariciresinol. The levels of lignans in all plant foods have not been comprehensively measured, but levels in a variety of plant foods have been determined using an *in vitro* fermentation model to measure mammalian lignan production (Thompson *et al.*, 1991). This model suggested that lignans are present in most fibre-rich foods (Table 8.3) and therefore could be more readily incorporated as a phytoestrogen source into UK and European diets than isoflavones (Table 8.3). Although the levels of lignans are generally low on an individual food basis, their ubiquity in the plant kingdom suggests that they may well be an important source of phytoestrogens, particularly to high consumers of plant-based diets (*e.g.* vegans, vegetarians). However, to date there are few data on the exposure of these population groups to this important class of compounds. In addition, to date interest in the biological effects of lignans in relation to human health has received little attention compared with the isoflavone class.

8.6.4 Stilbenes

Stilbenes (Section 2.4.3) are widely distributed in plants (Cassidy *et al.*, 2000). *trans*-Resveratrol (Figs 2.14 and 7.29), which is synthesised in the plant in response to microbial infection or stress,

has been identified as the major active compound and is the one on which the physiological activity of stilbenes has focused.

Recent quantitative data suggest resveratrol levels in peanut samples range from 1.3 to 3.7 µg/g (Sanders *et al.*, 2000) while more recently the 3-β-glucoside of *trans*-resveratrol, termed piceid, has been identified in peanut butter (Ibern-Gomez *et al.*, 2000). The potential health benefits of these compounds for humans have not yet been significantly investigated.

8.7 Absorption and metabolism of phytoestrogens

Over 20 years ago, it was established that the intestinal microflora played a key role in the metabolism of phytoestrogens from the lignan and isoflavone class. Antibiotic administration blocks metabolism and germ-free animals do not excrete the metabolites (Setchell & Cassidy, 1999). Although we know that after ingestion the phytoestrogens are absorbed and metabolised or biotransformed by the intestinal microflora (see Chapter 5), we currently have a limited understanding of factors that affect their bioavailability (see Chapter 6) and pharmacokinetic profile (Cassidy & Faughnan, 2000; Setchell *et al.*, 2001). Current data show wide variability between subjects in their metabolic profile of phytoestrogens following a known dose of a phytoestrogen-rich food or pure phytoestrogen compound. Not only is there wide individual variability in response to a phytoestrogen-rich diet, but also the bioavailability of phytoestrogens varies depending on the dose given and the food matrix used (*e.g.* supplement, soya drink, soya food). These data have implications for clinical studies, as it cannot be assumed that all phytoestrogens are comparable with respect to pharmacokinetics and bioavailability. For more details on the absorption and metabolism of phytoestrogens, see Section 6.4.1.

8.8 Potential health effects of phytoestrogens

The international variation in many diseases, including cardiovascular disease, osteoporosis and breast and prostate cancer, and menopausal symptoms, has stimulated interest in the role of isoflavones in the diet as potentially bioactive components. In Asia, where urine and plasma levels of these compounds are high, these conditions are rare. However, to date, studies that have examined the potential of isoflavones to cause physiological effects in humans have been limited to epidemiological studies, or to dietary intervention trials that have examined effects on menopausal symptoms, cardiovascular function and endocrine regulation of the menstrual cycle. Overall, these dietary studies have shown positive effects that may be interpreted as beneficial, but it is difficult to tease out the precise contribution that isoflavones play in the overall endpoints measured. In particular, we have insufficient data to ascertain the optimal dose of isoflavone necessary to exert potential health effects.

8.8.1 Menopausal symptoms

Studies in pre-menopausal women suggest that relatively low doses of phytoestrogens (fed as soya, 45–138 mg/day) can have significant effects on endocrine status (Cassidy & Faughnan, 2000). If these relatively low dietary intakes of isoflavones can affect women during their reproductive life, one would expect them to produce a magnified response in the post-menopausal period when endogenous oestrogen levels are low. Oestrogenic effects from daily isoflavone exposure have been reported and have led to the suggestion that these compounds may provide an exogenous source of oestrogen for menopausal women. Because isoflavones are biologically active in post-menopausal women, isoflavone-rich diets would be expected to reduce menopausal symptoms. This would be consistent with menopausal symptoms reportedly being much less common in countries where consumption of soya products is high. For example, the incidence of hot flushes ranges from 70 to 80% in menopausal women in Europe and is 18% in China. There have been 16 clinical studies of isoflavone-rich foods or supplements conducted in post-menopausal women to evaluate the effects on menopausal symptoms. The results and conclusions have been variable,

but in general, isoflavone supplements appear to be relatively ineffective in managing hot flushes, whereas isoflavone-rich foods appear to have a beneficial effect that exceeds that of a placebo. There is a well-established strong placebo effect on menopausal symptoms from hormone replacement therapy (HRT) studies, but the response is significantly less impressive than the effects observed with HRT. However, most of the studies were conducted over a short time-scale and used limited endpoint assessment (Setchell & Cassidy, 1999). In addition, frequently it is often difficult to define the dose administered. The question of whether consuming phytoestrogen-rich foods over the pre-menopausal years (similar to the Japanese experience of lifetime exposure) and prior to entering the menopause would abate menopausal symptoms remains to be addressed.

8.8.2 Breast cancer

The striking international variability in breast cancer incidence rates, together with the evidence from migrant studies, suggests the importance of environmental factors in the aetiology of breast cancer. Substantial epidemiological and experimental evidence shows that oestrogen plays a critical role in the aetiology of breast cancer and many of the established risk factors for breast cancer, such as early menarche and late menopause, may be attributed primarily to an increased duration and/or dose of oestrogen exposure. It has long been accepted that hormones can potentially promote cancer by increasing cell proliferation, but there is uncertainty as to the precise oestrogen environment that modulates risk and the causal role of many reproductive factors, or indeed diet (Key & Pike, 1988). Increased levels of oestrogens in serum and urine correlate with increased risk for breast cancer, and serum oestrogen levels are generally lower in women from low-risk areas (rural China, Japan) than high-risk population groups (UK, North America) (Goldin *et al.*, 1986; Key *et al.*, 1990).

Dietary intervention studies in healthy young women have shown that intakes of phytoestrogens in the region of 109–158 mg/day can decrease serum oestrogen levels and alter the metabolism of oestrogens to a more favourable profile (Nagata *et al.*, 1997; Lu *et al.*, 2000). Japanese women have higher urinary and blood levels of isoflavones than Western women and they also have significantly longer menstrual cycles. This would translate into an overall lower lifetime exposure to oestrogen, and may in part explain their reduced risk for breast cancer (Cassidy *et al.*, 1994).

Nonetheless, the risks versus the benefits of phytoestrogens in relation to breast cancer are one of the most debated issues in the field. Given their ability to bind to oestrogen receptors, particularly their stronger binding affinity to ERβ than to ERα, antagonist effects have been proposed from *in vitro* model systems. In addition, *in vitro* studies suggest that the pure compounds can induce differentiation and inhibit cell proliferation, albeit at pharmacological doses (Cassidy & Faughnan, 2000).

Although there are substantial animal and cell culture data to support an anticancer effect of soya isoflavones, there are limited data from human studies to support a protective effect. Few studies have been performed, although two clinical secondary prevention studies are under way in the USA and the data they produce will be helpful in attempts to draw any conclusions on the risks versus benefits of phytoestrogen-rich diets.

However, several studies have generated some data of potential concern. In one study, consumption of a 60 g soya supplement (45 mg of isoflavones) increased the number of breast epithelial cells in a group of pre-menopausal women (Petrakis *et al.*, 1996). In another study, consumption of a soya protein isolate (38 mg/day of isoflavones) was associated with increased secretion of breast fluid and the appearance of hyperplastic cells (McMichael-Philips, 1998). Both of these observations would be consistent with increased cell proliferation. In isolation these observations shed concern about the increased risk of tumour development in women consuming phytoestrogen-rich diets, even though this view is inconsistent with the epidemiological data. Data from animal models suggest that a lifelong diet rich in phytoestrogen-rich foods may confer the

greatest protective effects. This increased resistance to developing experimentally induced breast cancer was observed in neonatal and prepubertal rats, and also in the offspring of mothers who were fed isoflavones while lactating (Lamartinere *et al.*, 1995, 1998). Unquestionably, further studies are needed to address the potential safety issues, particularly for women who are at high risk for developing breast cancer. The data from secondary prevention trials should clarify this issue. However, it is possible that the lower incidence of breast cancers in populations consuming soya as a staple may be more a function of lifetime exposure to isoflavones (particularly from an early age) as this may programme adaptive responses and result in a lower susceptibility to breast cancer. The UK Government's Committee on Toxicity of Chemicals in Foods, Consumer Products and the Environment (COT) is currently reviewing the literature on the role of phytoestrogens in breast cancer.

8.8.3 Endometrial cancer

Another potential risk from the consumption of potentially oestrogenic compounds in the diet relates to endometrial cancer. However, in a multi-ethnic group of women in Hawaii, a high consumption of soya products and other legumes by women who had neither used oestrogens nor been pregnant was associated with a decreased risk of endometrial cancer (Goodman *et al.*, 1997). Studies in animals have found that whereas unopposed oestrogens increase uterine weight, the isoflavone genistein had the opposite effect (Foth & Cline, 1998). These findings would support a potential protective effect of soya isoflavones on the endometrium, but there have been no clinical studies to confirm this. The lack of ERβ receptors in the endometrium may well explain these antagonistic effects because isoflavones would be more readily available for competitive binding to ERα receptors, thereby antagonising the adverse effects of oestrogen.

8.8.4 Coronary heart disease

The hypocholesterolaemic effect of soya has been recognised from animal studies for almost a century. These studies have shown that substituting soya protein extracts for casein or other animal protein causes a reduction in total cholesterol and low-density lipoprotein (LDL) concentrations and an increased HDL cholesterol concentration (Anthony *et al.*, 1996). A meta-analysis of 38 studies in humans concluded that the mean reduction in serum total cholesterol was 9.3%, while LDL decreased by 12.9% with soya protein extracts (Anderson *et al.*, 1995). However, many of these studies used very large amounts of soya, considerably more than might be expected to be readily incorporated into a Western diet. An intake of 25 g/day of soya protein would be associated with a 0.23 mmol/L reduction in serum cholesterol (Anderson *et al.*, 1995). A 250 mL serving of soya drink typically contains about 8 g soya protein and soya desserts typically contain 4–5 g per serving (British Nutrition Foundation, 2002c). On the basis of this evidence and further clinical studies, the FDA approved a health claim in the USA for cholesterol reduction based on an intake of 25 g of soya protein per day (see Chapter 13). A similar claim has recently been approved in the UK (http://www.jhci.co.uk/).

This intake is higher than the current daily intake in Japan, but again it is unknown whether lifetime exposure to diets rich in these compounds accounts for the lower blood cholesterol and CHD rates in the Asian populations. The FDA drew no conclusions regarding the role of isoflavones in the cholesterol-lowering effect, but a recent study has shown that isoflavones play a significant role in lowering plasma LDL and their absence from soya renders the food ineffective in reducing cholesterol levels (Crouse *et al.*, 1999). The beneficial effects on lipid profiles may be only one component of any protective responses because isoflavones have also been shown to inhibit the process of coagulation (improve blood flow), exert anti-inflammatory effects and act as antioxidants, or may exert direct effects on the arterial wall (Setchell & Cassidy, 1999). See also Chapter 4. Further clinical trials need to be conducted to assess the potential therapeutic effects of isoflavones for coronary heart disease as the importance of dietary isoflavones in CHD prevention has not yet received adequate attention to permit a firm conclusion.

8.8.5 Osteoporosis

The weak oestrogenic action of isoflavones may offer some protection against bone loss. While the consensus of data from rodent studies clearly demonstrate that soya isoflavones are effective in reducing bone loss and increasing bone formation (Anderson *et al.*, 1998b), two long-term studies using ovaectomised monkeys have failed to show an effect of soya isoflavones on bone (Jayo *et al.*, 1996; Lees & Ginn, 1998). It is possible that the responsiveness to bone may differ between species, as it is known that there are significant species differences in the metabolic handling of these compounds.

Epidemiological evidence is consistent with a role of dietary isoflavones in preventing bone loss because the incidence of hip fractures is lower in Asia than in most Western communities. However these differences in osteoporosis-related fractures may be accounted for by other factors including, for example, skeletal size. To date only limited clinical studies have been conducted to examine the effects of isoflavone ingestion on bone density or bone biochemical markers in post-menopausal women. A number of short-term studies are suggestive of beneficial effects on biochemical markers of bone turnover; however, whether these data translate into long term effects on bone density remains to be established (Setchell & Cassidy, 1999).

8.8.6 Effects of phytoestrogens in men

To date, few studies have examined the effects of isoflavones and lignans specifically in men. The dietary intervention studies that have searched for evidence of hormonal effects of phytoestrogen-rich diets in men suggest only minimal effects. These findings are in contrast to the significant hormonal effects observed in women from similar intakes of isoflavone-containing foods and the reasons for this gender difference in responsiveness are still unclear.

Interestingly, isoflavone intake is higher in countries where the incidence rates of prostate cancer and other conditions linked to oestrogen exposure (hypospadia, testicular cancers) are low. Analysis of plasma and prostatic fluid from Asian men, who have a low risk for prostate cancer relative to European men, found high concentrations of the isoflavones (Morton *et al.*, 1997). These types of data have consequently led to speculation that dietary isoflavones may play a role in the reduced risk for prostate cancer evident from some epidemiological studies. However, in the absence of solid data from clinical studies, the existing evidence in support of this hypothesis (from *in vitro* and animal studies) must be regarded as circumstantial.

8.8.7 Infants

The role of phytoestrogens in infant health has been a controversial issue, but few studies have examined their potential biological effects. Soya infant formula contains high concentrations of isoflavones (40 μg/mL) and exposure levels for 4-month-old infants exclusively fed on soya infant formulae is about 6–11 mg/kg bodyweight (Setchell *et al.*, 1997). This is an order of magnitude higher than the amount (50 mg/day) consumed by oriental adults (<1 mg/kg bodyweight). Plasma concentrations in these soya formula-fed babies ranged from 654 to 1775 ng/mL which is again almost an order of magnitude higher than concentrations in Asian adults and 13 000–22 000 times higher than circulating levels of plasma oestradiol in infants (40–80 ng/mL) (Setchell *et al.*, 1997).

The safety of soya-based formulae has been under scrutiny because of their potential 'hormonal' effects at critical periods of development in several animal experiments. However, given the significant species differences that have been observed in the metabolism of these compounds, it is difficult to interpret these studies in the context of human consumption. Soya infant formulae have been in use for over 30 years with no obvious evidence of detrimental effects to health. There is some suggestion (albeit from animal experiments) that early exposure (through the lactating mother, neonatal, perinatal) may programme a resistance to cancer formation in later life (Lamartinere *et al.*, 1998). Concerns have been expressed about the effects of soya on thyroid function from *in vitro* data, but there is no clinical evidence to support this speculation (Divi & Doerge, 1996; Divi *et al.*, 1997). The few reports of thyroid disease in infants fed soya infant formula occurred prior to the time that these formulae were fortified with iodine. Assessment of the risks versus the benefits of soya infant formula is currently one of the key areas under discussion by COT.

8.9 Summary

In addition to their macronutrient content, cereals, nuts and pulses contain a number of potentially bioactive substances, in particular selenium, folates and other bioactive compounds from the phytoestrogen class. Given that the UK Department of Health (see Chapter 13) already recommends diets rich in cereals, nuts and pulses as an integral part of a healthy diet, the presence of bioactive substances in this food group adds further weight to their proposed beneficial effects for human health. However, further research is required, particularly in relation to the phytoestrogens (present in pulses), in order to define optimal intakes for specific health benefits.

8.10 Research recommendations

- Studies are needed on the bioavailability of constituents of cereals, nuts and pulses, and to define the factors which influence their absorption and metabolism.
- Studies are needed to identify other constituents present in cereals, nuts and pulses which may reflect the potential health benefits of these food groups.
- There is a need for furthering understanding of the risk versus benefit profile of novel compounds present in plant foods, in order to formulate safe and efficacious levels, and to ensure a balanced scientific view is available for consumers.
- Genomic and metabolomic technology should be embraced to allow further understanding of individual variability in response to the intake of specific foods and constituents of foods.

8.11 Key points

- In addition to their macronutrient content, cereals, nuts and pulses contain a number of potentially bioactive substances, in particular selenium, folates and other bioactive compounds from the phytoestrogen class. The presence of bioactive substances in this food group adds further weight to their proposed beneficial effects for human health. However, further research is required, particularly in relation to the phytoestrogens, in order to define specific health benefits and optimal intakes.
- High consumption of cereals, nuts and pulses may be associated with a decreased risk of diseases such as cardiovascular disease and some cancers, but so far many of the specific food constituents that might be responsible for these associations have yet to be identified. To date, research interest has concentrated on folate, selenium, phytoestrogens and fibre (which is not considered in detail in this report).
- Selenium is found in many plant foods, and both cereals and nuts can be important sources. In humans, it is an essential component of a number of enzymes, *e.g.* glutathione peroxidase, and recent research has been focused on cancer protection and cardiovascular benefits. Cereals and pulses are contributors to folate intake. This micronutrient has recently been recognised as important in protecting against neural tube defects in fetal life and as a potential influence on cardiovascular risk via an effect on reducing blood homocysteine levels.
- Phytoestrogens comprise a range of structurally dissimilar compounds with the common characteristic of being able to bind to oestrogen receptors in humans. The group includes isoflavones, lignans and stilbenes, which function as anti-fungal agents in plants.
- Relatively little is known about the factors that influence the bioavailability and the pharmacokinetic profile of phytoestrogens.
- Through their ability to bind to oestrogen receptors, it has been suggested that phytoestrogens may be beneficial in post-menopausal women in relation to menopausal symptoms, and risk factors for heart disease and osteoporosis. A role in breast cancer has also been suggested.
- The richest source of isoflavones is soya beans (although they are also present in chick peas and kidney beans). They are either present as the aglycone (genistein or daidzein) or as various glycoside conjugates (*e.g.* daidzin and genistin).
- Isoflavone supplements seem to be relatively ineffective in managing menopausal hot

flushes, whereas isoflavone-rich foods appear to have a beneficial effect that exceeds that of a placebo, although the impact is much less than that seen with HRT. A key issue is whether consumption needs to be life-long (as in Japan, where soya consumption is high) to be effective.

- Soya has a recognised modest ability to reduce plasma cholesterol levels. The cholesterol-lowering effect appears to be the result of a combination of components acting together; isoflavones together with soya protein appear to have a greater effect than soya protein alone. Other effects of isoflavones have also been proposed including a direct effect on the arterial wall. Clinical data to determine the effects of isoflavones in relation to osteoporosis are still lacking; however, recent short-term human data are not as supportive as the available mechanistic data and animal data for a positive effect of isoflavones on bone health. The data with regard to bone health are still unclear, and the risks versus benefits of phytoestrogens in relation to breast cancer are unresolved.

- The role of phytoestrogens in infant health has been a controversial matter, as isoflavones are present in high concentrations in soya infant formula. Assessment of this matter is currently being addressed by the UK Government's Committee on Toxicity of Chemicals in Foods, Consumer Products and the Environment (COT).

- In Europe, owing to the frequency of consumption, cereals, nuts and pulses makes a significant contribution to intake of many of these bioactive compounds. However, information on their absorption, metabolism and mechanisms of action at physiologically relevant levels is required to design appropriate human intervention studies to define optimal doses for health benefits.

9
Beverages

9.1 Types of beverages

Water is an essential part of the diet. It is needed to maintain tissue integrity and to provide optimum conditions for the complex biochemical reactions that occur within and between our cells (Saltmarsh, 2001). Possibly because it is a rather bland drink, many people prefer to consume water when flavoured with a wide range of natural and synthetic products. Such beverages include teas, coffee, cocoa, wines, spirits and beer in addition to a vast range of proprietary products and carbonated drinks that are available from the local supermarket. Unlike water, which has little nutritional value, beverages may contain significant quantities of nutrients and compounds capable of interacting with biochemical and cellular processes. This chapter will cover the commonly consumed hot (tea, coffee, cocoa) and cold (wine, spirits, beer) beverages. Fruit juices and herb teas are discussed in Chapters 1, 7 and 11.

9.2 Phenolic compounds in beverages

Beverages can contain a wide variety of macronutrients and essential trace elements and vitamins. Many also contain plant-derived phenolic compounds with a diverse range of effects *in vitro* suggestive of a putative role in the prevention of chronic diseases. In recent years, there has been a veritable explosion of research in this area. Therefore, a brief review of the relevant phenolic compounds is merited prior to discussion of potentially bioactive substances in individual beverages. See also Chapter 2.

9.2.1 Origin of phenolic compounds

Plants produce thousands of phenolic and polyphenolic compounds as secondary metabolites. The majority are either synthesised via the phenylpropanoid pathway or are derived from this pathway in which 4-coumaric acid is a key compound (see Chapter 2). Phenolic and polyphenolic compounds are essential to the plants' physiology, being involved in diverse functions such as structure, pigmentation, pollination, allelopathy, pathogen and predator resistance and growth and development (Croteau *et al.*, 2000; Pierpoint, 2000; Dewick, 2002). The main polyphenolics in plants are flavonoids, a structurally diverse group of C_{15} compounds arranged in a C_6–C_3–C_6 configuration (Fig. 9.1).

Other polyphenols include condensed tannins [$(C_6$–C_3–$C_6)_n$] and stilbenes (C_6–C_2–C_6) while the simpler phenolic compounds include phenolic acids (C_6–C_1) and hydroxycinnamates (C_6–C_3) (see Chapter 2). Most research to date on the possible nutritional role of phenolic compounds

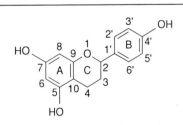

Fig. 9.1 General features of the flavonoid skeleton indicating the A, B and C rings and the numbering system.

Table 9.1 Classification of some common dietary flavonoids indicating major food sources.

Flavonoid	Major subclasses and food sources
Flavonols	Kaempferol (R_1 = H, R_2 = H), quercetin (R_1 = OH, R_1 = H), myricetin (R_1 = OH, R_1 = OH). Present as sugar conjugates in fruits, vegetables and beverages including apples, plums, cranberries, strawberries, grapes, kale, onions, broccoli, celery stalks, tomatoes, red wine, green tea, black tea, grape juice
Flavones	Apigenin (R = H), luteolin (R = OH). Present as sugar conjugates in celery, olives and sweet red peppers
Flavan-3-ols	(+)-Catechin (R_1 = H, R_2 = β–OH), (–)-epicatechin (R = α–OH). Present in apples, plums, green tea, black tea, red wine, grape juice and cocoa as monomers, gallate derivatives, dimers and oligomers
Flavanones	Naringenin (R_1 = H, R_2 = H), hesperitin (R_1 = OH, R_2 = OCH$_3$). Present in citrus fruit, including oranges, lemon and grapefruit as sugar conjugates
Anthocyanins	Pelargonidin (R_1 = H, R_2 = H), cyanidin (R_1 = OH, R_2 = H), delphinidin (R_1 = OH, R_2 = OH), malvidin (R_1 = OCH$_3$, R_2 = OCH$_3$). Found as mainly 3-*O*-glucose conjugates in black grapes, red wine, grape juice, strawberries, raspberries, blackcurrants, blueberries, blackberries, cranberries, plums. Aglycones referred to as anthocyanidins

Based on Duthie *et al.* (2000).

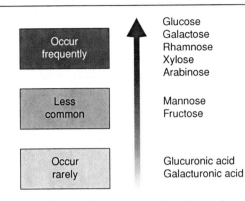

Fig. 9.2 Types of sugars found as flavonol and flavone conjugates ranked according to the frequency of their occurrence in plants (compiled by Janet Kyle, Rowett Research Institute).

Table 9.2 Some examples of the range of flavonol–sugar complexes found in common beverages and foods.

Food item	Flavonol and flavone form
Black tea	Quercetin-3-*O*-β-D-glucoside Quercetin-3-*O*-β-D-galactoside Quercetin-3-*O*-α-L-rhamnoglucoside Quercetin-3-*O*-α-L-rhamnodiglucoside Quercetin-3-*O*-β-D-glucorhamnogalactoside Myricetin mono- and diglycosides Kaempferol mono-, di- and triglycosides
Apples	Quercetin-3-*O*-β-D-galactoside Quercetin-3-*O*-α-L-arabinoside Quercetin-3-*O*-β-D-glucoside Quercetin-3-*O*-α-L-rhamnoside Quercetin-3-*O*-α-L-xyloside
Onions	Quercetin-3-*O*-β-D-glucoside Quercetin-4'-*O*-β-D-glucoside Quercetin-7-*O*-β-D-glucoside Quercetin-3,4'-di-*O*-β-D-glucoside Quercetin-7,4'-di-*O*-β-D-glucoside Isorhamnetin-4'-*O*-β-D-glucoside

has been focused on the flavonoids, around 8000 of which have been described to date. Major classes (Table 9.1), which are discussed in Chapter 2, include isoflavones (see Chapter 8), flavonols, flavones, flavan-3-ols, flavanones and anthocyanins.

There are numerous structural variations within these major flavonoid classes, which depend on the level of hydrogenation, hydroxylation, methylation and sulphation of the molecules. In addition, most flavonoids form complexes with sugars, lipids, amines and carboxylic and organic acids (Harborne, 1993). For example, more than 380 flavonol and flavone glycosides have been described (Fig. 9.2).

Individual foods can differ in the number and nature of glycosides associated with a particular flavonol. For example, the flavonol quercetin is found in onions in the form of glucose conjugates linked at the 3-, 7-and 4'-positions (Tsushida & Suzuki, 1995), whereas in apple peel it occurs as quercetin-3-*O*-conjugates of glucose, arabinose, galactose, rhamnose and xylose (Dick *et al.*, 1985) (see Table 9.2). See Section 6.3.2 for information on the effect of glycosides on absorption.

Although flavonoids are ubiquitous in foods of plant origin, accurate determination of dietary intakes is problematic owing to their immense diversity of form, a dearth of reference compounds and variations in analytical methodology. In addition, their concentrations in foods can vary by many orders of magnitude and are influenced by several factors, including species, variety, light, degree of ripeness, processing and storage (Peterson & Dwyer, 1998a). Consequently, calculated flavonoid intakes ranging from 3 mg/day in Finland to 65 mg/day in Japan (Duthie *et al.*, 2000) must be regarded as 'rough and ready' approximations. In general, however, dietary intakes of flavonols and flavones are quantitatively similar to those of many well-recognised micronutrients such as vitamins E and C and the overall flavonoid intake may be well in excess of that of the 'traditional' vitamins.

9.2.2 Effects in mammalian cells

Numerous cell culture and animal model studies indicate that plant phenolics can affect diverse processes in mammalian cells and it has also been shown that many of these compounds are potent antioxidants *in vitro* (for a review, see Duthie *et al.*, 2000). This is essentially due to the ease with which a hydrogen atom from an aromatic hydroxyl group of the polyphenol is donated to a free radical and the ability of the aromatic structure to support an unpaired electron due to delocalisation around the π-electron system. If such activity also occurs *in vivo*, phenolic compounds could inhibit oxidative reactions implicated in the development of clinical conditions including heart disease and cancer (see Chapter 4). In addition, certain phenolics may have potent anticancer effects by mechanisms that do not necessarily invoke antioxidant activity, such as enzyme modulation, gene expression, up-regulation of intercellular signalling and P-glycoprotein activation. They may also protect against heart disease by preventing platelet aggregation and by being potent vasodilators (Bravo, 1998). Such mechanisms are discussed in greater detail in Chapter 4. The available evidence linking dietary antioxidants and chronic disease has been reviewed recently by the EU-funded EUROFEDA project (Astley & Lindsay, 2002) and by the BNF on behalf of the Food Standards Agency (Buttriss *et al.*, 2002)

9.2.3 Bioavailability

Flavonoids and other phenolic compounds have to be absorbed from the gut if they are to exert a protective effect against heart disease and systemic cancers. Early animal studies (Das, 1969) appeared to indicate that flavonoids were absorbed only to a limited degree because gut micro-organisms preferentially destroyed the heterocyclic rings of the compounds before any absorption took place in the small intestine. However, an increasing number of studies have now detected selected flavonoids and their metabolites in plasma and urine of human volunteers following the consumption of pure compounds and polyphenol-rich extracts and beverages (Cao & Prior, 1999; Donovan *et al.*, 1999; Tsuda *et al.*, 1999; Watson & Oliveira, 1999). This may suggest that the bioavailability of polyphenols is greater than previously assumed.

However, increases in the concentrations of polyphenols and associated metabolites in plasma and urine do not necessarily mean that they have significant effects *in vivo*. As yet, few data are available on their intracellular location and mechanism of action. Consequently, clarification of the absorption, bioavailability and metabolism of the plethora of polyphenols in beverages will be an important research area in the future. See Chapter 6 for further discussion.

9.2.4 Toxicity

Although polyphenols may have potential health benefits, it should be noted that many function in plants to discourage attack by fungal parasites, herbivorous grazers and pathogens (see Chapter 7). Not surprisingly, many are also toxic and mutagenic in cell culture systems (Bruswick, 1993) and consumption to excess by mammals could possibly cause adverse metabolic reactions (see Section 13.6). However, the concentrations of polyphenols used in cell culture studies are likely to exceed that which is achievable in the body by diet alone. Hence, there is currently very little evidence that they are carcinogenic *in vivo*. Nevertheless, until further studies are undertaken, it may be unwise to contemplate excessive supplementation with polyphenol-rich products. Potential toxicity of bioactive compounds is discussed in Chapters 1, 6 and 13.

9.3 Tea

9.3.1 History

Tea arrived in Europe in the 18th century, having been drunk elsewhere for centuries, for example by the Chinese for probably 5000 years. Tea was initially sold in coffee houses (see Section 9.4.1) but became more popular than coffee, perhaps because of early Royal patronage, and by the 1750s tea houses and tea gardens were common in and around London. The popularity of tea was such that from the latter part of the 18th to the beginning of the 19th century a transition took place in the drink of the labouring class as tea replaced beer and gin (Cobbett, 1985).

Table 9.3 Main varieties of teas.

Green	Oolong	Black
Genmaicha (Japan)	Ti Kuan Yin (Mainland China)	Assam (India)
Gyokuro (Japan)	Formosa Oolong (Taiwan, many varieties)	Ceylon (Sri Lanka)
Spider Leg (Japan)	Pu-erh (Cpaulhina)	Darjeeling (India)
Mattcha (Japan, used in the Tea Ceremony)	Keemun (China)	Nilgiri (India)
Sencha (Japan)		Sikkim (India)
Hojicha (Japan)		Yunnan (China)
Longjing (China)		
Baozhong (China)		
Gunpowder (China)		

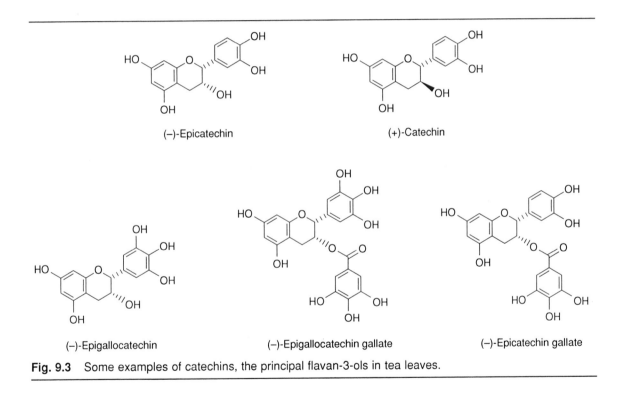

Fig. 9.3 Some examples of catechins, the principal flavan-3-ols in tea leaves.

9.3.2 Production and varieties

'Tea' is a drink made by infusing young leaves of the tea plant (*Camellia sinensis*) in hot water. From its origins in China, the tea plant is now cultivated in over 30 countries, major commercial producers being Japan, Taiwan, Sri Lanka, Kenya, Indonesia and India. Tea is the most widely consumed beverage in the world (Weisburger, 1997) and there are hundreds of varieties (Table 9.3).

The three main categories are green, oolong and black tea. These arise from differences in processing procedures. To produce green tea, which is consumed mainly in the Far East and North Africa, the leaves are chopped, rolled and quickly steamed or heated to minimise oxidation. However, the black teas consumed mainly in Western countries undergo several hours of oxidation in their preparation for market, being first dried and crushed prior to extensive peroxidase-mediated fermentation (as distinct from alcoholic fermentation) and firing. Oolong tea, which is produced in Taiwan and exported to Japan and Germany, involves a shorter fermentation period and is said to have taste and colour somewhere between the green and black teas. In addition, there are numerous scented and flavoured teas available such as Earl Grey (black tea with oil of bergamot), Lady Grey (black tea with orange and lemon peel and oil of bergamot), Lapsang Souchong (black, scented with smoke) and Jasmine (green, scented with jasmine flowers).

9.3.3 Composition of teas

(i) Polyphenols

Tea leaves contain, in quantities equivalent to 20–30% of the dry weight, a range of polyphenols,

particularly the flavan-3-ols, namely (+)-catechin and (–)-epicatechin and their gallate derivatives (Fig. 9.3).

The types and proportion of flavan-3-ols in the tea leaf varies with season, the age of the leaf, climate, and horticultural practices. In addition, major changes occur during processing. In the rolling and crushing used to manufacture oolong and black tea, polyphenol oxidase released from the leaf endoplasmic reticulum catalyses the condensation of the catechins to the yellow–orange coloured theaflavins. These undergo oxidation and randomly polymerise to form high molecular weight thearubigins, which are major components and impart the red–brown colour that characterises black tea (Fig. 9.4). These compounds are responsible not only for the colour of black tea but also for its astringent flavour. In comparison with green tea, black tea is low in monomeric catechins but high in oligomeric derivatives, most

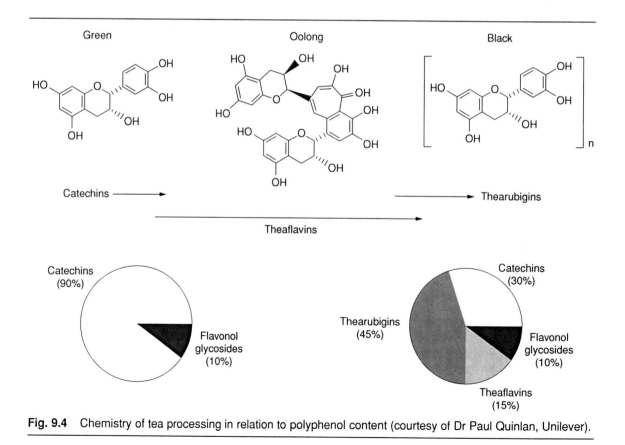

Fig. 9.4 Chemistry of tea processing in relation to polyphenol content (courtesy of Dr Paul Quinlan, Unilever).

notably thearubigins (Haslam, 1998). Fermentation, however, does not affect the level or composition of flavonol glycosides, which are similar in black and green tea (see Fig. 9.4).

The polyphenols in tea can react with divalent ions such as iron (Disler *et al.*, 1975). This could reduce the bioavailability of iron but this effect is not definitively associated with any increased morbidity (Nelson, 2001). The presence of catechins indicates that tea extracts have considerable antioxidant activity. In certain model systems, such antioxidant activity compares favourably with the antioxidant nutrient vitamin E (Fig. 9.5).

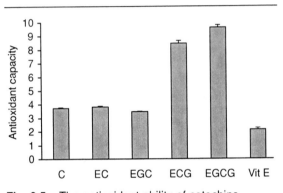

Fig. 9.5 The antioxidant ability of catechins compared with vitamin E. Key: (+)-catechin (C); (−)-epicatechin (EC); (−)-epicatechin gallate (ECG); (−)-epigallocatechin (EGC); (−)-epigallocatechin gallate (EGCG); α-tocopherol (Vitamin E). Adapted from Gardner *et al.* (1997).

(ii) Other components

Consumption of tea probably provides a negligible intake of macronutrients. For example, less than 2% of the hot-water-soluble solids of black tea are proteins, 4–5% are carbohydrates and 2–3% are lipids, mainly linoleic and linolenic acids (Stagg & Millin, 1975). However, macronutrient content is markedly increased by the UK habit of adding milk and sugar.

Tea also contains a range of micronutrients including manganese, potassium, niacin, riboflavin, folate and zinc (Table 9.4). However, the contribution of tea to the overall vitamin and mineral intake in the UK has declined in recent years. According to MAFF's National Food Survey statistics, tea consumption has decreased by more than 50% in the last 20 years to about 3.5 cups per person per day (one cup in the UK is typically 200 mL). Statistics on beverage consumption in the UK can also be found in Chapter 1. In addition, the tea drunk today may be less rich in micronutrients than in previous decades as infusion times have decreased from 5–6 min to 40–60 s.

All types of tea also contain significant quantities of the purine alkaloid caffeine (see Section 2.6) together with smaller amounts of theobromine (Fig. 9.6) (Ashihara & Crozier, 1999, 2001). About 80% of the purine alkaloids are extracted into the water-soluble phase during brewing. Typically, a 200 mL cup of black tea contains 50–100 mg of caffeine. The potential effects of caffeine on human metabolism are discussed in Section 9.4.

Table 9.4 Estimated contribution of black tea to UK Reference Nutrient Intakes (RNI).

Nutrient	Amount from average daily tea intake	% RNI
Riboflavin	34 μg	2.6
Niacin	262 μg	2.2
Folate	2.6 μg	1.3
Potassium	60 mg	2.0
Zinc	0.8 mg	9.4
Manganese	1.7 mg	Not determined

Data courtesy of Dr Paul Quinlan and Dr Peter Collier (Unilever). The figures are based on a current average adult tea consumption of 5.2 g leaf/day (equivalent to ~500 mL and 3 × 180 mL traditional cups).

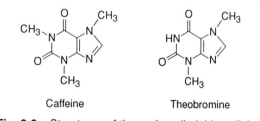

Fig. 9.6 Structures of the purine alkaloids caffeine and theobromine.

9.3.4 Health implications of tea

There are suggestions that tea and tea catechins may have a variety of health effects in man. Most interest has been focused on the possibility that tea may inhibit the development of heart disease and cancers, diseases that account for the majority of premature mortality in developed countries (see Chapters 3 and 13).

(i) Tea and heart disease

A number of epidemiological studies have suggested that consumption of tea *per se* or diets rich in the polyphenols found in tea are associated with decreased risk of heart disease and associated conditions (Fig. 9.7) (see Chapter 3). A recent

prospective study in the Netherlands (Geleijnse *et al.*, 1999) of 3454 men and women aged 55 years found a significant inverse association between tea intake and radiographically quantified aortic atherosclerosis. In addition, green tea consumption appears to be associated with about a 30% decrease in aortic lesion formation in hypercholesterolaemic rabbits (Tijburg *et al.*, 1997).

A recent meta-analysis of 10 cohort and seven case-control studies serves to emphasise the hetrogeneity in reported effects. The authors estimated an 11% decrease in the rate of myocardial infarction with an increase in tea consumption of around three cups a day. However, the possibility of publication bias and evidence of geographical differences (a decreased risk was consistently found in continental Europe but studies in the USA and UK showed little or no effect, or even an increased risk of CHD) urges caution in the interpretation of this finding (Peters *et al.*, 2001).

Another Dutch study (Arts *et al.*, 2001a) used data from the Zutphen Elderly Study (a prospective cohort of 806 men aged 65–84 years at baseline) to assess whether total catechin intake, which was 72 ± 47.8 mg/day at baseline, mainly from tea, apples and chocolate, influenced the risk of death from ischaemic heart disease or incidence or death from stroke. They report that

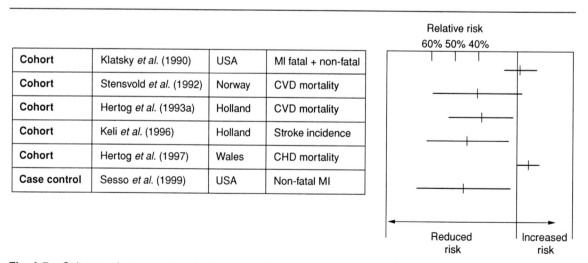

Fig. 9.7 Cohort and case-control studies implicating tea in reduced risk of myocardial infarction (MI), coronary heart disease (CHD), cardiovascular disease (CVD) and stroke (courtesy of Dr Paul Quinlan, Unilever).

catechins, whether from tea or other sources, may reduce the risk of ischaemic heart disease death but not stroke.

One possible mechanism by which tea may reduce heart disease risk is via the ability of catechins to prevent the oxidation of low-density lipoprotein cholesterol to an atherogenic form (see Chapter 4). *In vitro*, the oxidation of low-density lipoprotein by endothelial cells, macrophages and Cu^{2+} can be inhibited by a wide range of polyphenols and polyphenol-rich extracts (Duthie *et al.*, 2000). Such effects may be due to the direct scavenging by the polyphenols of the oxidising species or may result from the polyphenol-mediated regeneration of vitamin E in the low-density lipoprotein. However, whether such *in vitro* antioxidant effects also occur *in vivo* and translate into reducing the risk of developing heart disease is unclear at present (see Chapter 3).

The consumption of tea may also prevent atherosclerosis by mechanisms that do not necessarily involve the antioxidant properties of catechins (Duthie *et al.*, 2000). For example, *in vitro* studies suggest that tea extracts may prevent platelet adhesion and aggregation by inhibiting the cyclooxygenase pathway and reducing the cyclic 3′,5′-adenosine monophosphate (AMP) response of platelets to prostaglandin I_2. Moreover, reported vasodilatory effects of tea extracts and polyphenols may be due to their affecting enhanced nitric oxide generation, cyclic 3′,5′-guanosine monophosphate (GMP) accumulation and other endothelium-dependent relaxation factors. The relevance of these findings to normal human diets still needs to be established. Caffeine in tea may reduce blood coagulation by inhibiting thrombin-stimulated thromboxane formation. It has also been suggested that reported hypocholesterolaemic effects may reflect reduced cholesterol absorption from the intestine, caused by flavan-3-ol esters reducing the solubility of cholesterol in mixed micelles.

(ii) Tea and cancer

Epidemiological studies (see Chapter 3 for definitions) of black tea consumption and cancer have produced mixed results (for example, see Table 9.5). For green tea consumption, a review published in 1998 found that out of five studies on the incidence of colon cancer, three found an inverse association, one reported a positive association and one found no statistically significant association. For rectal cancer, of four studies one reported an inverse association and two reported an increased risk (Bushman, 1998). The inconclusive findings of these and other studies may reflect problems of measurement error (recall bias in case-control studies) and specificity of exposure (duration and amount not specified), or lack of control of potentially important cofounders (see Chapter 3). At the present time the epidemiological evidence is at best inconclusive as to whether there is any benefit from either black or green tea.

In contrast to human epidemiological studies, many *in vitro* and animal studies have demonstrated the inhibition of chemically induced cancer by tea and tea polyphenols. For example,

Table 9.5 Review of the results of some of the case control and cohort studies investigating black tea consumption and risk of cancer.

Type of cancer	No. of studies showing		
	Decreased risk	Increased risk	No association
Oesophageal	–	5	9
Stomach	–	2	16
Colorectal	5	4	23
Pancreas	4	1	11
Breast	4	–	6

Adapted from Blot *et al.* (1997).

rats fed a diet containing 1% green tea catechins have a significantly reduced mortality from mammary tumours following treatment with a chemical carcinogen compared with rats given the carcinogen alone (Hirose *et al.*, 1994). Hamsters fed green tea polyphenols display fewer hyperplastic pancreatic duct lesions after treatment with *N*-nitrosobis(2-oxopropyl)amine (Majima *et al.*, 1998). In a comprehensive study, Yang *et al.* describe the ability of both green and black tea infusions to inhibit *N*-nitrosodiethylamine-induced lung carcinogenesis in knockout mice (Yang *et al.*, 1998). Tea extract also significantly reduced the progression of chemically induced, non-malignant adenomas to malignant adenocarcinomas. Furthermore, the spontaneous formation of lung tumours and rhabdosarcomas was inhibited 50% in rats fed either black or green tea infusions.

There are a number of mechanisms by which tea may potentially influence both carcinogenic initiation and promotion (Duthie *et al.*, 2000). In brief, these include direct and indirect antioxidant protection of DNA, the modulation of enzyme systems such as cytochrome P450 complexes that metabolise carcinogens or procarcinogens to genotoxins and the modulation of malignant transformation, apoptosis and gene expression (see Chapter 4). Gut flora profiles could also be altered to decrease the formation of potentially carcinogenic compounds such as ammonia and amines (see Chapter 5).

9.3.5 Bioavailability of tea catechins

Consumption of a single dose of green tea extract results in a small but significant increase in plasma concentrations of total catechins (Fig. 9.8). The effect is less for black tea arguably because of the potentially poor absorption of high molecular weight thearubigens and theaflavins, which predominate in black tea (see Section 9.3.2). The presence of milk does not appear to affect the absorption of catechins from tea (van het Hof *et al.*, 1999). In addition, radiolabelling studies with primates suggest that significant quantities of (–)-epigallocatechin gallate or its metabolites can be found in tissues indicating that they may arrive at target sites within cells in peripheral tissues (Suganuma *et al.*, 1998). This is an essential requirement if consumption of the catechins found in tea is to exert effects similar to that observed in cell culture. See Chapter 6 for further information on the bioavailability of flavan-3-ols.

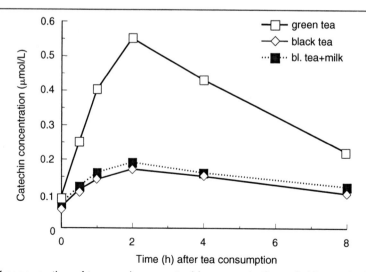

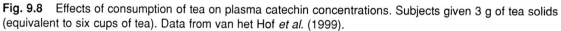

Fig. 9.8 Effects of consumption of tea on plasma catechin concentrations. Subjects given 3 g of tea solids (equivalent to six cups of tea). Data from van het Hof *et al.* (1999).

9.3.6 Summary of tea

In many biological systems, extracts of tea have a wide range of effects with potential health benefits. In cell culture and animal models they may inhibit oxidation of low density lipoproteins, prevent mutations and be anti-carcinogens. Much of this activity is ascribed to the polyphenolic components of tea, in particular the catechin-derivatives. More studies are required to establish the bioavailability of these compounds and their effects *in vivo* before any health benefits can be established with certainty. The impact of these compounds when consumed as part of a normal diet and in amounts normally consumed by humans is not yet clear.

9.4 Coffee

9.4.1 History

Coffee was cultivated certainly by the 15th century and arrived in Europe in the 17th century. On the continent the coffee houses became the great cafes – for example, Zimmerman's in Leipzig had a concert hall that could hold 150 people and held concerts twice a week and J.S. Bach wrote a coffee cantata for performance there. In England these places of refreshment developed differently and became more exclusive. The aristocracy patronised particular places according to their preference and politics. Lloyd's coffee house for seafaring men became a place where news about shipping and naval battles was first heard. It developed into an insurance brokerage. Jonathan's became the stock exchange. Others became gentlemen's clubs.

9.4.2 Production and varieties

In economic terms, coffee is the most valuable agricultural product exported by developing counties. *Coffea arabica* (Arabica coffee) is cultivated extensively and represents approximately 70% of the world market. The remaining 30% consists mainly of *Coffea canephora* (Robusta coffee). Small-scale cultivation of *Coffea liberica*, *Coffea racemosa* and *Coffea dewevrei* occurs in some African countries but the resultant beverages are of lower quality and most is sold locally rather than exported.

The major coffee producers are Brazil, Colombia, Indonesia, Ivory Coast, India and Angola. Most coffee is exported from these countries as 'green beans', the freshly picked cherries being either sun dried for 2–3 weeks, followed by mechanical removal of the dried husk, or alternatively soaked and fermented in water to remove the pulp prior to drying. The former method is called the dry process and the latter the wet process, producing respectively 'natural' and 'washed' coffee beans. The dried green beans are roasted at up to 220°C for 15 min to impart flavour and aroma and can be blended to produce various commercial grades. Although roasted beans can be bought for grinding at home, most coffee is purchased in vacuum packs pre-ground by metallic micrometric grinding cylinders. The beverage is often then prepared by percolation where steam passes through the grains or by passing hot water through the grains which are restrained by a filter (Table 9.6). However, more than 95% of coffee consumed in the UK is of the 'instant' type which merely requires the addition of hot water. Instant coffee is produced by extracting the ground and roasted coffee into hot water under pressure. The extract is concentrated and either lyophilised or spray-dried to produce a granular or powdered product which readily dissolves (Debry, 1994).

Worldwide, approximately 1.7×10^9 cups of coffee are drunk each day and on average in 1997 each person in the UK consumed about 1.8 kg of coffee (http://www.realcoffee.co.uk). Consequently, compounds found in coffee may have a considerable metabolic and nutritional impact. For more information about beverage intakes in the UK, see Chapter 1.

9.4.3 Composition of coffees

(i) Phenolics

Green coffee contains a large amount and variety of polyphenols, typically chlorogenic, caffeic, ferulic and 4-coumaric acids. Roasting markedly

Table 9.6   Brewing methods to produce coffee beverages.

Type	Procedure
Boiled coffee	Coarse grains are infused in boiling water for ~10 min. The infusion is consumed without removal of the grains. Method not widespread in UK
Espresso	Fine grains are extracted with water at 95 °C at a pressure of 8–12 bar for 15–25 s
Filtered	Extraction obtained by pouring boiling water over finely ground coffee usually in a paper filter
Infusion/cafetière	Infusion of coarse ground coffee in boiling water for a few minutes. The beverage is separated from the grounds by pouring through a metal strainer
Percolated	Coarse ground coffee is extracted by recirculating boiling water
Turkish coffee	Finely ground grains added to gently boiling water until it foams
Soluble or instant	Most common type in UK. Beverage prepared by dissolving 1.5–3 g of instant coffee powder in 150–200 mL of hot water

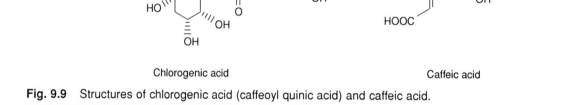

Chlorogenic acid   Caffeic acid

Fig. 9.9   Structures of chlorogenic acid (caffeoyl quinic acid) and caffeic acid.

affects the composition of the coffee polyphenols and this, and the caramelisation of carbohydrates (see Table 9.8), gives coffee its taste and aroma. About 40 phenolics are present in roasted coffee and most attention has been focused on chlorogenic acid, a hydroxycinnimate (see Section 2.4.2) which may be partially hydrolysed in the gut to caffeic acid (Figs 2.1, 2.13 and 9.9). A recent study with ileostomy volunteers indicates that 30% of ingested chlorogenic acid and almost all caffeic acid are absorbed in the small intestine of humans (Olthof *et al.*, 2001). Such phenolics contribute to the overall antioxidant activity of coffee, which in some *in vitro* systems is comparable to the catechin-rich teas (Table 9.7).

(ii) *Other components*

Green coffee contains sucrose, polysaccharides, proteins and minerals, and during roasting numerous reactions occur so that a cup of coffee contains many complex molecules (Table 9.8). For example, whilst the levels of chlorogenic acid decrease during the roasting process, the amounts of other organic acids such as malate, lactate and quinic acid may rise as a result of the degradation of polysaccharides and other components. However, the coffee brew can be regarded as being naturally low in digestible proteins, carbohydrates and fats, with the amounts being insufficient to contribute significantly to the average daily intake of macronutrients (Southgate, 2000).

Table 9.7 Comparison of the antioxidant activities of coffee and tea.

Beverage	Total phenols (μM)	TEAC value* (mmol/L)	CLT50[†] (μM)
Green tea	12	7.5	66
Black tea	17	7	67
Coffee	10	7	106

*TEAC value as Trolox equivalents (courtesy of Dr Paul Quinlan, Unilever).
[†]CLT_{50} is the concentration required to inhibit the oxidation of LDL by 50%.
Adapted from Vinson (1998).

Table 9.8 Approximate typical composition in mg of a cup* of brewed and instant coffee.

Component	Filter brew	Instant
Caffeine	11	58
Minerals	400	186
Organic acids	520	314
Reducing sugars	30	98
Polysaccharides	320	574
Proteins	200	244
Lipids	1	1
Caramelised compounds	460	578

*Assumes 10 g of roasted coffee and 2 g instant coffee used per cup.
Data adapted from Clarke and Macrae (1993).

Table 9.9 Estimated contribution of black coffee to UK Reference Nutrient Intake (RNI).

Micronutrient	Amount from average daily coffee intake	% RNI
Niacin	2800 μg	28
Riboflavin (B_2)	7 μg	0.5
Pantothenic acid (B_5)	280 μg	Not determined
Potassium	280 mg	9
Zinc	40 μg	0.5

The macronutrient impact of coffee can be enhanced by the habit of adding sugar and milk to the beverage. There are also specialised coffee beverages such as cappuccino (which contains frothy milk and chocolate sprinkles), mocha (which contains cocoa), Viennese (with whipped cream) and Irish (which contains sugar and whisky). Coffee can also be obtained blended with other plant extracts such as chicory.

More than 700 volatile compounds in roasted coffee have been identified to date including hydrocarbons, alcohols, ketones, furans, pyrroles and pyrazines. Among the micronutrients, niacin is present in relatively high amounts as it is produced from trigonelline during the roasting process. Consequently, an average consumption of 3.5 cups per day contributes significantly to an adult's reference nutrient intake (RNI) (see Table 9.9).

(iii) Caffeine and decaffeinated coffee

Caffeine (see Fig. 9.6) comprises more than 1 and 2% of the dry weight of mature beans of *Coffea arabica* and *Coffea canephora*, respectively. Since the early 1970s, sales of decaffeinated coffee have increased markedly and currently it accounts for 23% of sales in the USA and 9% in the UK. This is the result of a growing belief among consumers that ingestion of large amounts of caffeine can have adverse effects on health (see Section 9.4.4). Tea also contains caffeine (see Section 9.3.3) but sales of decaffeinated tea (3% in the UK and 13.2% in the USA) are lower than those of decaffeinated coffee.

Decaffeinated coffee is produced at the green coffee stage, generally by extraction of the whole beans with organic solvents (Debry, 1994). The latest decaffeination technology involves the use of supercritical fluid extraction with carbon dioxide to eliminate potential health problems posed by toxic residues from extraction solvents such as dichloromethane. However, this process is extremely expensive for a commercial scale operation and to discerning consumers flavours and aromas will still be lost. In the long term, it seems likely that the increasing demand for decaffeinated coffee could be better met by the use of *Coffea* species with beans that contain low levels of caffeine. Indeed there are *Coffea* species that have relatively small amounts of caffeine in their seed (Ashihara & Crozier, 1999). Unfortunately, they are not an attractive commercial option because the coffee trees are either difficult to grow, produce small numbers of beans or make a beverage with a bitter taste. Plant breeders' attempts to transfer the low caffeine trait to *Coffea arabica* have proved difficult because *Coffea arabica* is polyploid whereas most other species of *Coffea* are diploid. As a consequence, a breeding programme to establish and stabilise a low caffeine phenotype would probably take 20 years or more. In the circumstances an alternative approach would be the use of genetic engineering to produce transgenic caffeine-deficient *Coffea arabica* (Crozier, 1997). The recent cloning of genes that encode key enzymes in the caffeine biosynthetic

pathway (Moisyadi *et al.*, 1999; Kato *et al.*, 2000) has opened up the possibility of producing such plants through gene silencing with antisense mRNA or RNA interference technology (Ashihara & Crozier, 2001). However, current consumer concerns over the use of genetically modified products in the food chain will have to be addressed before such coffee becomes widely available.

9.4.4 Health implications of coffee

Until recently, much research into the health consequences of coffee has been focused on the potentially adverse effects of caffeine. Paradoxically, although tea also contains caffeine, most interest has been directed to its potential health benefits.

(i) Effects attributed to caffeine

Biological activities of coffee are generally attributed to caffeine, which is known to influence adenosine A1 and A2 receptors, phosphodiesterases and intracellular calcium homeostasis. As a consequence, coffee is a powerful stimulant of the central nervous system, respiration, and skeletal muscles; other activities include cardiac stimulation, coronary vessel dilation, cardiac smooth muscle relaxation and diuresis (Table 9.10). Abstinence by coffee drinkers appears to be associated with a decreased alertness although

Table 9.10 Some reported effects of coffee consumption by humans.

System	Apparent effects
Central nervous system	Slight improvement in mental performance, increased 'vigilance', improved mood, enhanced depression, potentiated pain relief of analgesics, enhanced anxiety, delayed sleep onset
Cardiovascular	Tachycardia, increased blood pressure
Digestive	Heartburn, increased gastric acid secretion, gall stone formation
Respiratory	Stimulated ventilation, aggravated asthma
Endocrine	Predisposition to goitre, stimulation of adrenaline and nor-adrenaline, enhanced pre-menstrual syndrome
Reproduction and fertility	Decreased placental blood flow, decreased female fertility, increased male fertility

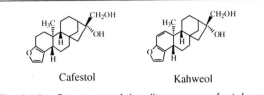

Fig. 9.10 Structures of the diterpenes cafestol and kahweol from boiled coffee.

this may be a psychological rather than pharmacological withdrawal effect (Chan, 1998). Reported unpleasant effects from caffeine include palpitations, gastrointestinal disturbances, anxiety, tremor, increased blood pressure and insomnia (Chou & Benowitz, 1994; Nurminen *et al.*, 1999). Coffee consumption has also been adversely linked to a range of conditions including cancers and heart disease. However, results from such studies have often been vehemently disputed.

(ii) Coffee and heart disease

A number of early epidemiological studies suggested that consumption of coffee was an independent risk factor for heart disease. This was ascribed, in part, to the apparent cholesterol raising abilities of the diterpenes, kahweol and cafestol (Fig. 9.10) in boiled coffee which is not widely consumed in the UK. More recent studies indicate that coffee raises plasma homocysteine concentration (Grubben *et al.*, 2000). This may be regarded as a putative risk factor for cardiovascu-lar disease (see Chapter 3). However, meta-analysis of cohort study data has suggested very little excess risk of coronary heart disease among habitual coffee drinkers, and the Scottish Heart Health Lifestyle and Risk Factor Study (Woodward & Tunstall-Pedoe, 1999) indicated that coffee consumption had mild beneficial effects on mortality and morbidity. Such apparent protection could be ascribed to the antioxidant properties of chlorogenic and caffeic acids. However, there appear to be no studies indicating that these phenolics prevent oxidation of low-density lipoprotein to an atherogenic form *in vivo*.

(iii) Coffee and cancer

Although an early ecological study (Armstrong & Doll, 1975) found statistically significant associations between coffee consumption and increased risk of cancers of the colon, rectum, breast, ovary, endometrium, prostate, kidney and testis, the majority of subsequent epidemiological studies indicated no relationship with cancer risk (Table 9.11). Of 17 studies that have assessed risk of colorectal cancer associated with increased coffee consumption, 10 indicated a possible protective effect, four no association and three an increased risk. The putative mechanisms for the reported chemopreventative effect is unclear although a number of animal models suggest that chlorogenic acid and caffeic acid inhibit chemically induced carcinogenesis of the large intestine (Morishita *et al.*, 1997). Such effects may be mediated by these phenolics inducing glutathione transferase activity,

Table 9.11 Summary of cohort and case control studies on coffee and cancer.

Type of cancer	No. of studies showing		
	Decreased risk	Increased risk	No association
Colorectal	10	3	4
Breast	0	3	22
Stomach	0	0	10
Pancreas	0	3	33
Kidney	1	1	8
Prostate	1	0	5

Data from WCRF (World Cancer Research Fund, 1997).

inhibiting the absorption of the carcinogens, modulating phospholipase A2-dependent signal transduction, and/or increasing cyclooxygenase and lipoxygenase activities.

(iv) Coffee and reproductive health

A number of animal studies have shown increased rates of fetal malformations, still births and miscarriages and decreased birth weight with high maternal caffeine intakes (10–50 mg/kg) (Christian and Brent, 2001). Some human cohort and case-control studies have also reported significantly increased risks of spontaneous abortion and intra-uterine growth retardation, generally with caffeine intakes greater than 300 mg/day (Fenster *et al.*, 1991, Fortier *et al.*, 1993, Dlugosz *et al.*, 1996, Cnattingius *et al.*, 2000). There is less consistent evidence for an association at lower caffeine intakes (150–300 mg/day). It is difficult to establish whether any association, even at high doses, is causal or might be due to potential confounders such as social factors. The assessment of caffeine intake is also difficult because of the wide variation in the caffeine content of food and beverages and this can interfere with obtaining valid interpretations from many human studies (Christian and Brent, 2001).

The Committee on Toxicology of Chemicals in Food, Consumer Products and the Environment (2002) recently reviewed the effects of caffeine consumption on reproduction and concluded that caffeine intakes above 300 mg/day may be associated with low birth weight and, in some cases, miscarriage. The evidence was insufficient, however, to define the association as causal. The current advice for pregnant women from the Food Standards Agency is to limit their intake to 300 mg/day, the equivalent of four average cups of instant coffee or six cups of tea per day.

9.4.5 Summary of coffee

Most studies on the health effects of coffee have been focused on the diverse actions of caffeine on cellular metabolism. There is little evidence that coffee exacerbates or decreases the risk of heart disease and cancer. However, animal models suggest possible anticarcinogenic activity of the coffee phenolics, chlorogenic and caffeic acid.

9.5 Cocoa

9.5.1 History

Cocoa was consumed by the Mayas before 1000 AD and the pods were used for their sweet pulp as much as 2000 years before that. As with tea and coffee, chocolate as a drink arrived in Europe in the 17th century. The first reference we have to chocolate in the UK is in an advertisement that states that 'in Bishopsgate Street, in Queen's Head Alley, at a Frenchman's house, is an excellent West India drink called Chocolate to be sold'. For more details about cocoa and chocolate, see Chapter 11.

The Western world first came into contact with cocoa at the beginning of the 16th century when Cortez visited Montezuma's court in 1519. However, the tree had already been cultivated in Central America for over 2000 years and cocoa was a major item of commerce for the Aztecs and their predecessors. The origin of the wild cocoa tree is believed to be the upper regions of the Orinoco and Amazon River systems but here the crop was never valued as it was by the Aztecs (Young, 1994). The first record of cocoa being consumed as a beverage appears to be that of Montezuma, leader of the Aztecs, who in the 16th century apparently imbibed copious quantities of a drink containing ground and roasted cocoa beans, maize meal, vanilla and chilli.

The chocolate that the Spanish found when they entered Mexico was a high-status product. Beans were both used as currency and processed into beverages, when mixed with maize flour, annatto and spices, especially chilli pepper. All these drinks were prepared by grinding the constituents together, mixing with cold water and beating to a raise a frothy head. The roasted beans were also ground to a liquid and allowed to set. The resulting block could then be transported and eaten or used as a medicine (see Chapter 11).

When Cortez revisited Spain in 1528 he took chocolate with him. The drink was at first not well received because it was too bitter but subsequently sugar and cinnamon were added and the resulting drink (still made with water) became the basis for a whole series of recipes with different spices. The Spaniards held on to the secret of chocolate for almost a century but once the secret was out its popularity spread rapidly.

The first chocolate house was opened in London in 1657, preceded by similar houses in Paris. Chocolate was so expensive that only the very rich could afford it and it was claimed to have a remarkable range of benefits, from cure-all to aphrodisiac. In 1727 Nicholas Sanders first added milk to chocolate, and the resulting drink was promoted by Dr Hans Sloane among others as healthy for both children and adults.

9.5.2 Production and variety

Cocoa is a tree that originated in the tropical regions of South America. The cocoa plant is now cultivated worldwide, major producers being the Ivory Coast, Ghana, Nigeria, Indonesia, Brazil and Cameroon. The main cultivated form is *T. cacao* var. forastero, which accounts for more than 90% of the world's usage. Other varieties such as criollo and trinitario are also grown and some regard these as providing better flavour qualities to cocoa-based products (Leung & Foster, 1996).

Ripe cocoa pods contain about 30–40 seeds, which are embedded in a sweet mucilagenous pulp comprised mainly of sugars. The pods are harvested and broken open and the pulp and seeds are formed into large mounds and covered with leaves. The pulp is fermented for 6–8 days. During this period sucrose is converted to glucose and fructose by invertase and the glucose is subsequently utilised in fermentation yielding ethanol, which is metabolised to acetic acid. As the tissues of the beans lose cellular integrity and die, storage proteins are hydrolysed to peptides and amino acids while polyphenol oxidase converts phenolic components to quinones, which polymerise yielding brown, highly insoluble compounds that give chocolate its characteristic colour (Haslam, 1998; Lass, 1999). After fermentation, the seeds are dried in the sun, reducing the moisture content from 55 to 7.5%. The resulting cocoa beans are then packed for the wholesale trade.

Cocoa beans are used extensively in the manufacture of chocolate. The nutritional implications of chocolate are considered in Chapter 11 and this chapter is confined to the use of cocoa as a beverage. To produce the cocoa powder used in the beverage, the beans are roasted at 150°C and the shell (hull) and meat of the bean (nib) are mechanically separated. The nibs, which contain about 55% cocoa butter, are then finely ground while hot to produce a liquid 'mass' or 'liquor'. This sets on cooling and is then pressed to express the 'butter' that is used in the manufacture of chocolate. The residual cake is pulverised to produce the cocoa powder traditionally used as a beverage. An alkalisation process is also often employed nowadays to modify the dispersability, colour and flavour of cocoa powders. This involves the exposure of the nibs prior to processing to a warm solution of caustic soda (Bixler & Morgan, 1999). Cocoa powder is also used extensively in products such as ice cream, cakes and biscuits.

9.5.3 Composition of cocoa

The manner in which cocoa powder is made into a beverage is very much a matter of individual taste. For example, it can be prepared using hot milk or water or combinations thereof. Sugar may also be added to allay bitterness. Consequently, assessment of the nutritional consequences of drinking cocoa is problematic. However, in general, cocoa as a beverage is a rich source of several nutrients and compounds with potential health benefit.

(i) Polyphenols and phenolics in cocoa

Polyphenols and phenolic acids comprise about 14% of dried unfermented cocoa beans (Jardine, 1999). As with tea, the dominant polyphenols in cocoa appear to be flavan-3-ol derivatives. The principle components in fresh beans are (–)-epicatechin, the dimeric procyanidins B-2 and B-5 (Fig. 9.11), the trimer C-1 and higher oligomers. During fermentation these components

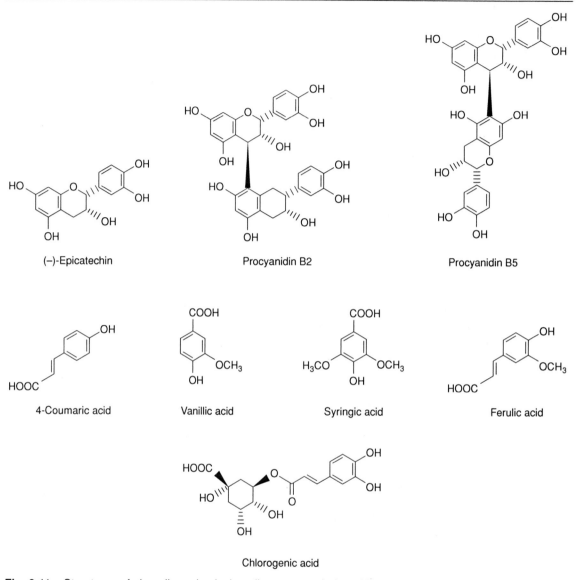

(−)-Epicatechin

Procyanidin B2

Procyanidin B5

4-Coumaric acid

Vanillic acid

Syringic acid

Ferulic acid

Chlorogenic acid

Fig. 9.11 Structures of phenolic and polyphenolic compounds found in cocoa.

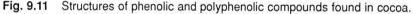

are converted to insoluble red–brown polymeric compounds of undetermined structure and as a consequence the level of soluble polyphenols falls by about 90% (Haslam, 1998; Hammerstone *et al.*, 1999; Jardine, 1999; Würsch & Finot, 1999). An 'average' home-made serving of hot cocoa has approximately 200 mg of catechin-type polyphenols (Vinson *et al.*, 1999). In addition, a considerable range of phenolic acids have been identified in cocoa, including vanillic acid, syringic acid, coumaric acid, caffeic acid, ferulic acid and chlorogenic acid (Fig. 9.11). However, there is little information on how these phenolics are affected by the production process used to manufacture cocoa powder. For example, as a result of fermentation, some conjugated phenolics may be hydrolysed by galactosidases liberating the aglycone.

Table 9.12 Composition of cocoa powder and a cocoa beverage prepared with milk.

Constituent	Cocoa, dry powder (per 100 g)	Cocoa as a beverage, prepared with whole milk	
		Per 100 mL	% RNI
Protein	18.5 g	3.4 g	6–8
Fat	21.7 g	4.1 g	–
Sugars	Trace	10.3 g	–
Starch	11.5 g	0.3 g	–
Sodium	950 mg	70 mg	4.4
Potassium	1500 mg	160 mg	4.6
Calcium	130 mg	110 mg	16
Phosphorus	660 mg	99 mg	18
Iron	10.5 mg	0.2 mg	2.3

Data adapted from Southgate (2000).

Despite possible chemical modification during preparation, cocoa does display antioxidant activity in several model systems (Sanbongi *et al.*, 1998). Such activity is comparable to that of green tea (Vinson *et al.*, 1999). In addition, consumption of cocoa is reported to delay the oxidation of low density lipoprotein *ex vivo*, which may indicate that some of the polyphenols in the beverage are bioavailable (Kondo *et al.*, 1998).

(ii) Other components

Consumption data for cocoa beverages are not readily available. For example, there is no mention of cocoa consumption in the Dietary and Nutritional Survey of British Adults. This indicates that cocoa powder as a reconstituted beverage is drunk less widely in the UK than tea and coffee and may not markedly contribute to dietary intakes of major macronutrients and micronutrients. However, cocoa powder is a significant source of several nutrients (Table 9.12).

Cocoa powder also contains zinc, copper, manganese and magnesium (Cheney, 1999). In addition, there are numerous beverage products available that contain cocoa mixed with cereals, milk solids or egg. Such products may also be fortified with vitamins. Cocoa beans, like tea and coffee, contain purine alkaloids but the major component is theobromine (Fig. 9.6) (2.5% of dry weight) with only traces of caffeine (Ashihara & Crozier, 1999).

9.5.4 Health implications of cocoa

Apart from a study in which no relationship was observed between cocoa consumption and bladder cancer (Pannelli *et al.*, 1989), there are few epidemiological studies relating consumption of cocoa as a beverage with incidences of major diseases. However, as mentioned above, consumption of 35 g of depilated cocoa delays the *ex vivo* oxidation of low-density lipoprotein (Kondo *et al.*, 1998). This may indicate that some of the polyphenols in cocoa have potentially anti-atherogenic properties (see Chapter 4) although whether such an effect is apparent using more nutritionally relevant quantities is unclear. In cell culture procyanidin oligomers from cocoa influence the transcription of interleukin-2, which could imply a potential clinical use of cocoa on disorders of activated immune function (Mao *et al.*, 1999). In addition, epicatechins in cocoa could have anti-carcinogenic properties in an analogous manner to those discussed in Section 9.3.3 for tea-derived polyphenols. However, whether effects in model systems reflect analogous responses *in vivo* remains unproven.

9.5.5 Summary of cocoa

Cocoa as a beverage is less widely consumed than tea and coffee and its nutritional impact is likely to be relatively small. Cocoa powder is a rich source of minerals and contains a range of polyphenols, in particular catechin-type polymers. Whether the antioxidant activity that these compounds confer to cocoa is translated into health benefits is not clear at present.

9.6 Wine

A source of sugar, preferably glucose, is necessary to make alcohol, so either a material that already contains a sugar is used or a source of starch is converted to sugars. Historically for the sugar route, grapes, dates, apples and pears were fermented, as were honey and sap from trees (*e.g.* coconut palm or maple) or from succulents such as agave. The starch route started from grain either using germination as in malt to provide the enzymes to split the starch. In early times, the choice of drink was determined by the type of crop available that would ferment, so the main drinks in Europe produced by these means were ale (see Section 9.8) and wine.

9.6.1 History

Wine making is as old or, if anything, older than ale production and started around the 4th millennium BC, although there are claims of evidence of wine making in the Stone Age, around 12 000 years ago. The wild grapevine originated in the Far East and Egypt and evidence for wine production dates from neolithic times. Wine was consumed by many ancient civilisations including the Mesopotamians, Egyptians, Greeks and Romans. Once the floods had receded, Noah appears to have over-indulged in wine (Genesis, Chapter IX, Verse 21) and St Paul apparently recommended the consumption of wine on health grounds (Timothy, Chapter V, Verse 23; Watkins, 1997). By the beginning of the Christian era, a great deal of wine was being produced in a number of countries and Roman authors describe the wine-

making process with appropriate advice to stop the wine going off. Pliny (who lived in the first century AD) mentions a vast range of wines, wines imported from several countries, wines from fruits and herbal wines. He estimated that there were 185 kinds of beverages available or, if varieties be reckoned with, almost twice that number. Pliny also mentioned the Greeks' habit of diluting wine. Roman vintners also knew they could recover some less than good wines, *e.g.* making it sweeter, changing the colour with potash and clarify it with egg white, alum, isinglass and gums. It is interesting to reflect on these additives and see which are now considered adulterants and which part of traditional practice. Much later, Galileo made and drank his own red wines right up to his death at the age of 78 in 1642 (Sobel, 1999).

During the Middle Ages, when the climate was warmer than it is now, vines were extensively cultivated in England, particularly in monasteries, but nevertheless most of the wine consumed was imported. The trade with Bordeaux, for example, goes back to at least 1154 when Henry II married Eleanor of Aquitaine, but wine was imported from a number of countries. Champagne was invented by Dom Perignon, the cellar-master of the Benedictine Abbey at Hautvilliers from 1668 to 1715. His contribution was not to make wines sparkling but to make sparkling wines clear. The sparkling wines that came before were generally cloudy, and not much appreciated.

9.6.2 Production and variety

'Wine' is basically fermented grape juice although the process of production can also be applied to most fruits and other plant products, *e.g.* nettles, elderflower, dandelion. This section is confined to wine manufactured from grapes.

Today, wines are produced from numerous varieties of grapes, including Cabernet Sauvignon, Merlot, Pinot Noir, Rondinella, Sangiovese, Grenache, Tempranillo and Carignan. The main commercial producers are located in France, Italy, Australia, New Zealand, Spain, Chile, Argentina, California, Bulgaria and Romania.

A wide variety of processes are used in the making of red wine. Typically, however, black grapes are pressed and the juice (must), together with the crushed grapes, undergo alcoholic fermentation for 5–10 days at about 25 °C. The solids are removed and the young wine is subjected to a secondary fermentation during which malic acid is converted to lactic acid and carbon dioxide. This softens the acidity of the wine and adds to its complexity and stability. The red wine is then matured in stainless-steel vats or, in the case of higher quality vintages, in oak barrels, for varying periods before being filtered and bottled.

White wines are produced from both black and white varieties of grapes. The berries are crushed gently rather than pressed to prevent breaking of stems and seeds. Solid material is removed and the clarified juice fermented typically at 16 °C for 5 days. The resultant must then undergoes malo-lactic fermentation, before maturation, filtration and bottling. Readers interested in obtaining further information on the procedures used for making red and white wines in different parts of the world are recommended to consult a readable and well illustrated book on the topic (*e.g.* Halliday & Johnson, 1992).

9.6.3 Composition of wine

Wines are produced from an assortment of grape cultivars grown under climatic conditions that can vary substantially not only in different geographic regions but also locally on a year to year basis. To complicate matters further, grapes at different stages of maturity are used and vinification and ageing procedures are far from uniform. It is hardly surprising, therefore, that wines are extremely heterogeneous in terms of their colour, flavour, appearance, taste and chemical composition (Singleton, 1982; Haslam, 1998).

(i) Phenolics and polyphenols

In general, red wines. and to a much lesser extent white wines, are an extremely rich source of a variety of phenolic and polyphenolic compounds (Fig. 9.12, Table 9.13). In the making of red wine, with prolonged extraction, the fermented must can contain up to 40% of the phenolics originally present in the grapes. Subtle changes in these phenolic components occur during the ageing of the wines especially when carried out in oak barrels or, as in recent years, during exposure to chips of oak wood. Consequently, there is a

Table 9.13 Major classes of phenolics in wines.

Phenolic class	Comments
Flavonols	Black grapes contain quercetin, myricetin, kaempferol and isorhamnetin as conjugates. Up to 5–50% of flavonols in red wine can be present as aglycones. White wines contain only trace amounts of flavonols
Flavan-3-ols	Red wine contains mainly (+)-catechin, (−)-epicatechin, proanthocyanidin dimers (B-1–B-4), the trimer C-1 and oligomers (tannins). Oligomeric forms increase with ageing of the wine. Small amounts only in white wine
Anthocyanins	Absent in white wines. Malvidin-3-*O*-glucoside is the main anthocyanin in most red wines and polymeric forms accumulate as wines age
Stilbenes	*trans*-Resveratrol is found in both free form and conjugated to glucose (conjugate referred to as polydatin or piceid)
Hydroxycinnamate	Wine does not contain chlorogenic acid but both red and white have substantial amounts of caftaric, coutaric and fertaric acids
Phenolic acids	Gallic acid is present in 10-fold higher concentrations in red than white wine and can be converted to ellagic acid and to pentagalloylglucose, which is the basic component of hydrolysable tannins

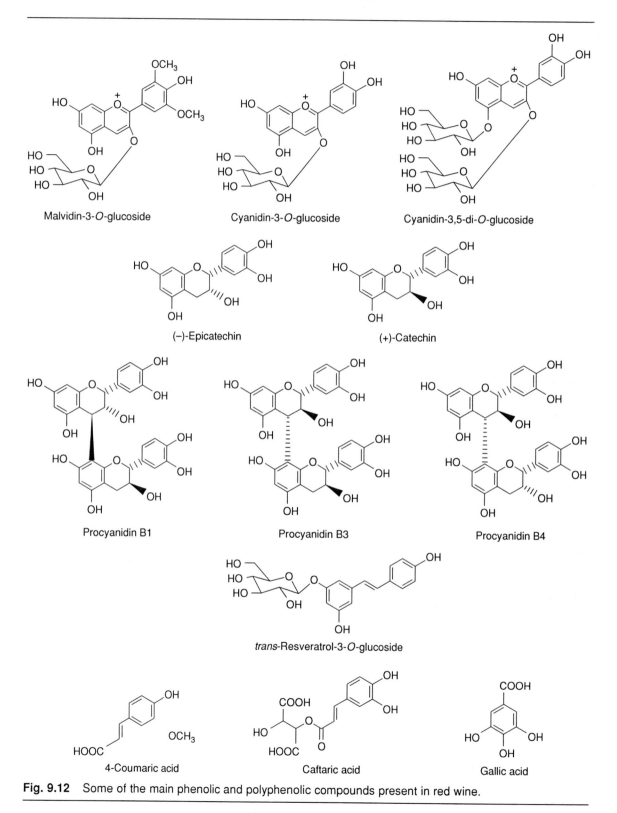

Fig. 9.12   Some of the main phenolic and polyphenolic compounds present in red wine.

wide range in the level of phenolics between different red wines, the concentration of flavonols, for instance, varying by more than 10-fold (Table 9.14).

The production of white wine results in either low levels or an absence of skin- and seed-derived phenolics, so the overall level of phenolics can be 10-fold lower than that found in many red wines (Waterhouse & Teissedre, 1997). Caftaric acid is

one of the main phenolics in white wines and the levels in Californian white wines are reported to range from 11 to 80 mg/L, with broadly similar concentrations in red wines (Nagel *et al.*, 1979).

The presence of phenolic compounds gives red wine considerable antioxidant activity *in vitro* (Fig. 9.13). This ability is closely related to the total phenol content measured in a number of assay systems, suggesting that hydrogen/electron donation from the extensive conjugated π-electron systems of the phenolic constituents is the major antioxidant mechanism. Antioxidant activity is mainly ascribed to gallic acid, anthocyanins and catechin components, with less than 1.5% being due to flavonols such as quercetin and myricetin (Gardner *et al.*, 1999; Burns *et al.*, 2000).

Table 9.14 Range of concentrations of phenolic components of red wines of different geographical origin.

Phenolics	Range (mg/L)
Total flavonols	5–55
Total stilbenes	1–18
Gallic acid	8–71
Total hydroxycinnamates	66–124
(+)-Catechin and (−)-epicatechin	8–60
Free and polymeric anthocyanins	41–150
Total phenolics*	824–4059

*Based on colorimetric Folin–Ciocalteau assay, data expressed as gallic acid equivalents.
Based on Burns *et al.* (2000).

(ii) Other components

In addition to phenols, more than 500 other compounds are present in wine. These include sugars (mainly glucose and fructose), alcohol (mainly ethanol but also propanols and butanols), volatile acids (mainly acetic acid) and carboxylic acids (such as tartaric, malic, lactic, succinic, oxalic,

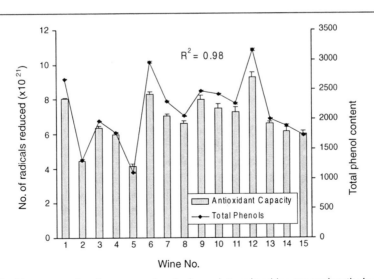

Fig. 9.13 The antioxidant capacity of a range of red wines determined by assessing their ability to reduce Frenny's radical. Capacity is closely related to total phenol content expressed as mg gallic acid equivalent per litre (based on Burns *et al.*, 2000).

Table 9.15 Typical composition (% weight) of wines.

Component	White wine	Red wine
Water	87	87
Ethanol	10	10
Other volatiles	0.04	0.04
Sugars	0.05	0.05
Pectins	0.3	0.3
Glycerol	1.1	1.1
Acids	0.7	0.6
Phenols	0.01	0.2
Amino acids	0.25	0.25
Lipids	0.01	0.02

Adapted from Singleton (1982).

Table 9.16 Content of some minerals and trace elements in wine*.

Micronutrient	Amount per glass (mg)	% RNI[†]
Calcium	4–18	0.6–2.6
Copper	0.05–0.13	4–10
Iron	0.5–1.25	5–15
Magnesium	7.5–19	2.5–6.3
Potassium	82–145	2.3–4.1
Sodium	0.6–17.5	0.03–1.1
Zinc	0.12–0.43	1.3–4.5
Pantothenic acid	0.06–0.15	0.9–2.0[‡]
Pyridoxin (B_6)	0.012–0.06	0.8–4.3
Riboflavin (B_2)	0.007–0.04	0.5–3.1
Thiamin (B_1)	0.0006–0.045	0.07–5.0
Vitamin C	1.25–1.87	3.8–4.7

*Data for red and white wines combined as there is no clear difference between the two types.
Data from several sources assuming a 125 mL glass.
[†]Adult males, 18–55 years.
[‡]This value based on US RDA.

citric and fumaric acid) (Table 9.15). Both red and white wines also contain several trace elements including iron, potassium, copper and sodium. The total concentration of minerals in wine can be as high as 1 g/L. In previous eras many wines also had potentially toxic levels of lead. This is now limited to 0.3 mg/L by the Office Internationale de la Vigne et du Vin, although levels as high as 4 mg/L have occasionally been reported in contaminated wines.

Wine consumption in the UK has increased in recent years (see Chapter 1 for trends). Consequently, wine may contribute to the daily intakes of certain micronutrients. The amounts of vitamins and trace elements in wine vary considerably (Table 9.16) and depend on numerous factors such as grape type, year of harvest and wine preparation method. For example, vitamin C is added to wine in order to stabilise the product. However, because vitamin C is very sensitive to oxygen and light it is subject to storage losses (see Chapter 12). Older wines contain at best only trace amounts. Similarly, the concentration and type of B vitamins in wine depend to a large extent on the yeast varieties used in the fermentation process.

9.6.4 Health implications of wine

Aided by popular articles and books, there is now the widespread perception that 'Wine will help you live longer. It's as simple as that' (Jones, 1995).

However, any potential health benefits must be balanced against the fact that wine contains alcohol. Excessive consumption of alcohol is a major public health problem and alcohol-containing drinks in general are identified by the International Agency for Research on Cancer as carcinogenic.

(i) Wine and heart disease

In the last decade, there have been numerous epidemiological studies and also clinical studies (measuring CVD risk factors) which indicate that light to moderate consumption of alcoholic beverages reduces the risk of developing coronary heart disease. Such protective effects have been ascribed to ethanol *per se* inducing favourable changes in high-density lipoprotein and low-density lipoprotein cholesterol, platelet aggregation and fibrolytic activity (see Chapter 4). However, strong inverse cross-country relationships between red wine consumption and heart disease mortality (Fig. 9.14) may indicate additional protective benefits in addition to that from ethanol intake, although superiority of wine

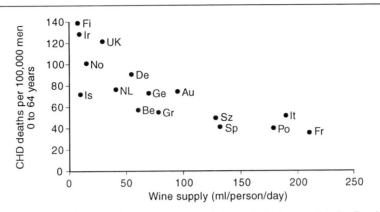

Fig. 9.14 The strong (*r* = 0.8, *P* = 0.001) cross-country relationship between standardised mortality rates for coronary heart disease calculated as an average from 1985–1987 and total wine supply. Au, Austria; Be, Belgium; De, Denmark; Ge, Germany (former West); Fi, Finland; Fr, France; Gr, Greece; Ic, Iceland; Ir, Ireland; Is, Israel; It, Italy; Ja, Japan; NL, Netherlands; No, Norway; Po, Portugal; Sp, Spain; Sz, Switzerland; UK, United Kingdom; US, United States. Data courtesy of Dr Mary Bellizi, Rowett Research Institute.

per se or red wine over white wine has not yet been satisfactorily established (see Section 1.4.8). Furthermore, several potential confounding factors remain to be excluded, *e.g.* social class (Leger *et al.*, 1979; Rimm *et al.*, 1996c; Watkins, 1997).

These 'added' benefits of wine have been ascribed in part to the antioxidant properties of the polyphenolic compounds. In particular, their ability to inhibit the oxidation of low density lipoprotein *in vitro* (see Chapter 4) has been suggested as the mechanistic explanation for the epidemiological associations relating moderate red wine consumption to a lowered risk of coronary heart disease (Frankel *et al.*, 1993). However, whether such effects occur *in vivo* is unclear as trials with human volunteers have given totally contradictory results (de Rijke *et al.*, 1996; Nigdikar *et al.*, 1998). Other proposed protective mechanisms (see Chapter 4) include the ability of wine polyphenols to inhibit platelet aggregation (Pace-Asciak *et al.*, 1995), inhibit 5-lipoxygease (Soleas *et al.*, 1997a) and induce endothelium-dependent relaxation of blood vessels, mediated by the NO–cGMP pathway (Fitzpatrick *et al.*, 1993). Although such *in vitro* results are suggestive, the health benefits of wine are unclear because large-scale intervention trials with wine or wine-based supplements and morbidity as

the end-point have not as yet been conducted. Furthermore, it will be important to exclude potential confounding factors, such as social class, in the design of future studies.

(ii) Wine and cancer

Epidemiological studies which relate red wine consumption to cancer incidence give variable results. Although many indicate that, in general, consumption of ethanolic beverages increases risk of cancer, some emphasise that this relationship is weak for red wine alone. In addition, some studies have suggested that there might be beneficial effects of wine drinking in reducing risk of some cancers (Table 9.17). Again, there is considerable potential for confounding factors to influence the association.

The inconclusive nature of the epidemiological studies may reflect, in part, potential biases in recall and the difficulty of separating effects of red wine from those of alcohol (see Chapter 3). However, some *in vitro* studies do support a role for wine in protecting against cancer. For example, red wine concentrate has dose-dependent anti-proliferative effects on breast cancer cell lines (Damianaki *et al.*, 2000) and consumption of dehydrated, dealcoholised red wine (wine solids)

Table 9.17 Epidemiological studies which consider wine in relation to cancer risk.

Reference	Cancer	Type of study	Authors' wine-related conclusion
Nanji & French, 1985	Hepatocellular	Cross-country	Intake of wine greatest in countries with highest cancer rates
Thomas *et al.*, 1983	Bladder	Case-control	No evidence that risk of cancer related to wine
Barra *et al.*, 1990	Upper digestive tract	Case-control	Wine greatly enhances cancer rate in areas with high wine consumption
Riboli *et al.*, 1991	Colorectal	Case-control	Consumption of wine not associated with cancer
Mesquita *et al.*, 1992	Pancreas	Case-control	Total wine consumption not associated with risk. Consumption of white wine inversely associated with risk
Klatsky *et al.*, 1989	Colorectal	Prospective	No relationship between wine consumption and cancer
Gronbaek *et al.*, 1998	Upper digestive tract	Prospective	Moderate wine intake does not increase risk
Chiu *et al.*, 1999	Non-Hodgkin's lymphoma	Prospective	Inverse association between alcohol intake, particularly red wine and risk
Prescott *et al.*, 1999	Lung	Prospective	Wine intake may be protective
Schuurman *et al.*, 1999	Prostate	Prospective	White wine but not red wine positively associated with risk
Putnam *et al.*, 2000	Prostate	Prospective	Wine consumption (as well as beer and liquor and total alcohol intake) was associated with an increased risk

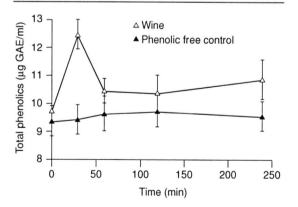

Fig. 9.15 Effects of consuming 500 mL of red wine on total phenol content (as gallic acid equivalents) in plasma of human volunteers. Adapted from Duthie *et al.* (1998).

delays tumour onset in transgenic mice that spontaneously develop externally visible tumours without carcinogen pretreatment (Clifford *et al.*, 1991). Moreover, there are now numerous papers indicating potential anticarcinogenic effects of the wine polyphenol resveratrol, which among other effects induces significant dose-dependent inhibition of proliferation and DNA synthesis in a number of cancer cell lines (Elattar & Virji, 1999).

9.6.5 Bioavailability of wine polyphenols

The ingestion of red wine results in a rapid and transient increase in total phenol content of plasma (Fig. 9.15). As yet, it is unclear which of the many polyphenols in wine are most bioavailable.

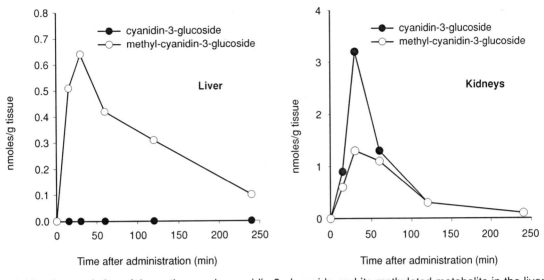

Fig. 9.16 Accumulation of the anthrocyanin cyanidin-3-glucoside and its methylated metabolite in the liver and kidneys of rats after oral administration of cyanidin-3-glucoside. Redrawn from Tsuda *et al.* (1999).

However, there is now a significant body of evidence supporting the view that flavonol conjugates are preferentially absorbed and that the nature of the conjugation may be important (Hollman *et al.*, 1995; Aziz *et al.*, 1998) (see Chapter 6). There is one report on the low level accumulation of conjugated quercetin in plasma following red wine consumption (Crozier *et al.*, 2000). The presence of (+)-catechin metabolites, mainly sulphate and glucuronide conjugates, has also been demonstrated in human plasma after the consumption of red wine (Donovan *et al.*, 1999). However, as with flavonols, the overall levels were relatively low compared with the flavan-3-ol content of the red wine itself.

Cyanidin-3-*O*-glucoside (see Fig. 9.12), a minor anthocyanin in red wine, also appears rapidly in plasma of orally dosed rats along with its degradation product protocatechuic acid. Cyanidin-3-*O*-glucoside and a methylated metabolite both accumulated in kidney tissue while only the methylated metabolite was detected in much lower concentrations in liver extracts (Fig. 9.16). In contrast to other flavonoids, no glucuronide and sulphate derivatives of cyanidin-3-*O*-gluco-

side were detected in plasma and tissue extracts (Tsuda *et al.*, 1999).

Similar data have been obtained with humans where 30 min after oral ingestion of cyanidin-3-*O*-glucoside and cyanidin-3,5-di-*O*-glucoside (see Fig. 9.12), both compounds were detected in plasma and there was an absence of sulphate, glucuronide and methylated derivatives (Miyazama *et al.*, 1999). There is, therefore, plausible evidence that these cyanidin glucosides can be absorbed from the digestive tract and incorporated into body tissues without undergoing structural modification.

trans-Resveratrol (see Fig. 9.12) appears in plasma after administration of this stilbene to rats (Juan *et al.*, 1999) and both *trans*- and *cis*-resveratrol levels in plasma, kidneys, liver and heart of rats increase following ingestion of red wine (Bertelli *et al.*, 1996). However, there are no reports on the absorption of other non-flavonoid phenolic components in red wines although the hydroxycinammates 4-coumaric acid, caffeic acid and ferulic acid have been detected in human urine after a high intake of fruit (Bourne & Rice-Evans, 1998). There is also evidence that caffeic acid is absorbed in the small intestine (Olthof *et al.*, 2001) (see Section 6.6).

9.6.7 Summary of wines

Any health benefits arising from red wine have to be considered within the context of the well-known adverse affects of excessive alcohol consumption. With this caveat, there is substantial evidence that low to moderate intakes of red wine may reduce the risk of heart disease. Although such effects have generally been attributed to ethanol *per se*, additional benefits may be linked to the many polyphenols in wine, some of which are absorbed through the gut and have been demonstrated to have potentially promising effects *in vitro*.

9.7 Spirits

9.7.1 History

Distilled drinks – spirits – were made at least 2800 years ago but in very small quantities. The technique of distillation was known to the Romans, Greeks and Arabs and even the British were distilling spirits before the Romans arrived. However, all this was on a very small scale, because the vessels were small and the process was initially used in the West mainly for perfumes or medicines. Distilling for drinks started towards the end of the 15th century. Scotch whisky was being made at least as early as 1494 when a document records that enough malt was issued to Friar John Cor to produce 1500 bottles of whisky. The name whisky comes from the Gaelic *uisge beatha* – the water of life. Rye whisky is made from malted rye, and bourbon from malted barley or wheat with maize. One difference between Irish, Scotch and Bourbon whisky is the number of times the spirit is distilled. Irish is distilled three times, Scotch twice and Bourbon only once. In addition, some whiskies are filtered through charcoal (see Table 9.18).

In 1512 a Dutch merchant decided that if he could reduce the volume of his wine by removing water he could save on shipping costs. He would then add back the water at the destination and all

Table 9.18 Basic process involved in the production of selected spirits.

Spirit	Basic process
Brandy	Distillation of wine and at least 2 years' storage in oak casks
Rum	Distillation of fermented sugar cane and storage in oak barrels
Gin	Distillation of fermented grain and addition of extracts of juniper berries
Tequila	Distillation of the fermented sap from the heart of the blue species of the agave plant
Vodka	Distillation of fermented grain followed by filtering through charcoal
Scotch whisky	Distillation of fermented barley followed by ageing in oak casks

would be well. The product he made did not turn out quite as he intended. It was called burnt wine (*Brandewijn* in Dutch), or brandy. There are now many such distilled wines, made not only from grapes but also from cider and various fruit wines, particularly plum and cherry. Cognac, probably the most famous brandy, started in the 17th century. The discovery of brandy had an impact on other wines. It was recognised that stronger wines stood up to sea journeys better than weak ones, so during the 17th century brandy was added to a wines from Jerez and the Douro, making Sherry and Port. These are the fortified wines we mainly recognise but there are others made, for example, in the south of France and in Spain.

Of the other spirits, rum is made from cane sugar and is a useful by-product for the sugar industry. Rum was first made in about 1640 and became a naval ration by 1655. In rum, brandy and whisky the source of the grain and the barrel make a contribution to the taste but in vodka the barrel seems to make all the contribution as vodka is distilled to make a neutral spirit. Vodka was invented around the beginning of the 12th century in Poland or Russia. It is distilled to high proof and then filtered through charcoal so it has precious little flavour left, other than the alcohol. Gin is also based on a neutral or tasteless spirit. It was invented as a medicinal material, an alcoholic extract of juniper and other herbs, to provide an inexpensive medicine having the diuretic properties of juniper. A Dutchman invented it and named it after the juniper berry, Geneva bess. The word gin comes from Geneva, nothing to do with the city. In 1734 over 6 million gallons of gin were consumed in England. Hogarth painted *Gin Lane* to highlight the deprivation that excess consumption caused and he contrasted it with *Beer Street*. Gin Lane was run down with drunken and dissolute people whereas the inhabitants of Beer Street were very prosperous, happy and contented.

9.7.2 Production and variety

A spirit is a beverage of high alcoholic content obtained by the distillation of fermented fruits or grains. The major difference between a spirit and other alcoholic beverages such as beer and wine is the distillation process whereby the water content is reduced by heat to prepare a liquid with a greater proportion of alcohol. Because alcohol boils at a lower temperature than water, it evaporates first and the vapour is collected and then cooled to a liquid form. The resulting 'neutral spirit' is the raw material for the production of distilled drinks such as whiskies, rums, vodkas, gins, tequilas and brandies. These beverages obtain their various characteristics through a combination of storage conditions and the addition of flavoured extracts (Table 9.18) and as a result they can contain a highly complex mixture of bioactive compounds. For the purposes of this chapter, the example used will be Scotch whisky.

9.7.3 Scotch whisky

It is believed that whisky was first produced first by the Ancient Celts. Over the years *uisge beatha* ('water of life') has been ascribed many medicinal and health-promoting properties including the relief of colic, palsy and even smallpox. Both malt and grain whiskies are produced in Scotland. Scotch malt whisky is made from malted barley, water and yeast. The barley is steeped in tanks of water for 2–3 days before being spread out on the

floors of the malting house to germinate. The plant hormone gibberellic acid is added to the germinating seed to increase α-amylase synthesis, which speeds up the hydrolysis of starch and the accompanying accumulation of sugars. To arrest germination when sugar levels are high, the malted barley is dried in a kiln, often over a peat-fuelled fire, the smoke ('peat reek') imparting a distinctive aroma to the final spirit. Subsequent mashing and mixing of the malted barley produces a wort which is transferred to a fermenting vat, where added yeast converts the sugar to alcohol. The resulting 'wash' containing about 10% alcohol is then distilled twice in copper stills and the distillate containing about 65–70% alcohol is aged in sherry casks for at least 3 years (Piggott *et al.*, 1993).

Scotch grain whisky is made from unmalted wheat, rye, oats or maize, which is first gelatinised by cooking under pressure to convert the cereal starches into fermentable sugars. A proportion of malted barley is then added to the sugar-rich 'wort'. Following fermentation, distillation is carried out in a continuously operating, two-columned Coffey still and the distillate is then aged in oak casks. Although unblended single malts are commonly drunk, most Scotch whisky bought in shops is a blend of malt and grain whiskies.

9.7.4 Composition of whisky

A blended whisky can be a combination of anything from 15 to 50 single whiskies of varying ages. Producers tend to have their own secret formula for the blending process so each whisky brand will differ in its profile of bioactive substances. Consequently, data in the following sections are approximate.

(i) *Phenolic compounds and heterocyclic oxygen compounds*

Scotch malt whiskies contain complex mixtures of phenolic compounds (Fig. 9.17) which are extracted from the wooden casks in which the maturation process takes place. The phenolic profile is influenced by several factors, including

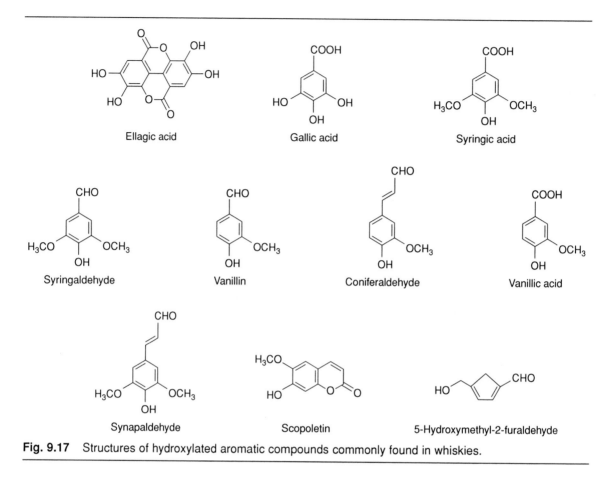

Fig. 9.17 Structures of hydroxylated aromatic compounds commonly found in whiskies.

the length of maturation, the species of oak from which the casks are made, the pretreatment of the cask by charring of the wood, prior usage of the cask for Bourbon or sherry storage and the number of times the cask has been used for maturation (Rous & Aldersen, 1983; Singleton, 1995). Simple phenolics in whisky may arise from the thermal degradation of benzoic acid derivatives from malt and peat smoke. Phenolic aldehydes such as vanillin, syringaldehyde, coniferaldehyde and synapaldehyde are formed from the breakdown of wood lignin during cask charring and maturation. Of the polyphenols, ellagic acid is generally present in highest concentration although some studies have also detected flavonoids such as myricetin, quercetin, naringenin and hesperidin. Heterocyclic oxygen compounds such as

furaldehydes (Fig. 9.17) and lactones are also present, formed from hexoses during mashing and distillation.

The presence of phenolics conveys considerable antioxidant activity to whisky *in vitro*. For example, the ability of ethanolic extracts of whiskies to quench a synthetic free radical exceeds that of white wine and is similar to that found in red wines (Fig. 9.18). In this assay system, ellagic acid, gallic acid, syringic acid and syringaldehyde account for 31–53% of the total antioxidant capacity of the whisky residues (McPhail *et al.*, 1999). This suggests that unidentified compounds, such as flavonoids from the sherry casks, or oligomer breakdown products of lignin, also contribute to the total antioxidant activity of the whiskies.

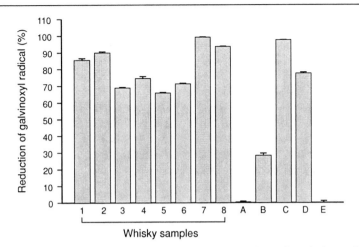

Fig. 9.18 Reduction of a 0.5 mM solution of galvinoxyl radical by ethanolic solutions of whisky residues (1–8) compared with (A) new make, which is the raw spirit prior to maturation in oak barrels; (B) white wine; (C) red wine; (D) 0.1 mM ethanolic solution of quercetin; and (E) ethanol–water control. Source: McPhail *et al.* (1999).

(ii) Other components

According to food composition tables (McCance & Widdowson, 1991), whisky contains negligible amounts of proteins, fats and carbohydrate and therefore nutritionally the alcohol is the only source of energy. Similarly, whisky is virtually free of trace elements and vitamins so consumption makes no significant contribution towards any RNIs. Although the raw spirit 'new make' contains significant quantities of copper (about 2.0 mg/L) derived from the copper stills, this tends to decrease substantially during the maturation process, presumably by chelation with the wood phenolics in the casks.

9.7.5 Health implications of whisky

As with wine, any potential health benefits of whisky must be balanced against the recognition that alcoholic drinks in general are identified by the International Agency for Research on Cancer as carcinogenic. Unlike wine, there appear to be few epidemiological studies that have attempted to relate whisky consumption *per se* to the incidences of heart disease and cancer. Therefore, it is not clear whether any perceived benefit of moderate whisky consumption is due solely to the effects of alcohol or reflects an additional therapeutic benefit from the phenolic constituents, or other characteristics of the diet. As with wine, consumption of a glass of whisky causes a transient increase in the total phenol content and antioxidant capacity of plasma, suggesting that some whisky phenolics are bioavailable and could therefore have antioxidant function *in vivo* (Duthie *et al.*, 1998). In addition, ellagic acid, a major polyphenol found in whisky, is reported to reduce significantly the incidence and number of tumours in rat medium term multi-organ carcinogenesis model (Akabi *et al.*, 1995). However, whether such potential anti-carcinogenic effects arise from moderate consumption of whisky is not established.

9.7.6 Summary of whisky

Scotch whisky contains many phenolic compounds extracted from the wood during maturation in casks. The antioxidant potential of the whisky is similar to wine and its consumption transiently raises antioxidant activity of plasma. However, there are few data to suggest that this translates into an overt health benefit.

9.8 Beer

9.8.1 History

There is evidence that the Sumerians were making ale from the end of the fourth millennium BC. Hammurapi, the king in about 2000 BC, had a code of laws inscribed upon an ebonite pillar and law 119 relates to ale and appears to describe a penalty for making ale too weak. The Sumerians used two grains for fermentation, barley and wheat. There is evidence for eight kinds of ale from barley, another eight from wheat and three from mixed grains, so there was a choice even then. However, the ale was not the crystal clear liquid we would expect today. It appears to have been a thick brew drunk with a straw directly off the grains. It has been described as the 'ferment for a day, keep for a week' variety, rather like some African brews now. The Egyptians were equally keen brewers.

Ale had a much shorter shelf-life than wine so it was brewed more frequently and more locally. In the Middle Ages every monastery or great house had its brewhouse. There were public houses and certainly after the Stuart period it was not unusual for labourers to brew their own. People drank considerable quantities of ale and it would have comprised a good proportion of the daily energy intake of labourers, who would have consumed between 4 and 8 pints a day. To combat the short shelf-life, great efforts were made to preserve ale using a whole range of herbs. It was generally agreed that ale is made without hops and beer made with hops, but recently the terms seem to have become synonymous (see below). Hops were used in Babylon around 200 BC but are first mentioned in Europe in 736 AD and then it took until the 16th century before the manufacture of beer rather than ale was common throughout Europe. On the Continent a mixture of herbs known as *Gruit* was the alternative to hops. The word is the Dutch name for the bog myrtle, but it was applied to a mixture of herbs.

There were, of course, a variety of beers. All were made from malt, but this could be from wheat or barley, and then were three extractions of the malt, giving strong beer, table beer and small beer. Strong beer could have an alcohol content as high as 9%. The flavour of ale and beer was affected by the degree of malting of the barley and the extent to which the barley was then dried or roasted – or burnt in the case of one popular beverage. Thus ale or beer and wine, with some mead and cider, were almost the sole drinks in Europe until the great explorations of the medieval period.

9.8.2 Production and variety

Beer is an alcoholic beverage made from malted grains (usually barley or wheat), hops, yeast and water. Typically, in the first stage of beer manufacture, the cereal is allowed to germinate in a warm atmosphere to activate the amylolytic diastases in the grain, thus initiating the enzymatic hydrolysis of the starches. The sprouted grains are then heated to inactivate the enzymes and the dried malt is ground and mixed with water to produce the 'wort'. Hops, which are the dried flower heads of the female hop plant (*Humulus lupulus*), are added to convey a characteristic bitter flavour to the beer. The cooled 'wort' is then inoculated with yeast to begin the fermentation process. The fermented wort is allowed to stand to flocculate the yeast. Some beers are filtered and pasteurised prior to bottling or canning. However, the clarity and stability of traditional beers is often achieved by racking and skilled cellar management.

Originally the terms 'beer' and 'ale' referred to different beverages, ale by tradition being made without using hops. Since virtually all commercial products now use hops, the term 'beer' now encompasses two broad categories: ales and lagers. Ales are brewed with 'top-fermenting' yeasts such as *Saccharomyces cervisiae* at around room temperature and the term 'ale' encompasses a broad range of beer styles including bitters, pale ales, porters and stouts. Lagers are brewed with 'bottom-fermenting' yeasts such as *S. carlsbergensis* (uvarum) at colder temperatures (10 °C) over much longer periods of time (months) and include bocks, doppelbocks, Munich- and Vienna-style, Märzen/Oktoberfest and pilsners.

Table 9.19 Summary of the characteristics of some UK and Irish beers.

Type	Country	Comments
Bitter ale	England	Most common in UK. Typically produced from malted barley and English hops
Pale ale	England	A premium bitter ale which tends to be bottled
Mild ale	England	Darker, less bitter in taste, colour derived from caramel
Scots ale	Scotland	Relatively low bitterness, creamy
Bitter stout	Ireland	Black beer with creamy head, using roasted or black malted barley

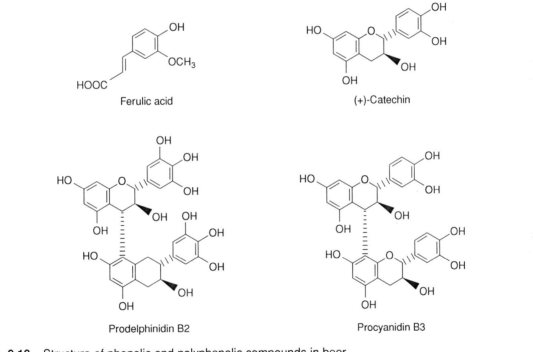

Ferulic acid

(+)-Catechin

Prodelphinidin B2

Procyanidin B3

Fig. 9.19 Structure of phenolic and polyphenolic compounds in beer.

9.8.3 Composition of beer

There are numerous varieties of beer whose character depends on the fermentation conditions, strain of yeast used and post-fermentation processing (Table 9.19). Consequently, as with wines, beers are not of uniform composition and therefore the following sections give generic rather than specific information.

(i) Phenolics and polyphenols

Beer contains a range of phenolic and polyphenolic compounds, which come partly from the barley and partly from hops. Total phenolic concentrations are at least comparable to those found in white wine and may approach levels found in phenolic-rich red wines. Major phenolics include ferulic acid, (–)-catechin, prodelphinidin

Table 9.20 Estimated contribution of 1 pint (568 mL) of beer to the UK Reference Nutrient Intake (RNI).

Micronutrient	Bitter		Lager		Stout	
	Amount	% RNI	Amount	% RNI	Amount	% RNI
Sodium (mg)	51	3	23	1	131	8
Potassium (mg)	210	6	193	5	256	7
Calcium (mg)	45	6	23	3	45	6
Magnesium (mg)	40	13	34	11	45	15
Phosphorus (mg)	62	11	68	12	96	17
Riboflavin (mg)	0.2	13	0.1	8	0.2	13
Niacin (mg)	1.7	10	1.9	12	1.5	9
Folate (µg)	23	11	23	11	23	11

RNI relates to males 55 years and over.
Data adapted from McCance & Widdowson (1991).

B-3 and procyanidin B-3 (Andersen *et al.*, 2000) (Fig. 9.19). Consequently, beer exhibits considerable antioxidant activity in model systems (Fantozzi *et al.*, 1998). Moreover, some of the phenolics such as ferulic acid appear to be readily absorbed and as a result the antioxidant capacity of plasma increases after consuming beer (Bourne *et al.*, 2000; Ghiselli *et al.*, 2000), although the relevance of this to health remains unclear.

(ii) Other components

The alcohol content of beer usually ranges from 3 to 7 g/100 ml, the strength being determined by the concentration of carbohydrates in the wort. Negligible amounts of vitamins A, C, D and E are present in beer. However, it contains numerous other micronutrients so that consumption of a pint per day contributes significantly to the overall the daily intake of, for example, magnesium, folate and riboflavin (Table 9.20).

9.8.4 Health implications of beer

As with other alcoholic beverages, possible health benefits arising from potentially protective substances in beer must be weighed against the known detrimental consequences of excessive alcohol consumption. *In vitro*, beer appears to prevent mutagenesis and DNA adduct formation against several heterocyclic amines, suggesting potential anti-cancer effects (Arimoto-Kobayashi *et al.*, 1999). In contrast, some epidemiological studies indicate that moderate to excess consumption of beer is associated with an increased risk of cancer of the lung and upper digestive tract (Gronbaek *et al.*, 1998; Prescott *et al.*, 1999). Many studies have shown a link between moderate alcohol consumption and reduced incidence of coronary heart disease (see Section 1.4.8). For example, consumption of up to 1 L of beer per day is associated with a reduced risk of heart disease (Bobak *et al.*, 2000). However, it is less clear whether this protective effect is ascribed to the phenolics in beer or to ethanol alone or other factors. Additional benefits from the bioactive compounds in beer are suggested by *in vitro* studies indicating that phenolics extracted from beer and ferulic acid, a phenolic present in beer, inhibit the oxidation of low-density lipoprotein (Abu-Amsha *et al.*, 1996; Bourne & Rice-Evans, 1997). It is unclear whether such anti-atherogenic effects occur *in vivo*.

9.8.5 Summary of beer

Beer contains phenolic compounds and its antioxidant potential is similar to that of wine. Consumption of beer transiently increases the antioxidant activity of plasma, and phenolics in beer inhibit the oxidation of low-density lipoprotein and DNA damage *in vitro*. Whether these effects result in protection from heart disease and cancer is not clear. However, when consumed in moderation beer will contribute to the RNI for several essential micronutrients.

9.9 Research recommendations

- Studies are needed to establish whether the *in vitro* effects identified for tea are of biological relevance *in vivo*, in particular whether absorbed polyphenols reach and are active in target tissues. The same applies to coffee and cocoa polyphenols.
- For alcohol-containing beverages, there is a need to establish the extent to which the beneficial effects of low to moderate intakes on heart disease risk are attributed to plant-derived bioactive substances. The bioavailability of these substances and their mode of action also need to be established.
- There is also a need to understand more clearly the balance between risks and benefits of alcohol-containing beverages.

9.10 Key points

- In many biological systems, extracts of tea have a wide range of effects with potential health benefits. In cell culture and animal models they may inhibit oxidation of low-density lipoproteins and prevent mutations and have been shown to be anti-carcinogens. Much of this activity is ascribed to the polyphenolic components of tea, in particular the catechin derivatives. More studies are required to establish the bioavailability of these compounds and their effects *in vivo* before any health benefits can be established with certainty. The impact of these compounds when consumed as part of a normal diet and in amounts normally consumed by humans is not yet clear.
- Most studies on the health effects of coffee have been focused on the diverse actions of caffeine on cellular metabolism. There is little evidence that coffee exacerbates or decreases the risk of heart disease and cancer. However, animal models suggest possible anti-carcinogenic activity of the coffee phenolics chlorogenic and caffeic acid.
- Cocoa as a beverage is less widely consumed than either tea or coffee, and its nutritional impact is likely to be relatively small. Cocoa powder is a rich source of minerals and contains a range of polyphenols, in particular catechin-type polymers. It is not yet clear whether the antioxidant activity of these compounds confer health benefits.
- Any health benefits arising from alcoholic beverages have to be considered within the context of the well-known adverse affects of excessive alcohol consumption. With this caveat, there is evidence that moderate intakes of alcoholic beverages may reduce the risk of heart disease. Although such effects have generally been attributed to ethanol *per se*, additional benefits may be linked to the many polyphenols in red wine, some of which are absorbed through the gut and have potentially promising effects *in vitro*.
- Scotch whisky contains many phenolic compounds extracted from the wood during maturation in casks. The antioxidant potential of whisky is similar to that of wine and its

consumption transiently raises the antioxidant activity of plasma. However, there are few data to suggest that this translates into an overt health benefit.

• Beer contains phenolic compounds and its antioxidant potential is similar to that of wine. Consumption of beer transiently increases the antioxidant activity of plasma, and phenolics in beer inhibit the oxidation of low-density lipoproteins and DNA damage *in vitro*. Whether these effects result in protection from heart disease and cancer is not clear. Beer also contributes to the intake of several essential micronutrients.

10
Plant and Plant-derived Lipids

10.1 Introduction

Plant lipids or oils have been an important part of the human diet since time immemorial. In addition to nutrients and other constituents that plants contain, lipids are also important because they add flavour to, and enhance the palatability of, foods. Fat in small amounts is an essential component of the diet. Fat provides energy, carries vitamins (see Chapter 1) and contains essential fatty acids (α-linolenic acid and linoleic acid, see Sections 10.6.2 and 10.6.3). These are particularly important in the formation of cell membranes, maintaining their function and integrity. They also participate in the regulation of cholesterol metabolism and they are precursors of eicosanoids (20 carbon-derived lipids including prostaglandins, thromboxanes and leukotrienes), which act as local hormones and are involved in wound healing, inflammation and platelet aggregation and also in signal transduction mechanisms within cells (see Section 10.6.7).

Much of the interest in plant lipids and health is because of the effects of different fatty acids on CVD and associated risk factors (see Section 10.4).

There are also other lipids derived from plants and found in animal cells. These lipids include conjugated linoleic acid, CLA (unsaturated fatty acids derived from linoleic acid but with a conjugated double bond) (Section 10.7), columbinic acid (a trienoic *trans*, *cis*, *cis* fatty acid from columbine), sphingolipids (Section 10.8) and plant stanols and sterols (Section 10.9). These plant-derived lipids are generating much interest

for their possible beneficial effects particularly with respect to CVD and cancer.

10.2 Structure and function of lipids

Lipids in foods are known as fats or oils depending on whether they are solid or liquid at room temperature. Most of the fat in food is in the form of triacylglycerol or triglyceride (TAG). This is made up of three fatty acids attached (esterified) to a glycerol backbone. There are many types of fatty acids; all are composed of a hydrocarbon chain of varying length with a methyl group (CH_3) at one end (ω or *n*-end) and a carboxylic acid group (COOH) at the other (Δ-end). The acid group is able to combine, in an ester bond, with the hydroxyl (OH) groups of glycerol. The physical properties of fats and oils are influenced largely by the nature (chain length and degree of unsaturation) of their constituent fatty acids.

Phospholipids, which contain a variety of phosphoryl head groups (*e.g.* phosphatidylcholine, phosphatidylethanolamine, phosphatidylserine, phosphatidylinositol) attached to the *sn*-3 position of the glycerol backbone with fatty acids attached to the *sn*-1 and *sn*-2 positions, are also important complex structural lipids (or fats) present in mammalian cell membranes including muscle. Meat can therefore provide significant amounts of fatty acids to a balanced diet, including polyunsaturated fatty acids, which predominate in membrane phospholipids. Similarly, phospholipids with sphingosine as a backbone in place of glycerol also play important roles in plant and animal metabolism. Sterols are an essential component of the membranes of all eukaryotic organisms. They are either synthesised *de novo* or are taken up from the environment. Their function appears to be to control membrane fluidity and permeability, and in animals they are also precursors of hormones and bile acids. Some plant sterols have a specific function in signal transduction.

10.3 Classification of fatty acids

Fatty acids differ according to:

- chain length (**C18**:2 *n*-6, has 18 carbon atoms)
- number of double bonds (C18:**2** *n*-6, has two double bonds)
- positioning of the bonds (C18:2 *n*-**6**, first double bond is six carbons away from the methyl or omega end of the chain)
- positioning of double bonds (**9,12**-18:2 *n*-6 means double bonds are between carbons 9–10 and 12–13 from the Δ or carboxyl end)
- positioning of hydrogen atoms around the double bond (*c*9,*c*12-18:2 or *c*9,*tr*11-18:2, where *c* is the short-hand form for *cis* configuration and *tr* is for *trans* double-bond configuration).

The major fatty acids in biology form a homologous series from C_2 (acetic acid) with C_2 additions to chain lengths of C_{26}. When a C_2 or C_4 unit (acetate or butyrate) is the primer in the synthesis, the series consists of even carbon numbers (C16:0, C18:0), but when propionate (C_3 unit) is the primer, the series is odd-numbered (C17:0, C19:0). Fatty acids can be saturated or unsaturated. When each of the carbon atoms (except the two at the ends of the chain) is bonded to two hydrogen atoms, the fatty acid is saturated – all the bonding capacity of the carbons is saturated with hydrogen. Examples of saturated fatty acids (SFA) include lauric (C12:0), myristic (C14:0) and palmitic (C16:0) acids (Gurr & Harwood, 1991).

When each of two adjacent carbon atoms in the chain (except the two at the ends of the chain) is bonded to only one hydrogen, a double bond exists between the pair of carbons, and the fatty acid is unsaturated. This results from the removal of two hydrogen atoms from the acyl chain.

Monounsaturated fatty acids (MUFA) (*e.g.* oleic acid, 18:1; see Section 10.5) contain only one double bond. Polyunsaturated fatty acids (PUFA) (see Section 10.6) have two or more double bonds. The major fatty acids and their metabolic derivatives in mammalian biology can be categorised into three families: the *n*-9 (ω-9) family, *e.g.* oleic acid, 18:1*n*-9; the *n*-6 (ω-6) family (*e.g.* α-linoleic acid, C18:2 *n*-6) and the *n*-3 (ω-3) family (*e.g.* α-linolenic acid, C18:3 *n*-3,). Derivatives from the parent members of these families are not interconvertible (see Section 10.6.6 and Gurr & Harwood, 1991).

There are isomers, molecules with the same atoms but differently arranged, of unsaturated fatty acids. Geometric isomers have the hydrogen atoms on the same side (*cis* configuration) or on opposite sides of the double bond (*trans* configuration). Stereoisomers have the double bonds in different positions along the hydrocarbon chain. The most important fatty acids in the diet are in the *cis* configuration, but there are some notable exceptions. An example is conjugated linoleic acid (CLA), a dienoic fatty acid with a *trans* double bond conjugated to a *cis* double bond, which is discussed in more detail in Section 10.7. Also, certain trienoic fatty acids in plants have similar *cis/trans* conjugated double bonds, *e.g.* columbinic acid, and are known to interfere with eicosanoid formation (Gurr & Harwood, 1991).

10.4 Fatty acids and health

Dietary fatty acids are important modulators of a number of physiological processes involved in atherosclerosis and so also influence risk for CVD. They are also implicated in the aetiology and prevention or amelioration of cancer (see below).

10.4.1 Cholesterol

A raised blood cholesterol concentration is a risk factor for CVD. Determining the proportion of total cholesterol found in LDL and HDL particles is an important index of overall CVD risk. High levels of HDL cholesterol reduce the risk of atherosclerosis and heart disease, whereas high levels of LDL cholesterol increase the risk. This is because cholesterol is transported from tissues back to the liver in HDL particles (clearing the blood of cholesterol), whereas cholesterol moves to and from the general tissues of the body in LDL particles (increasing the cholesterol content of the blood).

A high fat intake, and in particular a high intake of SFA, has been associated with a raised blood cholesterol level. However, some SFA present greater risks than others: stearic (C18:0) acid (see Chapters 9 and 11) seems to be relatively neutral in its effect, whereas palmitic acid (C16:0) and myristic acid (C14:0) tend to raise cholesterol concentration (Williams *et al.*, 1999b).

Increasing the proportion of unsaturated fatty acids in the diet can modify both blood cholesterol levels and TAG levels. For example, substitution of SFA with MUFA or PUFA has been found to lower LDL but not HDL cholesterol (Mensink & Katan, 1992). Diets in which SFA are partially replaced by MUFA, and to a greater extent PUFA, can achieve significant reductions in total and LDL cholesterol concentrations, even when total fat and energy intakes are maintained (Williams *et al.*, 1999b). The cholesterol-lowering effects of the plant-derived lipids stanol and sterol esters are discussed in Section 10.9.

10.4.2 Triacylglycerol

Plasma triacylglycerol (TAG) has emerged as an important and independent risk factor for CVD. A large meta-analysis showed that for every 1 mmol/L increase in plasma TAG, CVD increased by 14% in men and 37% in women (Hokanson & Austin, 1996). TAG levels can be significantly reduced by *n*-3 PUFA (British Nutrition Foundation, 1999). There is also evidence of a direct relationship between the magnitude of the post-prandial TAG response and the development of atherosclerosis (Groot *et al.*, 1991; Patsch *et al.*, 1992), although the mechanism is not clear.

10.4.3 LDL oxidation

There is much interest in the potential health effects of diets that provide a high intake of MUFA (see Section 10.5). With respect to oxidation, MUFA are less susceptible than PUFA (see Section 10.6). Thus, high MUFA diets may decrease the susceptibility of the LDL particle to oxidation (Reaven *et al.*, 1991; Aviram & Eias, 1993). This in turn may reduce the atherogenicity of the LDL particle, and the development of coronary heart disease (see Chapter 4). However, care must be taken when interpreting data from *in vitro* LDL oxidation studies. For example, consumption of *n*-3 PUFA as fish oil increases the susceptibility of the extracted LDL to oxidation by copper and ascorbate, yet these *n*-3 PUFA are regarded as anti-atherogenic.

10.5 Monounsaturated fatty acids

The most abundant monounsaturated fatty acid in foods is oleic acid (18:1 *n*-9). Rapeseed oil (known as canola oil in North America) contains 58 g of oleic acid per 100 g and is a component of many blended vegetable oils and spreads. Olive oil is the richest major source of oleic acid comprising 72 g/100 g. Although some nut oils, for example hazelnut and peanut (groundnut) oils, also contain high amounts of oleic acid (76 and 43 g/100 g, respectively) (MAFF, 1998), they make a much lower contribution to total intake.

Particular attention has focused on olive oil because it is a major component of 'the Mediterranean diet', which is associated with a lower incidence of CVD (see Chapter 3). However, this dietary pattern also provides plant foods (fruits, vegetables, grains, legumes) and fish, is relatively low in meat.

10.5.1 Olive oil

The high intakes of oleic acid from olive oil and the concomitant low intakes of saturated fatty acids, compared with the higher consumption of the latter in northern Europe and the USA, has been proposed as an important factor in the favourable health effects of the 'Mediterranean diet' (Visioli & Galli, 1998c). It should be noted that oleic acid is not necessarily the only component responsible for these beneficial effects. In addition to its fatty acid profile, unrefined olive oil contains bioactive constituents including many phenolic compounds in the non-glyceride fraction which have antioxidant and/or gene regulatory properties which may also explain its health benefit (Wanasundara *et al.*, 1997; Visioli & Galli, 1998b,c, 2001). There are also many aspects of diet and lifestyle (for example physical activity) which could be acting as confounders, rather than a specific benefit of olive oil itself (see Chapters 1 and 3).

10.5.2 History and production of olive oil

There is archeological evidence of olive trees dating back to 6000 BC and there are frequent Biblical references. Olive oil is obtained from the olives or drupes (fruits) of *Olea europea*, a tree that is best grown between the 30th and 45th parallels (see Section 7.5.1*xi*). The total world production of table olives between 1 November 2000 and 31 October 2001 was estimated to be 1342.5 thousand tonnes. The total world production of olive oil in the same period was estimated to be 2565.5 thousand tonnes (International Olive Oil Council 2002). Mediterranean countries produce more than 95% of the world's olive oil supply, 75% of which comes from the European Union. Around 8 million hectares in the Mediterranean region are dedicated to olive production, and this crop produces about 1 800 000 tons of oil (European Commission, 2000). Consumption of olive oil is increasing, albeit slowly, in non-Mediterranean areas such as the USA, Canada and Australia because of the interest in the reported health benefits of the Mediterranean diet. The worldwide consumption of olive oil increased from 1 508 000 tonnes in 1970–1 to 1 777 000 tonnes in 1995–6.

Extra virgin olive oil contains a variety of minor components that are responsible for its particular aroma and taste. In contrast to vegetable oils that are extracted from seeds by solvents, extra virgin olive oil is obtained from the whole fruit by means of physical pressure (cold pressings) without the use of chemicals. During this procedure the components of the drupe are transferred to the oil. Extra virgin olive oil contains considerable amounts of phenolic compounds and tocopherols (Ryan & Robards, 1998) and thus is more

stable than other edible oils against oxidation. Refined olive oil is processed in a similar way to other vegetable oils and has a much lower phenolic content. Refining also reduces the tocopherol content of vegetable oils.

10.5.3 Phenolic composition of olive oil

The polyphenolic compounds in olive oil are highly diverse both in chemical structure and proposed biological activity. The phenolic composition of both olive pulp and oil constitutes a complex mixture, the complete chemical nature of which has not been fully elucidated.

The phenolics in olive oil are responsible for its high stability (Tsimidou, 1998). The concentration ranges from 100 to 1000 mg/kg of olive oil, and varies according to climate, cultivar and stage of maturation of the olives, and is highest in the first-pressed oil, the so-called extra virgin olive oil (Montedoro *et al.*, 1993). The phenolic compounds in olive oil can be classified into two major sub-classes: simple and complex. The simple phenolics include hydroxytyrosol (3,4-dihydroxyphenylethanol), tyrosol and phenolic acids such as vanillic and caffeic acid. The complex group includes tyrosol esters, hydroxytyrosol esters, oleuropein and its aglycone. Other phenolics which have been identified are syringic acid, 4-coumaric acid, 2-coumaric acid, protocatechuic acid, sinapic acid, 4-hydroxybenzoic acid, 4-hydroxyphenylacetic acid and homovanillic acid (see Chapter 2). Oleuropein is responsible for the bitter taste of olives and for the browning of the olive skin (Visioli *et al.*, 1998a). It is a heterosidic ester of elenolic acid and hydroxytyrosol and on hydrolysis gives rise to hydroxytyrosol (see Figure 7.2.6).

The composition of olive oil (see Table 10.1) is very complex because the polyphenols are conjugated, and can be hydrolysed during storage, yielding aglycones. For example, 2-(3,4,4-dihydroxyphenyl)ethanol (DHPE) is one of the most abundant components of olive oil, and it accumulates during storage as a consequence of progressive hydrolysis of oleuropein. Tyrosol is derived from ligstroside, hydroxytyrosol from oleuropein, and hydroxybenzoic and hydroxycinnamic acids

Table 10.1 Major and minor components (ppm) of virgin and refined olive oil.

Component	Virgin olive oil	Refined olive oil
Phenolics and related substances	350	80
Hydrocarbons	2000	120
Squalene	1500	150
β-Carotene	300	120
Tocopherols	150	100
Esters	100	100
Aldehydes and ketones	40	30
Fatty alcohols	200	10
Terpene alcohols	3500	2500
Sterol alcohols	2500	1500

Table 10.2 Free radical-scavenging activity according to DPPH quenching test.

Compound	EC_{50}
Vitamin C	1.31×10^{-5}
Vitamin E	5.04×10^{-6}
BHT	1.05×10^{-4}
Hydroxytyrosol	2.60×10^{-7}
Oleuropein	3.63×10^{-5}

A 15 µM ethanolic solution of DPPH was added to the compounds under investigation. After 15 min of incubation, absorbance was read at 517 nm.

from the hydrolysis of flavones, flavonoids and anthocyanins (see Chapter 2). Phenolic acids present in virgin olive oil are almost completely destroyed during the refining process because they are polar compounds and removed by water.

10.5.4 Biological activities of olive oil phenolics

The uncontrolled production of free radicals is thought to be involved in a series of pathological conditions (see Chapter 4). The onset of atherosclerosis, in particular, may be exacerbated by free-radical induced oxidation of low-density lipoprotein. The phenolic constituents, oleuropein and hydroxytyrosol, have been shown to inhibit LDL oxidation *in vitro* (Visioli *et al.*, 1995). However, whether the antioxidant effects also occur *in*

vivo, and translate into reduced disease risk is unclear at present. Olive oil polyphenols have considerable antioxidant activity (Wanasundara *et al.*, 1997). In certain model systems, the radical scavenging properties compare well with antioxidants such as vitamins C and E (see Table 10.2). The relevance of such systems to *in vivo* activity is yet to be established.

The chemical constituents of olive oil may have beneficial effects that may be unrelated to antioxidant effects. Other beneficial effects that are reported are the inhibition of platelet aggregation (Petroni *et al.*, 1994), reduced eicosanoid production by leukocytes, and potentiation of the nitric oxide mediated macrophagic immune response (Visioli *et al.*, 1998a). The phenolics may modulate thrombus formation and inflammation but also play a role in host defence against parasites. Most of the *in vitro* assays of biological activity have examined the aglycone derivatives.

10.5.5 Absorption and bioavailability of olive oil phenolics

As for many of the phenolics (see Chapter 6), there is a lack of information on the absorption and bioavailability of the different phenolics in olive oil. Tyrosol and hydroxytyrosol are absorbed dose dependently in humans after ingestion and are excreted in urine as glucuronide conjugates. An increase in the dose of phenolics administered increased the proportion of conjugation with glucuronide (Visioli *et al.*, 2000). More work is required on the intestinal hydrolysis, absorption, distribution and serum levels, examining both the conjugate forms found in the oil and the aglycone forms.

10.5.6 Summary of olive oil

Although it has been proposed that the unique antioxidant properties of the phenolic compounds present in olive oil may contribute to the beneficial effects of the Mediterranean diet, it seems unlikely, given their concentration and their daily intake in countries other than Mediterranean, that they play a key role in promoting health. It is questionable whether olive oil consumption will

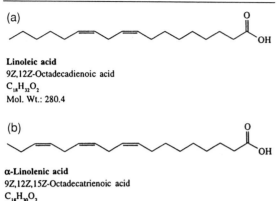

(a)

Linoleic acid
9Z,12Z-Octadecadienoic acid
$C_{18}H_{32}O_2$
Mol. Wt.: 280.4

(b)

α-Linolenic acid
9Z,12Z,15Z-Octadecatrienoic acid
$C_{18}H_{30}O_2$
Mol. Wt.: 278.4

Fig. 10.1 Structure of the essential fatty acids (a) linoleic acid and (b) α-linolenic acid. Source: The Oily Press. Reproduced with permission of P.J. Barnes and Associates 2000.

provide adequate amounts of phenolics for effects *in vivo* on platelet aggregation and LDL oxidation to be seen. Calculations from data in the literature on olive oil consumption indicate that 15–20 mg of total phenols may be supplied by the daily diet in the Mediterranean areas. However, it is not yet clear as to the bioavailability of these phenols in olive oil and their likely bioactivity *in vivo*. It is conceivable that both the high oleic acid intake, which reduces incorporation of PUFA into LDL, and the intake of phenolic antioxidants from olive oil, including tocopherol, confer health benefits, but that other components of the 'Mediterranean' diet such as fruit, vegetables and fish also have their part to play in the overall benefit to human health. Health benefits are multifactorial and are generally derived from a variety of foods in a mixed diet, not just one dietary component.

10.6 Polyunsaturated fatty acids

10.6.1 Essential fatty acids

Certain components of plant lipids are essential for the maintenance of mammalian, including human, health. Linoleic acid (LA; 18:2*n*-6, see Fig. 10.1a) and α-linolenic acid (ALNA; 18:3*n*-3, see Fig. 10.1b) are the only truly essential fatty

acids because they cannot be synthesised in the body and have to be provided by the diet. The two most important families of PUFA in mammalian physiology are derived from the parent LA and ALNA; *n*-6 (or ω-6) and *n*-3 (or ω-3) respectively. As mentioned above, the two families cannot be interconverted (see also Section 10.6.6). All other nutritionally and functionally important PUFA in mammalian metabolism, *e.g.* arachidonic acid (AA; 20:4*n*-6), eicosapentaenoic acid (EPA; 20:5*n*-3) and docosohexanoic acid (DHA; 22:6*n*-3), can be derived from the two precursors (LA and ALNA) (see Fig. 10.2) (Gurr & Harwood, 1991), although the extent to which they can be generated may be limited (*e.g.* DHA from ALNA in humans).

10.6.2 α-Linolenic acid

ALNA (C18:3*n*-3, see Fig. 10.1b) is the parent fatty acid of the *n*-3 family. It is a true essential fatty acid that needs to be ingested by mammals to ensure proper development and health (British Nutrition Foundation, 1999). It is present in varying concentrations in the leaves and seed oils of various plants and plant components, *e.g.* oils (such as walnut, rapeseed, soya and linseed oils) and some nuts (*e.g.* walnuts, peanuts, almonds), and small amounts are present in dark, green leafy vegetables (*e.g.* spinach). It is also present in oil-rich fish (*e.g.* kippers, mackerel, herring, salmon), meat (particularly from grass-fed ruminants), eggs and meat products. It is derived without modification from the land and marine plants and plankton eaten by the animals. Cereal products and milk are also quantitatively important sources, particularly where intake of oily fish is low (see Chapter 1). In humans, the synthesis of long-chain *n*-3 PUFA such as EPA from dietary ALNA occurs but the rate is low. The formation of DHA from ALNA in humans also appears to be negligible or very low. This could be because of competition for the desaturase enzymes between the LA and ALNA (British Nutrition Foundation, 1999). It is conceivable that the rate of synthesis of DHA from ALNA may be inadequate when the requirement for this PUFA is high, *e.g.* in pregnancy. It has been suggested that

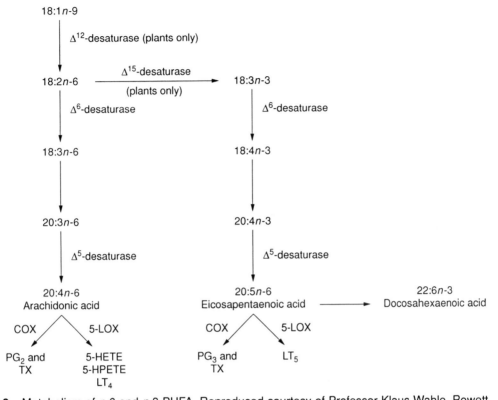

Fig. 10.2 Metabolism of *n*-6 and *n*-3 PUFA. Reproduced courtesy of Professor Klaus Wahle, Rowett Research Institute.

DHA deficiency occurs in the last trimester of pregnancy (Al *et al.*, 1994).

10.6.3 Linoleic acid

LA (C18:2 *n*-6, see Fig. 10.1a) is found in greatest natural abundance in vegetable and seed oils (*e.g.* safflower, sunflower, soya and corn oils, and in the spreads and shortenings commercially derived from them). These are the richest sources, but it is also found in nuts (*e.g.* walnuts, brazil nuts, peanuts, almonds) and seeds (*e.g.* sunflower, sesame, poppy), meat and eggs, and dairy products provide small amounts (see Chapter 1). LA was the first fatty acid to be identified as essential more than 70 years ago (Burr & Burr, 1930). Over the past 20–30 years, LA intake has been encouraged by nutritionists and the medical profession because of its essential role in healthy

development, its ability to lower blood cholesterol levels and its importance in eicosanoid production (see Section 10.6.8). Recent evidence suggests that the intake of LA may now be too high (see below).

10.6.4 Changes in intakes of ALNA and LA

Changing dietary patterns have led to a substantial change in the balance of intakes of *n*-6 and *n*-3 fatty acids (Table 10.3). Vegetable oils with a high ratio of LA to ALNA, *e.g.* sunflower and corn oils, are now widely used throughout the food industry in place of fats such as butter and lard. Meat from ruminant animals can make a substantial contribution to ALNA intake. However, the consumption of lamb and beef has fallen over the past two decades and changes in animal feeding practices, away from grass, have

Table 10.3 Trends in intake in the UK of *n*-3 and *n*-6 fatty acids.

PUFA	Intake g/day	
	1991	1995
Total *n*-3	**1.61**	**1.8**
18:3 *n*-3	1.39	1.55
18:4 *n*-3	<0.01	0.02
20:2 *n*-3	<0.01	0.03
20:4 *n*-3	0.06	0.07
20:5 *n*-3	0.04	0.06
21:5 *n*-3	0.06	0.02
22:5 *n*-3	0.01	0.05
22:6 *n*-3	0.07	0.1
Total *n*-6	**10.66**	**10.2**
18:2 *n*-6	10.48	10.04
Ratio of *n*-6 to *n*-3 fatty acids	**6.62:1**	**5.67:1**

Source: MAFF (1997).

led to lower concentrations of ALNA in meat and dairy products (British Nutrition Foundation, 1999). It has been suggested that the current high ratio of *n*-6 PUFA to *n*-3 PUFA (including the long-chain *n*-3 from fish oil) in the UK and US diets may actually have adverse rather than beneficial effects on health (see Section 10.6.8).

10.6.5 Eicosapentaenoic acid (EPA) and docosohexanoic acid (DHA)

The very long chain *n*-3 fatty acids, EPA (C20:5 *n*-3) and DHA (C22:6 *n*-3) can be synthesised *in vivo* from ALNA (see Fig. 10.2) albeit at an attenuated rate, especially for DHA synthesis. The reason why ALNA conversion to DHA is so low in healthy humans is not yet clear, but could relate to the competition for the desaturases and elongases by the high intakes of LA in current diets (British Nutrition Foundation, 1999). These long-chain *n*-3 PUFA are always associated with fish oil consumption but it should be remembered that they are also of plant origin because they derive mainly from marine algae and phytoplankton consumed by the fish (Sargent, 1997). Thus, they are provided in abundance in fish liver oils, and they are also present in the flesh of oil-rich fish (see Chapter 1). Fish have the ability, albeit

rather low, to desaturate further and elongate preformed *n*-3 PUFA such as ALNA to form DHA and EPA, but like humans, they cannot synthesise these fatty acids *de novo* (Sargent, 1997).

The possibility of producing long-chain *n*-3 PUFA from marine algae, which are thus suitable for vegetarians, is of great commercial interest at present. Such products may be particularly beneficial to pregnant vegetarian women and their infants because of the low capacity to synthesise these PUFA from ALNA in humans.

10.6.6 Synthesis of PUFA

The ω- or *n*-nomenclature describes the position of the double bonds from the methyl end (CH_3) of the hydrocarbon chain, whilst the delta- or Δ-nomenclature describes their position from the carboxyl end (COOH) (see Section 10.3). Similarly, the desaturase enzymes responsible for introducing a highly specific double bond into the fatty acyl chain are named according to the position of the double bond they introduce (see Fig. 10.2). The reason why mammals can no longer synthesise the two essential PUFA is because they have lost the ability to desaturate the acyl chain between the methyl end and a pre-existing double bond. Mammalian systems can only introduce the first double bond into a saturated acyl chain, *e.g.* of stearic acid (18:0) (synthesised *de novo* or obtained from the diet), at position Δ-9 (which is also *n*-9) which is catalysed by the Δ-9 desaturase. Subsequent desaturations can only occur between this double bond and the carboxyl end. This means that 18:1*n*-9 (oleic acid) will never be converted to an *n*-6 or *n*-3 product *in situ*. Similarly, 18:2*n*-6 can never be converted to 18:3*n*-3; the families of PUFA derived from these precursors are not interchangeable. The main desaturases in PUFA metabolism are Δ5 and Δ6. Desaturation in the Δ4-position to produce 22:6*n*-3 (DHA) is believed not to occur by a specific 4-desaturase but through a combination of elongation and desaturation of 22:5*n*-3 to 24:6*n*-3 in microsomes and then chain shortening to 22:6*n*-3 in peroxisomes. A similar pathway pertains for 22:5*n*-6 formation from 22:4*n*-6 (British Nutrition Foundation, 1999; Sprecher, 2000).

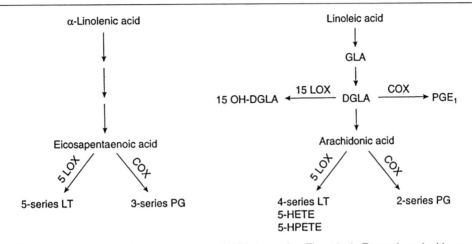

Fig. 10.3 Eicosanoid synthesis from *n*-6 and *n*-3 PUFA (see also Fig. 10.4). Reproduced with permission (British Nutrition Foundation, 2001b).

The three main families of fatty acids compete for the same desaturase enzymes with an affinity order of *n*-3 > *n*-6 > *n*-9 and consequently their relative concentrations in the diet and tissues can influence the rate of their metabolism (British Nutrition Foundation, 1999). Although both essential PUFA (ALNA and LA) and their desaturation/elongation products and products of the *n*-9 family have structural roles in cell membrane architecture, the essentiality of the essential PUFA relates primarily to their 20-carbon derivatives. These are 20:3*n*-6 (dihomo-γ-linolenic acid), 20:4*n*-6 (arachidonic acid, AA) and 20:5*n*-3 (EPA), which are themselves precursors of the 1-, 2- and 3-series prostaglandins, respectively (see Figs 10.3 and 10.4).

10.6.7 Eicosanoids

Eicosanoids are biologically active substances that are synthesised from the long-chain metabolites of LA (*n*-6) and ALNA (*n*-3). Similar substances are produced from each of the two essential fatty acid families and the two systems compete for the same enzymes (see Figs 10.3 and 10.4). Eicosanoids derived from the *n*-3 fatty acids tend to have less potent inflammatory and immunological effects than those derived from

n-6 fatty acids. Consequently, an increase in *n*-3 long-chain PUFA would be expected to reduce the inflammatory response, and an increase in *n*-6 PUFA to enhance this response (see Fig. 10.4).

The double bond positions within the chain, and the chain length of the products, are crucial for the conversion to prostaglandins (PG). These are regarded as lipid-derived second messengers in cell signalling and are responsible for regulating a multiplicity of cell functions involved in diseases such as cardiovascular disease, cancer, asthma and rheumatoid arthritis (Smith, 1992). High intakes of *n*-6 PUFA have been associated with increases in tissue AA concentrations and in the subsequent production of both 2-series PG and 4-series leukotrienes (LT) in response to various normal immune–inflammatory and oxidative stress stimuli (Wahle & Rotondo, 1999). It has been suggested that high availability of AA can result in an over-response in inflammatory eicosanoid production (Wahle & Rotondo, 1999). Such an increased production of eicosanoids may influence the risk of some diseases, *e.g.* atherosclerosis, which is increasingly regarded as an inflammatory disease (see Section 10.6.8). In particular, it is the balance between intakes of the two families of PUFA, rather than the individual levels of intake of the two families, that is a

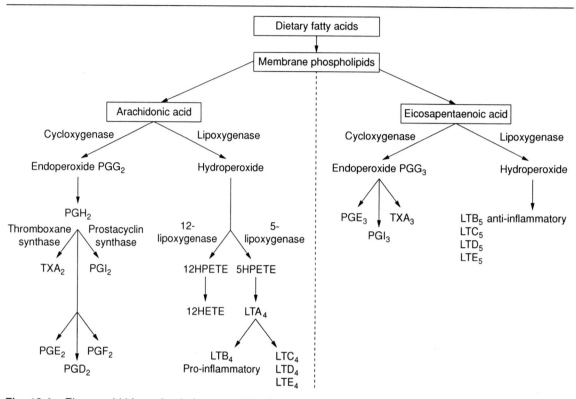

Fig. 10.4 Eicosanoid biosynthesis from arachidonic acid (AA) and eicosapentanoic acid (EPA) illustrating the COX and LOX pathways in more detail. Reproduced courtesy of Professor Klaus Wahle, Rowett Research Institute.

specific and controversial focus of scientific interest. This is because of the knowledge that the two families compete metabolically, and that a shift in their ratio may influence the types and potency of eicosanoids formed.

10.6.8 Health effects of PUFA

(i) CVD risk factors

EPA and DHA are the principal long-chain *n*-3 PUFA found in fish oils, but derived from marine plants, and are effective at lowering both fasting and postprandial TAG levels (Roche & Gibney, 1999). Furthermore, these types of fatty acids influence, in a beneficial manner, a number of other physiologically relevant mechanisms, especially those concerned with blood clotting, heart

arrhythmias, initiation of atherosclerosis, and inflammation. This may partly explain why *n*-3 PUFA intake is inversely related to CVD mortality.

(ii) Trends in intake of n-3 and n-6 PUFA

Fish and fish oils, which are rich in EPA and DHA, have been important components of the human diet throughout evolution (see Fig. 10.5). Studies of existing hunter–gatherer populations and of archeological dietary information suggests that the ratio of *n*-6 to *n*-3 long-chain fatty acids from vegetable and fish origins was about 1:1. These ratios changed little until the advent of the agricultural and industrial revolutions when cheap and plentiful vegetable oils (*n*-6 fatty acids) were included in the diets of humans

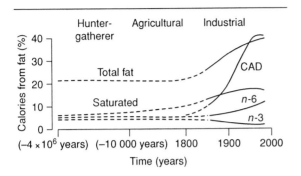

Fig. 10.5 Diagram of *n*-3 and *n*-6 intakes over eons. The figure illustrates a hypothetical scheme of the relative percentages of fat and different fatty acid families in human nutrition as extrapolated from cross-sectional analyses of contemporary hunter–gatherer populations and from longitudinal populations and their putative changes during the preceding 100 years in relation to the recent increase in the frequency of coronary artery disease (CAD) (Leaf & Webber, 1987). Reproduced with permission by the American Journal of Clinical Nutrition. © *Am. J. Clin. Nutr.* American Society for Clinical Nutrition.

and their livestock. This has now resulted in *n*-6 :*n*-3 fatty acid ratios in the human diet closer to 10–20:1 (Leaf & Webber, 1987).

The reported health benefits of high olive oil consumption in people from certain regions of the Mediterranean has been attributed in part to the concomitant lower intake of linoleic acid in these populations (Trichopoulou *et al.*, 1995). Olive oil phenolics (see Chapter 7 and Section 10.4.2) (hydroxytyrosol, tyrosol, caffeic acid, apigenin) and the well-documented high intakes of fruit and vegetables (see Chapter 3) may also contribute to the health benefits of the diets in these regions (Trichopoulou *et al.*, 1995).

(iii) Inflammatory disease

A number of diseases, including heart disease (British Nutrition Foundation, 2004), appear to involve inflammatory responses of the immune system; inflammatory cytokines such as TNF-α

and IL-1 and eicosanoids such as PGE2 and various leukotrienes are produced. High dietary *n*-6 intakes (from plant oils such as corn, sunflower and soya) are thought to result in overexpression of the inflammatory arm of the immune system (increased inflammatory cytokine and eicosanoid production), whilst EPA and DHA attenuate inflammation and inflammatory cytokine formation (see Fig. 10.4) (Calder, 1995; Rotondo, 1995). This is consistent with the observation that increased marine oil consumption may help to reduce or ameliorate the incidence and severity of diseases such as psoriasis, rheumatoid arthritis, ulcerative colitis, inflammatory bowel disease, Crohn's disease, cancer cachexia and asthma. However, whilst there are some trial data for rheumatoid arthritis, the evidence for effects in other conditions is much weaker (British Nutrition Foundation, 1999), although supportive evidence is accumulating. An in-depth discussion of the potential beneficial effects of marine oils on CVD and cancer is outside the remit of this chapter, but findings can be found in the literature (Brown & Wahle, 1990; Collie-Deguid & Wahle, 1996).

The *n*-6:*n*-3 ratios may influence risk of a number of diseases, particularly those with an inflammatory background. Ratios of *n*-6 to *n*-3 fatty acids in the diet of industrialised populations vary from 10:1 to about 20:1, and, consequently a number of expert panels have recommended a reduction in *n*-6 and an increase in *n*-3 PUFA to give ratios closer to the suggested ideal of 4–5:1 [see summary (British Nutrition Foundation, 1999)]. It has been hypothesised by some that the current high ratio of *n*-6 PUFA to *n*-3 PUFA intake in countries such as the UK and USA may contribute, at least in part, to risk of heart disease, cancer, a number of inflammatory disorders and allergies (Simopoulos, 1999). One of the outcomes of a recent workshop was the suggestion that an *n*-6:*n*-3 ratio of about 4–5:1 might be 'optimal' or desirable (Simopoulos *et al.*, 2000). However, others have recommended that much more research is needed, particularly with respect to potential mechanisms and optimum intakes of these fatty acids (British Nutrition Foundation, 1999).

(iv) Fetal and infant health

ALNA is the main form of *n*-3 PUFA in vegetarian and omnivorous diets, and there is still debate about the adequacy of dietary ALNA in providing optimum tissue concentrations of longer chain *n*-3 PUFA (British Nutrition Foundation, 2001b). This is particularly important for DHA in pregnant women because this fatty acid is crucial for the structure and function of the fetal brain and retina. It is conceivable that the high intake of LA in Western diets could reduce ALNA conversion to its longer chain derivatives through substrate competition at the level of the desaturase enzymes (see Sections 10.6.5 and 10.6.6). This point awaits experimental verification. Recent findings suggest that conversion of ALNA to EPA occurs at a significant rate but that DHA formation is negligible from ALNA (Sanderson, 2002a,b). It has been reported that supplementation of pre-formed long-chain fish oil *n*-3 PUFA to pregnant mothers prolongs gestation slightly, increases birthweight and elicits developmental benefits to the newborn infant (Olsen *et al.*, 1992). More studies on this topic are required to corroborate these findings.

The current balance of *n*-6 and *n*-3 fatty acids in the diet may influence growth and development, including brain and vision development, of the unborn and newly born infant, at least in the short to medium term (Carlson *et al.*, 1994; Uauy-Dagach *et al.*, 1994; British Nutrition Foundation, 1999; Innis *et al.*, 1999; SanGiovanni *et al.*, 2000). Global figures suggest that, on average, about 0.35% of the fatty acids in breast milk is DHA and 0.3–0.55% is AA. However, these values have wide ranges: values in the USA are 0.1–0.15% DHA and 0.1% AA, whereas in Japan average values are 1.9 and 3.0% respectively.

Grandmother's adage that fish is good for the brain appears to have gained scientific backing. Some national and international committees are now recommending increased fish or fish oil intakes in pregnant mothers and the inclusion of DHA in infant milk formulas. There is good evidence in relation to preterm infants who are less able than term infants to elongate the parent ALNA to longer chain PUFA (LC-PUFA)

(Simmer, 2001a,b). Published studies of randomised trials examining LC-PUFA status and functional outcomes were critically reviewed recently. After a workshop, international experts working in the field concluded that breastfeeding (which supplies preformed LC-PUFA) is the preferred method of feeding, and that infant formulas for term infants should contain at least 0.35% DHA and 0.4% AA. The workshop participants also recommended that because higher levels might confer additional benefits, these should be further investigated, because optimal intakes for preterm and term infants remain to be defined. It was considered premature to recommend specific intakes for pregnant and lactating women, but that it was prudent for them to include some food sources of DHA in view of the assumed increase in LC-PUFA demand and the relationship between maternal and fetal DHA status (Koletzko *et al.*, 2001).

10.7 Conjugated linoleic acid and its isomers

Conjugated linoleic acid (CLA) (see Fig. 10.6) is an intermediate in the conversion of forage linoleic acid to oleic acid by rumen bacteria (particularly *Butyrivibrio fibrisolvens*) and is found in milk, dairy products and the meat of ruminant animals. The acronym CLA is a collective term used to describe a mixture of positional and geometric isomers of linoleic acid (9*c*, 12*c*-18:2). CLA has the same chain length as linoleic acid, but the double bonds are conjugated, that is, attached to adjacent carbon atoms separated by a single carbon bond (thus 9*c*, 11*c*-18:2), rather than separated by two or more such bonds. The bonds in CLA can be either *trans* (*t*) or *cis* (*c*) configuration (see Section 10.3). In recent years, conjugated linoleic acids (CLA, *cis*, *trans* isomers of conjugated octadecadienoic acid; 18:2), derivatives of plant-derived linoleic acid, have aroused a great deal of interest because of their reported beneficial effects in reducing indices of disease, particularly cancer, in cell culture, in animal models (Pariza, 1999; Parodi, 1999), and possibly in humans (Calder, 2002; Majumder *et al.*, 2002).

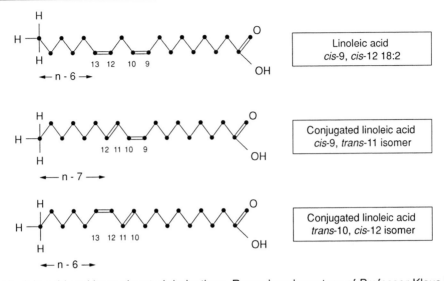

Fig. 10.6 Linoleic acid and its conjugated derivatives. Reproduced courtesy of Professor Klaus Wahle, Rowett Research Institute.

10.7.1 Occurrence of CLA

A wide range of fatty acids containing natural conjugated double bonds occur in plant lipids, mainly in seed oils, *e.g.* columbinic acid (a *trans, cis, cis*-trienoic fatty acid) from columbine seeds. However, the more common dietary vegetable oils only contain conjugated fatty acids, mainly CLA isomers, as a result of refining and processing (Hopkins, 1972). Heating, bleaching and deodorisation can contribute slightly to CLA formation, but the major process that can result in CLA contents ranging from 0.3 to 1.9% of total fatty acids, is partial catalytic hydrogenation or hardening (used in the commercial preparation of various margarines and shortenings) (Parodi, 1999). It should also be mentioned that this process produces *trans*-monoenoic, *trans, trans*-dienoic and various *cis, trans*- and *trans, cis*-dienoic isomers of mainly carbon-18 fatty acids (Pariza, 1999; Parodi, 1999). *trans*-Fatty acids are regarded as being detrimental to human health owing to their adverse influence on plasma lipids and inhibitory effects on EFA metabolism, although this is still somewhat controversial (British Nutrition Foundation, 1995b). Consequently, the evidence for potential health effects of CLA (see Sections 10.7.4, 10.7.5 and 10.7.6) is somewhat inconsistent and their mechanisms of action are unclear at present.

10.7.2 Sources

The richest natural source of CLA in the human food chain is ruminant tissue derivatives, particularly dairy products such as milk and cheese, but also meat (Mulvihill, 2001). The presence of CLA in milk was shown in the early 1930s. The CLA content of milk and meat can be enhanced by feeding programmes, although there is considerable individual variation in the response among cows (Pariza, 1999). Work is under way in the UK to determine if variations in feeding regimens can affect the ratios in ruminant meat and milk (Shepherd, 2001).

10.7.3 Intakes

Earlier estimates of the average daily consumption of CLA ranged from 0.5 to 1.5 g/day (Chin *et al.*, 1992; Fritsche & Steinhart, 1998), but a study in Sweden suggests that intakes there are much lower at around 0.16 g/day (Jiang *et al.*, 1999). Williams, from published reports on CLA, calculated that intakes effective in reducing tumorigenesis, atherogenesis and lipogenesis in experimental animals varied between 40 mg and 4 g/kg body weight (Williams, 2000). This equates to a range of 3–400 g/day in humans. Clearly, feasible intakes in humans would be at the lowest level of this range. Intakes of 2–3 g/day in human volunteers have elicited significant effects on immune function (Mohede *et al.*, 2001), and body composition (see below).

10.7.4 Effects of CLA on body composition

(i) Animal species

Evidence that dietary CLA can alter body composition is well documented in a variety of animal species including pigs, mice, rats and chicks (Pariza, 1999; Blankson *et al.*, 2000). Recent research clearly shows that the two major CLA isomers (*cis*-9,*trans*-11 and *trans*-10,*cis*-12) elicit markedly different and distinct physiological effects in animals. Feeding the *trans*-10,*cis*-12 isomer, but not the *cis*-9,*trans*-11 isomer, resulted in marked body composition changes (reduced body fat, increased body water, body protein and body ash) in mice and hamsters (De Deckere *et al.*, 1999; Park, 1999).

(ii) Humans

The effect of CLA on human body composition is not as convincing as in animals, and this may relate to the stage of growth. Most studies with animals that have shown a positive effect of CLA on body composition were conducted in growing animals and the concentrations of CLA used were comparatively high on a body weight basis. Most studies in humans are with adults and some have been reviewed recently (Calder, 2002). Supplementing the diets of obese and overweight volunteers for 12 weeks with a mixture of CLA isomers (0.0–6.8 g/day), with equal concentrations of the two main isomers, significantly reduced the body fat mass but not body weight or body mass index at supplementation levels of 3.4 and 6.8 g/day (Blankson *et al.*, 2000). A study with trained athletes showed that CLA reduced body fat content to a greater extent than in non-athletes and authors suggested that CLA prevented adipose 'refilling' (Thom *et al.*, 2001). A 1.2% reduction in body fat was also obtained when non-obese volunteers were given 4.2 g/day of a CLA mix (Riserus *et al.*, 2001). However, no differences were observed between obese volunteers receiving either 2.7 g/day of CLA or a placebo supplement (Atkinson, 1999). In this study, a sub-population of the 80 obese volunteers exhibited a statistically significant reduction in body fat with CLA and some showed increased lean body mass. Although the dose of CLA and the number of subjects was small this study indicated the possibility that certain sub-sections of the population were more sensitive or responsive to the effects of CLA than were others. Higher doses of CLA using weight gaining or growing subjects need to be investigated before a definitive statement regarding the effects of CLA on human body composition can be made. The efficacy of different isomers of CLA also requires investigation under similar conditions.

10.7.5 Effects of CLA on atherosclerosis

(i) Animal models

CLA have been implicated as dietary factors capable of reducing atherogenesis. The observations to support this suggestion are largely derived from animal studies and human cells in culture. Rabbits and hamsters fed hypercholesterolaemic diets with CLA exhibited lower plasma total and LDL cholesterol, lower LDL:HDL ratios and lower triglyceride levels, and had markedly fewer atherosclerotic lesions (Nicolosi *et al.*, 1997; Kritchevsky *et al.*, 2000).

However, the attenuation of cardiovascular disease by CLA is not clear cut and the evidence for the anti-atherogenic effects of CLA is equivocal. For example, in mice, despite a similar reduction in atherogenic lipoproteins and plasma lipids, and an increase in HDL cholesterol, to that observed in rabbits and hamsters, CLA feeding induced the development of fatty streaks (Munday *et al.*, 1999). Divergent results obtained with different animal species might be explained by different susceptibilities to the atherogenic diets used. It is difficult to extrapolate between animals and humans for obvious reasons and to date reported effects of CLA on atherogenesis are almost entirely from animal models.

(ii) Cell culture experiments

Human cells in culture have also shown increased prostaglandin formation when supplemented with CLA. Increased prostacyclin (PGI_2) production in primary human umbilical vein endothelial cells (HUVEC) can, however, be regarded as a beneficial effect of CLA on vascular function (Khaza Ai, 1997). Further studies with HUVEC in primary culture have clearly shown that CLA can elicit other apparently beneficial effects on cell function. The induction of intrinsic glutathione redox enzymes at the level of gene expression and enzyme activity and attenuation of inflammatory cytokine-induced up-regulation of adhesion molecules by CLA (both mixtures and individual isomers) are mechanisms that are considered potentially beneficial in the prevention of atherosclerosis (Crosby *et al.*, 1996; Wahle *et al.*, 2001; Wahle & Heys, 2002).

(iii) Human studies

CLA are known to be susceptible to lipid peroxidation and this has been suggested as a possible mechanism for their effects, at least on cancer amelioration in animal models (see Section 10.7.6). A recent report showed that CLA induced lipid peroxidation in human volunteers, which was determined principally as an increase in enzymatically produced prostaglandin or non-enzymatically produced isoprostanes (Basu *et al.*, 2000). This is in contrast to the majority of reports suggesting that CLA reduce prostaglandin formation in animal models. Although preliminary observations are encouraging, clearly further work in humans at the level of the vascular cells and *in vivo* is required before CLA and its isomers can be definitively regarded as anti-atherogenic components of the diet.

10.7.6 Effects on cancer

The interest in CLA stems from studies reported over 20 years ago indicating that fatty acids present in raw beef exhibited anti-tumour effects and that grilled minced beef extract had anti-carcinogenic properties (Pariza *et al.*, 1979; Pariza & Hargraves, 1985). The active component was a mixture of CLA isomers. The observations kindled the present intense interest in the health benefits of these fatty acids, and their anti-cancer properties appear to be their most reproducible and consistent effect. Anti-cancer effects of CLA and its major isomers in animals have been reported by various authors (Kritchevsky, 2000; Williams, 2000).

(i) Animal models

In animal models, dietary CLA significantly suppress chemically induced tumours of the skin (Pariza & Hargraves, 1985) and forestomach in mice (Ha *et al.*, 1990) and mammary tumours (Ip *et al.*, 1991, 1994; Banni & Martin, 1998) and colon tumours (Liew *et al.*, 1995) in rats. CLA elicit these anti-tumour effects when fed as either free fatty acids or triacylglycerols (Ip *et al.*, 1995). Of major significance is the observation that the anti-tumour effects are not influenced by the amount or type of fatty acids present in the diets (Ip & Scimeca, 1997). Significant anti-tumour effects of CLA have been found in animals inoculated with human breast cancer cells which produce both focal and metastatic tumours; tumour weights and sizes were reduced and metastasis was inhibited (Visonneau *et al.*, 1997). In a similar animal host study with human prostate cancer cells, mice were fed either CLA or the parent LA from which it is derived. Tumour volume and mass were significantly decreased in the CLA group, but increased in the LA group; lung metastases occurred in 80–100% of the control (normal diet-fed) and LA group, but in only 10% of the CLA group (Cesano *et al.*, 1998).

(ii) Cell culture experiments

Studies with various human breast and prostate cancer cells in culture have also reported strong anti-proliferative effects of CLA compared with LA and some other PUFA (Schulz *et al.*, 1992; Durgam & Fernandes, 1997). CLA induced apoptosis in human breast and prostate cancer cells by up-regulating apoptotic oncogenes and down regulating anti-apoptotic genes (Majumder *et al.*, 2002; Ochoa *et al.*, 2002).

10.7.7 Summary of CLA

Care must be taken when seeking to extrapolate between rodents and humans. Many findings in animals need verification in humans before claims concerning the beneficial effects of CLA on human health can be made. Potential detrimental effects of these fatty acids also need to be elucidated. To date, the reported effects of CLA on atherogenesis are almost entirely from animal models. Research findings support an anti-tumorigenic and, to some extent, an anti-athero-genic effect of CLA in animal models of the disease and in malignant cells, but little is known about the effects of these fatty acids on atherogenesis or tumorigenesis in human subjects *in vivo*. With the exception of body fat reduction, the lack of significant health-related benefits of CLA and the lack of consistency of results between studies are most probably due to the doses and the mix of isomers used, and the characteristics of the subjects studied. There may also be synergism or antagonism between different CLA isomers. The current sources and purity of CLA differ from those used in earlier studies (Banni *et al.*, 2002; Calder, 2002). Research on health benefits of CLA in human volunteers is developing rapidly and recent findings on effects on immune function (Mohede *et al.*, 2001) look promising. The rapid developments in CLA research have led

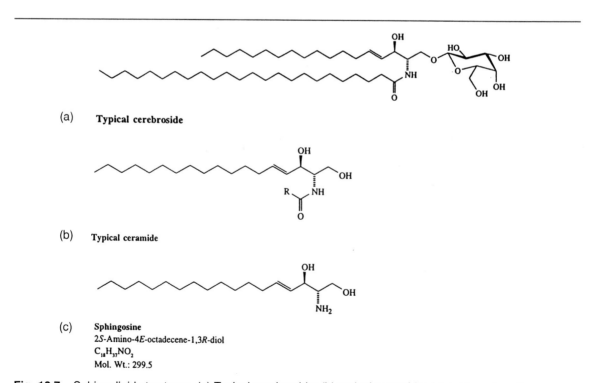

(a)   **Typical cerebroside**

(b)   **Typical ceramide**

(c)   **Sphingosine**
2*S*-Amino-4*E*-octadecene-1,3*R*-diol
$C_{18}H_{37}NO_2$
Mol. Wt.: 299.5

Fig. 10.7   Sphingolipid structures. (a) Typical cerebroside; (b) typical ceramide; (c) sphingosine. Source: The Oily Press. Reproduced with permission of P.J. Barnes and Associates, 2000.

to the establishment of a website that lists the scientific literature dating back to 1987 (www.wisc.edu/fri/clarefs.htm).

10.8 Sphingolipids

Sphingolipids are a structurally diverse class of complex, polar lipids present in all eukaryotic and some prokaryotic cell membranes and consequently they are ubiquitous in human foods of both animal and plant origin. Their contribution to the diet and reported health benefits have been reviewed recently (Vesper *et al.*, 1999; Schmelz, 2000). Sphingolipids are similar in structure to glycerophospholipids but utilise sphingosine as the 'backbone' of the diacyl ester rather than glycerol. The 'sphingosine' backbone was so named over 100 years ago because of its enigmatic or 'sphinx-like' properties (Merrill *et al.*, 1997).

10.8.1 Sources and intake

Sphingolipids are present only as minor components in most foods and their estimated average intake of 0.3–0.4 g/day in humans does not add in any meaningful way to overall energy intake. Eggs contain 2250 µmol/kg, milk and cheese 160 and 1300 µmol/kg, respectively, and meat products 400–500 µmol/kg, but soya beans at 2410 µmol/kg have the highest content (Vesper *et al.*, 1999). However, because of the actual volume/weight consumed per capita, the greatest intake of sphingolipids is from milk and dairy products, closely followed by meat products (Vesper *et al.*, 1999).

10.8.2 Structure

The structure of sphingolipids varies according to the type of food. Most sphingolipids found in plants are cerebrosides (see Fig. 10.7a) (mono- and oligohexosylceramides) such as glucosylceramides (the major sphingolipids in soya beans). Foods derived from animals (meat, dairy products and eggs) also contain lactosylceramide, sphingomyelins and gangliosides (as well as cerebrosides). Sphingomyelin is a source of dietary choline. The structural diversity achieved with the various 'headgroups' is greatly amplified by the variations in the sphingosine 'backbone' which can contain a variety of double bonds, hydroxylations and an array of amide-linked fatty acids of chain length C_{16}–C_{30} (Vesper *et al.*, 1999; Schmelz, 2000).

10.8.3 Metabolism

Sphingomyelinases, glucosylceramidases and ceramidases are enzymes that degrade complex sphingolipids in the small and large intestine but not the stomach. The resulting metabolites include free fatty acids, ceramides (see Fig. 10.7b), sphingosine (see Fig. 10.7c), sphingosine-1-phosphate and sphingamine, products which are potent regulators of cell function (Schmelz, 2000) and choline. Studies in rodents have shown that the digestion of complex sphingolipids is mostly incomplete. In similar studies with cerebrosides, the major sphingolipids in plants, 43% was excreted, with 40–70% remaining as the intact molecule and 25–60% as ceramide (Nilsson, 1969a,b; Nyberg *et al.*, 1997). These findings suggest that sphingolipids from plant foods may have a lower digestibility and might be less available, even in the intestinal tract.

Compounds not digested in the small intestine are further metabolised by colonic bacteria, resulting in partial or complete hydrolysis and increases in the bioactive ceramides and free sphingoid bases (Duan *et al.*, 1995). The observation that germ-free mice exhibit a drastic reduction in sphingolipid hydrolysis suggests that the intestinal microflora play an important role in this process (Duan *et al.*, 1995; Duan, 1996). Studies in rats and mice have shown that most of the sphingolipid metabolites are retained in the intestinal mucosa, often reincorporated into complex sphingolipids, suggesting that any beneficial effects of these polar lipids are elicited mainly in the intestinal mucosa. Only a small proportion of the metabolites is transported into the systemic circulation through lymph and blood, and so may exert their effects elsewhere (Schmelz *et al.*, 1994; Duan *et al.*, 1995). Intestinal lymph can contain about 1 nmol/mL of sphingolipid, about 40% of which is ceramide (Merrill *et al.*, 1995). It is not clear whether this is of endogenous or exogenous origin or both. For example, sphingosine-1-phosphate is also found in plasma and serum but appears to be derived from platelets (Yatomi *et al.*, 1995). Endothelial cells have a high affinity receptor for sphingosine-1-phosphate, which suggests that the presence of this sphingolipid in plasma is not an artefact (Brocklyn *et al.*, 1998).

The extent and site of sphingolipid digestion may differ between different species depending on whether the sphingolipid derives from animals or plants, and its relative transit time through the intestine (Schmelz *et al.*, 1999). The effects of metabolites of digestion may be greater in humans (who have longer gut transit times than rodents), but this has not been investigated.

Mammalian cells are able to synthesise sphingolipids *de novo* from serine and palmitic acid (Hanada *et al.*, 1992; Nagiec *et al.*, 1996). The availability of precursors might be a limiting factor in synthesis *de novo* and this needs to be investigated in humans. Long-term feeding with high concentrations of sphingolipids did not elicit any detrimental effects in animals (Kobayashi *et al.*, 1997). Incorporation of radiolabelled serine into sphingolipids is partially suppressed by sphingoid bases suggesting a degree of feedback or product inhibition of synthesis *de novo* (van Echten *et al.*, 1990).

10.8.4 Dietary sphingolipids as possible anti-cancer agents

Sphingosine and ceramide are potent modulators of cell growth, differentiation and apoptosis in most types of cells in culture (Vesper *et al.*, 1999). Both metabolites induce growth arrest and apoptosis but sphingosine-1-phosphate has the opposite effect and increases proliferation and inhibits apoptosis (Vesper *et al.*, 1999). Because dietary sphingolipids are digested to mainly sphingosine and ceramide, which is largely retained in the intestinal tract, it has been hypothesised that these metabolites, despite their low production rate *in vivo*, might be able to reduce the risk of colon cancer.

One of the earliest detectable changes in colon cancer is a defect in sphingomyelinase activity. This reduces the concentrations of available ceramide and sphingosine from endogenous cell membrane sources (Dudeja *et al.*, 1986). Dietary derived ceramide and sphingosine would bypass the requirement for sphingomyelinase activity in intestinal mucosa and mask the defect. The observation that sphingomyelin purified from milk and fed to tumour-bearing mice elicits a reduction of about 70% in aberrant colonic crypt foci, an early marker of colonic carcinogenesis, supports this hypothesis (Vesper *et al.*, 1999). A similar but larger study reported that sphingomyelin feeding suppressed the conversion of adenomas (benign tumours) to adenocarcinomas (malignant tumours) although the total number of tumours did not differ (Schmelz *et al.*, 1996). The range of sphingolipid intakes used in these studies represented 0.025–0.1% of the diet. This is greater than the estimated average consumption in human diets (300–500 mg/day for an average 70 kg person) and suggests that an increase in consumption of sphingolipid-rich foods could reduce the risk of colon cancer in humans.

Sphingosine and ceramide induce apoptosis in human adenocarcinoma cell lines HT29 (Schmelz & Merrill, 1998) and reduce tumour number in mice that have a genetic defect similar to human familial adenomatous polyposis (Powell *et al.*, 1992). The latter finding along with observations that sphingolipids can inhibit transplanted human and chemically induced tumours in mice *in vivo* suggest that these compounds can inhibit cancers at sites other than the colon (Vesper *et al.*, 1999). The reports that dairy products, which are rich sources of sphingolipids, can reduce the incidence of aberrant crypt foci in mice (Abdelali *et al.*, 1995) and reduce aberrant colonic epithelial cell proliferation, whilst restoring a normal differentiation profile (Holt *et al.*, 1998) in humans are also consistent with a reduced risk of human colon cancer (Glinghammar, 1997; van der Meer *et al.*, 1997) and support the suggestion that these compounds are also active in preventing or ameliorating colon cancer risk. The consumption of dairy products has also been implicated in reduced breast cancer risk in Finnish women (Knekt & Jarvinen, 1999). Whether this is due to milk sphingolipids, CLA or other factors requires further investigation.

(a)

(b)

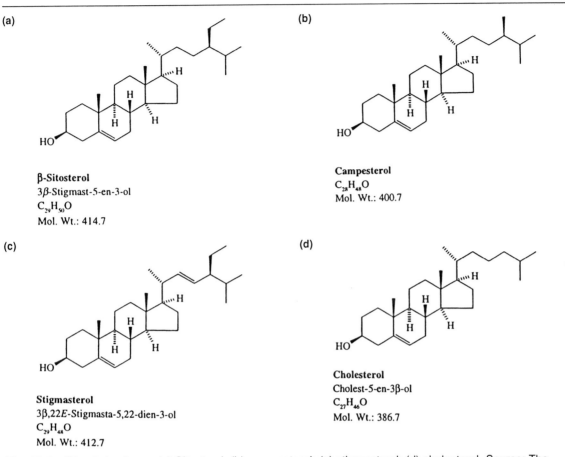

β-Sitosterol
3β-Stigmast-5-en-3-ol
$C_{29}H_{50}O$
Mol. Wt.: 414.7

Campesterol
$C_{28}H_{48}O$
Mol. Wt.: 400.7

(c)

(d)

Stigmasterol
3β,22E-Stigmasta-5,22-dien-3-ol
$C_{29}H_{48}O$
Mol. Wt.: 412.7

Cholesterol
Cholest-5-en-3β-ol
$C_{27}H_{46}O$
Mol. Wt.: 386.7

Fig. 10.8 Sterol structures. (a) Sitosterol; (b) campesterol; (c) stigmasterol; (d) cholesterol. Source: The Oily Press. Reproduced with permission of P.J. Barnes and Associates, 2000.

10.9 Plant sterols and stanols

10.9.1 Introduction

Sterols are an essential component of the membranes of all eukaryotic organisms. They are either synthesised *de novo* or are taken up from the environment. Their function appears to be to control membrane fluidity and permeability, and in animals they are also precursors of hormones and bile acids. Some plant sterols have a specific function in signal transduction. Over 250 different sterols have been isolated from plant and marine materials (Akihisa *et al.*, 1991). The most

abundant are β-sitosterol, campesterol and stigmasterol in plants and cholesterol in animals (see Fig. 2.2 in Chapter 2 and Fig. 10.8a–d).

Stanols are saturated sterols. They are less abundant in nature than sterols, but can be produced by hydrogenating sterols. 'Sterols' is sometimes used as a generic term that includes unsaturated sterols and saturated stanols.

Plant sterols are potentially atherogenic, like cholesterol, but atherogenesis does not occur because so little of the plant sterols is absorbed. The nutritional interest derives from the fact that plant sterols and stanols have a similar structure to cholesterol and some have a capacity to reduce the levels of total plasma cholesterol and LDL cholesterol. There has been a dramatic reduction in the morbidity and mortality from cardiovascular diseases using hypolipidaemic drugs (statins) and the interest in plant sterols and stanols lies in their potential to reduce blood cholesterol levels (Law, 2000; Jones & Raeini-Sarjaz, 2001).

The sterols and stanols are thought to act to lower serum concentrations of cholesterol through their ability to limit the uptake of cholesterol from the gut by competing for space in mixed micelles, and to increase cholesterol excretion. This knowledge has led to the development of specific foods with cholesterol-reducing abilities (see Section 10.9.8).

10.9.2 Structure

The sterol ring is common to all sterols; the differences are in the side chain (see Fig. 10.8). Plant sterols (phytosterols) have a similar structure to cholesterol with a 3-hydroxyl group and a double bond between carbons 5 and 6. They also contain a hydrocarbon chain at the C-24 position. They are sometimes referred to as Δ-5-sterols. They are distinguished from 'zoosterols', those present in animals (such as cholesterol which is exclusively an animal sterol), by the presence of the alkyl group at C-24 in the sterol side-chain.

Stanols are saturated sterols (*i.e.* they have no double bonds in the carbon ring). They are less abundant in nature than sterols, but can be produced by hydrogenating sterols. For example, sitostanol is a hydrogenated phytosterol, obtained as a by-product from the wood pulp industry.

10.9.3 Sources

(i) Oils

The principal natural sources of plant sterols in the diet are vegetable oils (Weihrauch & Gardner, 1978; Chan *et al.*, 1994). In plant oils the three most common sterols are β-sitosterol, campesterol and stigmasterol (see Table 10.4 and Fig. 10.8). Other sterols present include Δ-5-avenosterols, Δ-7-avenosterol and Δ-7-stigmasterol. Brassicasterol is typically found in rapeseed (canola) oil and other Cruciferaceae. Plant sterols may be present as the free sterol, conjugated as glucosides or present as acylated steryl glycosides (Wojciechowski, 1991). The esters can be found in the cell cytosol and in the storage vesicles, and are believed to provide a reservoir for the growth of new cells and shoots during the germination of seeds. Thus vegetable oils are rich sources of the sterol esters. The proportion of free sterols and steryl fatty acid esters varies

Table 10.4 Concentrations of the three most common phytosterols in some commonly consumed plant oils (mg/100 g).

Source	β-Sitosterol	Campesterol	Stigmasterol
Cocoa butter	138	22	61
Corn (maize) oil	595	179	51
Olive oil	102	2	1
Peanut oil	179	29	26
Rapeseed oil	129	95	4
Safflower oil	231	49	40
Sesame seed	430	164	60
Soya oil	194	65	71
Sunflower oil	210	32	35
Wheat germ oil	370	122	Trace

Source: Chan *et al.* (1994). The sterol contents of other oils and foods can be found in Weihrauch & Gardner (1978).

widely amongst the different oils. Free sterols dominate in soya bean, olive and sunflower oils but in rapeseed (canola), avocado and corn oils, free sterols account for only around 30% of the total (Phillips *et al.*, 1999a). Olive oil is an exception with low levels (100 mg/100 g) whereas the squalene content is high (see Section 10.5). This suggests the biosynthesis is limited to the squalene stage. Oil refining leads to a sterol loss of 10–70% depending on the oil and the processing conditions employed (Weihrauch & Gardner, 1978; Kochhar, 1983). As temperature and processing time are increased there is a further loss of sterols and some partial isomerisation particularly to the Δ-7-sterols. Campesterol and stigmasterol are less stable than sitosterol.

Only small amounts of plant stanols are found naturally in plants (Seitz, 1989; Dutta & Appelqvist, 1996) with highest amounts in bran oils. Hydrogenation of plant sterols causes the saturation of the 5,6-double bond to produce stanols. Thus, these compounds are present whenever margarines are prepared by hydrogenation of plant oils.

(ii) Cereals and nuts

At the level of the total diet, cereals are the next most important source of sterol intake, accounting for some 36% of the total intake of sitosterol and Δ-5-avenosterol and 50% of the intake of Δ-7-avenosterol (Morton *et al.*, 1995). There are considerable differences in both total sterol contents and sterol composition in terms of individual sterols and sterol-bound classes. They are also unevenly distributed within the kernel, leading to varying sterol contents in milled products. These differences are influenced by genetic background, but not apparently by the environment (Määttä *et al.*, 1999). Levels of total sources vary between 0.5 g and 1.8 g/kg sterols with sitosterol predominating. Nuts are also a good source of sterols ranging in content from 0.3 to 2.2 g/kg (USDA, 1999).

(iii) Fruits and vegetables

Fruits and vegetables are relatively poor sources of sterols. The median values of sterols in vegeta-

bles are around 100–120 mg/kg in the edible portion. Fruits show a median level of 120–160 mg/kg in the edible portion (Weihrauch & Gardner, 1978; Normén *et al.*, 1999). The lower values reported in the earlier study probably reflect the fact that an acid hydrolysis step was not included to liberate the free sterols. The predominant sterol is β-sitosterol (see Fig. 10.8a). Cooking (see Section 12.5) does not make an appreciable difference to the levels in most vegetables although, in the case of broccoli, there is a 35% decrease in levels on a dry weight basis (Normén *et al.*, 1999).

(iv) Fat spreads

It was recognised in the 1950s that plant sterols lower serum concentrations of cholesterol (see Section 10.9.6). By the 1980s it was recognised that as naturally occurring substances, plant sterols and stanols could be added to foods. Fats are needed to solubilise sterols and so fat spreads are ideal vehicles. More recently, other foods such as cream cheese, salad dressings and yogurt have also been developed. The esterification of plant sterols and stanols with long-chain fatty acids increases their lipid solubility and facilitates their incorporation into these foods (Law & Morris, 1998). The use of these 'functional foods' is discussed in Section 10.9.7.

10.9.4 Intake

The diet usually provides an intake of sterols of about 140–400 mg/day (Morton *et al.*, 1995; de Vries *et al.*, 1997; Phillips *et al.*, 1999b; Schothorst & Jekel, 1999). It has been estimated that consumers with a high intake of vegetable oils could have an intake of up to 1000 mg/day (Mattson *et al.*, 1977). Intakes are very dependent on the type of food consumed. It cannot be assumed that vegetarians are likely to have the highest sterol intake. However, it has been shown that on a diet rich in fibre (cereals, fruit and vegetables), patients with ileostomies excreted 350 mg/day of sterols (Ellegård & Bosaeus, 1991). A diet rich in shellfish (*e.g.* clams, oysters and scallops) can contain marine sterols such as brassicosterol, isofucosterol, 22-

dehydrocholesterol and 24-methylene cholesterol, thereby providing an intake which is comparable to the usual sterol intake (Lin *et al.*, 1983; Phillips *et al.*, 1999b). Plant stanol intake has been assessed to be about 10% of the sterol intake (Czubayko *et al.*, 1991). Sterols are secreted into human milk (Jensen, 1989) but at low levels compared with cholesterol.

10.9.5 Bioavailability

An important factor that determines the uptake of the plant sterols is their solubility. Many of the early experiments utilised free plant sterols, which are poorly soluble. They are also difficult to consume and variable results were produced. The dietary vehicle in which the sterols (or stanols) are incorporated is extremely important for consistent availability results to be obtained.

The intestinal hydrolysis of the conjugated plant sterols has not been studied in much detail. Intubation studies show that about 50% of the esterified sterols and stanols are hydrolysed in the upper intestine and transferred to the micellar phase (Gylling & Miettinen, 1999). The higher the free stanol content in the micellar phase, the more cholesterol remains in the oil phase, retarding its absorption. The effect is not confined to cholesterol; serum levels of plant sterols and cholestanol are also reduced. Feeding of sitosterol-rich sterols to humans lowers serum levels of campesterol but increases the serum content of sitosterol, whereas stanols lower the serum content of both campesterol and sitosterol (Vanhanen & Miettinen, 1992).

Elimination of plant sterols, mostly unchanged, occurs through bile. Biliary plant sterol secretion can be determined indirectly by multiplying their ratio to cholesterol by the daily biliary cholesterol secretion. This latter factor is calculated from faecal cholesterol elimination (including coprostanol and coprostanone).

The absorption efficiency of plant sterols can be determined using the unabsorbed marker sitostanol (Heinemann *et al.*, 1991, 1993). Other methods include the use of labelled sterols and recovery in faeces. Some 10% of campesterol is absorbed compared with 5% of sitosterol.

The absorption of campestanol has been determined to be 5% whereas only 1% of sitostanol is absorbed. Stanols have been shown to be virtually unabsorbable in intestinal infusion studies (Lutjohann *et al.*, 1995). At higher plant sterol intakes the absorption is lowered. Changes in the ratio of plant sterols to cholesterol reflect the changes in cholesterol absorption (Vanhanen & Miettinen, 1995).

Plant sterols have been reported to constitute less than 1% of the sterol in vascular walls and tissues (Mellies *et al.*, 1976). Unabsorbed sterols and their bacterial conversion products (methyl- and ethylcoprostanones and coprostanols) can be detected in faeces, mostly unconjugated (Miettinen *et al.*, 1964). Even in colorectomised patients, less than 10% are conjugated, implying that hydrolysis occurs in the small intestine. Colonic bacteria convert sterols to 5-β-coprostanes whereas 5-α-coprostanols are hardly formed. Less than 10% of faecal plant sterols are stanols from the diet (Czubayko *et al.*, 1991; Gylling & Miettinen, 1999b). The sterol nucleus is hardly degraded and since the faecal recovery of dietary plant sterols can be considered complete, they have been used as a measure of dietary intake.

Infants on formula diets that contain 300–400 mg/day of plant sterols increased their serum campesterol and sitosterol by 3–5 times higher than infants on low sterol intakes. Serum levels were similar to those seen in phytosterolaemia, suggesting that in young children absorption is high (Patel *et al.*, 1998).

10.9.6 Cholesterol-lowering effects

(i) Mode of action

Plant sterols and stanols lower serum concentrations of cholesterol by competing for space in mixed micelles. These are the packages in the intestinal lumen that deliver mixtures of lipids for absorption into mucosal cells. The added plant sterols or stanols in spreads and other products reduce the absorption of cholesterol in the gut, both dietary and endogenous (*i.e.* excreted in bile), by about 50% from the normal proportion of about half the total cholesterol to about one quarter. This reduced absorption lowers serum cholesterol despite the compensatory increase in cholesterol synthesis.

(ii) Use of free sterols and stanols

Plant sterols have been used since the early 1950s to lower serum cholesterol in hypercholesterolaemic patients (Pollak & Kritchevsky, 1981; Ling & Jones, 1995). Although perfusion experiments showed that increasing amounts of perfused sitosterol resulted in a corresponding decrease in cholesterol absorption (Grundy & Mok, 1977), it was not possible to obtain consistently similar effects from dietary administration. The early studies were performed on few patients and gave variable results. By the 1970s, the interest in using sterols had waned, partly because of these variable effects, and because studies led to an increase in serum sterol levels to those that are seen in the clinical condition of sitosterolaemia. The development of other hypocholesterolaemic agents, particularly statins, also reduced the interest in the sterols.

Early studies in humans, feeding the free stanols alone, led to a reduction in plasma cholesterol levels of around 15% after 4 weeks (Heinemann *et al.*, 1986). Later studies using relatively high doses of homogenised free stanols produced virtually no effect on serum total or LDL cholesterol in mildly hypercholesterolaemic men (Denke, 1995).

(iii) Use of sterol and stanol esters

The suggestion that poor solubility of the free stanols might be an explanation for these findings led to the development of the plant stanol esters in the early 1990s (Vanhanen & Miettinen, 1991; Gylling & Miettinen, 1992; Vanhanen *et al.*, 1993; Miettinen *et al.*, 1995). A consistent 10–15% reduction in serum total cholesterol was seen in a variety of patients when the esters were consumed in margarine or mayonnaise (Miettinen & Gylling, 1998).

This knowledge led to further studies into the effects of the sterol esters. Sitostanol esters were first used to lower serum cholesterol in small groups of mildly hypercholesterolaemic diabetic and non-diabetic people (Vanhanen & Miettinen, 1991; Gylling & Miettinen, 1992). Phytosterols added to a butter-rich diet significantly lowered serum cholesterol in normocholesterolaemic humans (Pelletier *et al.*, 1995). More recently, it has been found that phytosterols significantly reduce both total and LDL cholesterol but have no effect on serum campesterol levels or cholesterol synthesis (Jones *et al.*, 1999). The amounts of plant sterols in the diets of normal human subjects are negatively correlated with cholesterol absorption and serum total and LDL cholesterol (Gylling & Miettinen, 1997, 1999b).

10.9.7 Functional foods

The importance of utilising esters of sterols to reduce serum cholesterol has been exploited in the development of three brands of products to date: Benecol®, Take Control® and Flora Proactiv®). The former is based on a preparation of stanol esters whereas the latter products are based on sterol esters.

(i) Spreads containing stanol esters

The stanol ester margarine is reported to lower serum total cholesterol by 10–15% and LDL cholesterol by up to 20% in several studies of patients with mild or familial hypercholesterolaemia, individuals with type 2 diabetes, postmenopausal women with myocardial infarction and colorectomy, and alone or in combination with statins, neomycin and cholestyramine (Miettinen & Gylling, 1998; Andersson *et al.*, 1999; Hallikainen & Uutsitupa, 1999; Miettinen, 1999; Nguyen, 1999; Plat *et al.*, 1999; Puska *et al.*, 1999; Williams *et al.*, 1999a; Gylling & Miettinen, 1999b; Miettinen *et al.*, 2000; Plat & Mensink, 2000).

The effects are also observed in individuals with normal plasma cholesterol levels (Niinikoski *et al.*, 1997). There appear to be few effects on triglyceride or VLDL levels in plasma. An increase in HDL levels is observed only occasionally. Even with a low dietary intake of cholesterol the stanol esters also lower serum cholesterol, suggesting that the plant stanols not only inhibit cholesterol uptake from the diet but also result in an increased secretion of biliary cholesterol. The stanols are also effective when taken with a butter-rich diet.

The decrease of serum cholesterol is usually highest in people with a high cholesterol level. The sterol and cholestanol ratios to cholesterol are decreased in serum for as long as stanol ester consumption is continued. The increase in plasma sitostanol or campestanol is minimal even after long term consumption, probably because of the rapid biliary secretion of stanols. Fat soluble vitamin concentrations are unchanged, after correction for changes in plasma cholesterol, except for a decrease in β-carotene content. There have been no harmful or adverse effects reported from a careful review of clinical studies (Plat & Mensink, 1998; Plat *et al.*, 1999).

Cholesterol absorption efficiency was decreased by 45% in 52 patients studied for sterol balance on intakes of 0.8–3.0 g/day. The respective faecal level of sitostanol was 2.3 g/day, which indicates a total recovery of the dietary intake. Faecal fat or bile acids were unchanged but the reduced absorption efficiency reduced the faecal output of cholesterol by 32%, cholesterol synthesis by 15% and turnover by 10%. Precursor sterol ratios to cholesterol, which are indicators of cholesterol synthesis and were increased in serum in proportion to the synthesis and were inversely related to the ratios of cholestanol and plant sterols and cholesterol absorption. The greater the decrease in LDL cholesterol, the higher were the increments of the precursor sterol ratios and cholesterol synthesis and the decrements of the sterol ratios, reflecting cholesterol absorption, or the cholesterol absorption percentage.

(ii) Spreads containing sterol esters

Two studies have been reported using the sterol ester margarine (Weststrate & Meijer, 1998; Hendriks *et al.*, 1999). Serum cholesterol was significantly decreased by sterol ester consumption but serum sterol concentrations were increased, in contrast to the use of the stanol esters. An intake of 1.6 g/day was found to decrease serum cholesterol levels by 5–10% without seriously affecting plasma carotenoid concentrations.

Preliminary data from a large human study, in which subjects were randomised to consume a low-fat spread or up to 2.2 g/day plant sterol esters, reduced LDL cholesterol by up to 8%. Apo B levels were decreased by up to 8.4% and ratios of total to HDL cholesterol were 8% lower. Serum triacylglycerol levels decreased by up to 10%. Serum plant sterol concentrations increased by up to 48%. Serum concentrations of fat-soluble vitamins and carotenoids were generally within reference ranges (Maki *et al.*, 2001).

A study of 3 weeks duration in 15 subjects showed similar reductions of 10–13% in serum cholesterol, from a daily consumption of 1.8 g of sterol or stanol esters, versus 6% in a low-fat spread control group (Jones *et al.*, 1999). Cholesterol absorption efficiencies were decreased by 36% for the sterol ester and by 26% for the stanol ester, whereas the synthesis increased by 53 and 38%, respectively, without any change in cholesterol turnover.

(iii) Summary of effects of spreads containing sterol or stanol esters

Figure 10.9 summarises the findings of a review, conducted by Law, of randomised double blind trials in adults that compared the ability of polyunsaturated margarines with and without added plant sterols to lower cholesterol (Law, 2000). There was a continuous dose–response relationship up to about 2 g of plant sterol or stanol per day, with no further reduction in LDL cholesterol apparent at higher doses. The reduction in the concentration of LDL cholesterol was significantly greater in older people. At doses of 2 g per day the average reductions in serum LDL cholesterol were 0.54 mmol/L (equivalent to a 14% reduction) in subjects aged 50–59 years, 0.43 mmol/L (equivalent to a 9% reduction) in those aged 40–49 years and 0.33 mmol/L (equivalent to an 11% reduction) for those aged 30–39 years. The reductions in total cholesterol and LDL cholesterol were similar, with little change in serum concentrations of HDL cholesterol or triglyceride. Law also concluded that there was little differ-

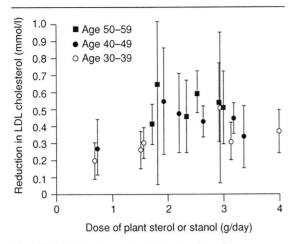

Fig. 10.9 Placebo-adjusted reductions in serum LDL cholesterol in randomised double blind trials using PUFA margarines with or without added sterols or stanols. The figure shows the mean reduction of LDL cholesterol (with 95% confidence intervals) achieved in each trial plotted against the daily dose of plant sterol or stanol used. Reproduced with permission of the BMJ Publishing Group from M. Law, *British Medical Journal*, 2000, 320, 861–4.

ence in the extent to which sterols or stanols lower LDL cholesterol concentrations, but that the confidence intervals (see Fig. 10.9) were consistent with the evidence that stanols are better.

10.9.8 Other considerations

(i) Toxicity

Rats fed 5% β-sitosterol in the diet showed no evidence of toxicity after long-term administration. Dogs fed 0.5 and 1.0 g/kg of β-sitosterol also showed no signs of toxicity after administration for up to 22 months. A similar lack of toxicity was seen in rabbits chronically fed 4% β-sitosterol or 4% soya sterols. Data on the effects of phytosterol administration have been reviewed and no effects, other than occasional diarrhoea, have been reported in people who metabolise phytosterols normally (Ling & Jones, 1995). The clinical entity of hereditary sitosterolaemia was discovered in 1974 (Bhattacharyya & Connor, 1974). The disorder was shown to be strongly atherogenic, probably due to markedly increased serum sitosterol and campesterol levels, and myocardial infarction can occur at an early age (Björkhem & Boberg, 1995).

(ii) Effects on fat-soluble vitamins

The main concern about the addition of plant sterols and stanols to foods is the potential effect on the absorption of fat-soluble vitamins. In his review of randomised trials, Law found that plant sterols and stanols lower blood concentrations of β-carotene by about 25%, α-carotene by about 10% and vitamin E by about 8% and had no effect on vitamin D (Law, 2000). Because the antioxidant vitamins help protect LDL cholesterol from oxidation, and because sterols and stanols reduce LDL cholesterol, after adjustment for this there was no effect on vitamin E, but β-carotene concentrations were reduced by between 8 and 19% (Law, 2000). Law suggested that an increase in intake of fruit and vegetables would counter the decreased absorption.

10.10 Research recommendations

• The reason why ALNA conversion to DHA is so low in healthy humans is not yet clear, but could relate to the competition for the desaturases and elongases by the high intakes of LA in current diets. This is an area requiring further research to elucidate the mechanisms involved and the conditions that give optimum conversion of ALNA to EPA and DHA. This would be of particular importance in determining intakes for vegetarian and vegan women contemplating pregnancy.

• As for many of the phenolics, there is a lack of information on the absorption and bioavailability. Further work is required on the intestinal hydrolysis, absorption, distribution and serum levels of the different phenolics in olive oil, examining both the conjugated forms found in the oil and the aglycone forms.

- Controlled dose–response studies of pure isomers of CLA are required so that their potential beneficial and adverse effects on health-related outcomes can be clearly defined. Studies investigating any synergism or antagonism between active isomers can then be conducted. Other PUFA with various conjugated double bonds also occur in plants and the study of their likely benefit in nutrition and their potential use in functional foods needs to be actively pursued.

- Complex phospholipids, such as plant and animal derived sphingolipids (sphingosine-1-phosphate and ceramides), have also been shown to regulate the function of cancer cells and endothelium *in vitro*. The relevance of this needs to be established through future research.

- For a complete understanding of the bio-availability of the plant sterols and stanols, studies are required on the intestinal hydrolysis and distribution to the micellar phase, their absorption and serum levels.

- Information is needed about the distribution of sterols to vascular and other tissues, their biliary secretion, and their excretion in faeces. Further work on determining these parameters is still required. Studies of the combined effects of sterols and PUFAs in unrefined versus refined vegetable oils on the reduction of plasma cholesterol would be useful

- Plant sterol and stanol esters are already marketed as functional foods and the claims of reduced cholesterol levels are based on solid scientific evidence. As a preventative health policy, the potential to provide an effective dose of plant sterol esters in the normal diet should be examined. This will require a more complete understanding of the bioavailability of natural plant sterols and their ability to lower cholesterol.

10.11 Key points

- Plant lipids provide energy, carry vitamins and contain essential fatty acids.

- Plant and plant-derived lipids are important for maintaining the function and integrity of cell membranes. They also participate in the regulation of cholesterol metabolism and they are precursors of eicosanoids which act as local hormones and are involved in wound healing, inflammation, platelet aggregation and signal transduction mechanisms within cells.

- Dietary fatty acids are important modulators of a number of physiological processes involved in atherosclerosis and so also influence risk for CVD. They are also implicated in the aetiology and prevention or amelioration of cancer. A number of plant and plant-derived fatty acids and lipids are reported to have beneficial, ameliorating or preventative effects on biomarkers of various disease states in animals and humans.

- A raised blood cholesterol concentration is a risk factor for CVD. Determining the proportion of total cholesterol found in LDL and HDL particles is an important index of overall CVD risk. High levels of HDL cholesterol reduce the risk of atherosclerosis and heart disease, whereas high levels of LDL cholesterol increase the risk. A high fat intake, and in particular a high intake of SFA, has been associated with a raised blood cholesterol level. However, some SFA present greater risks than others.

- Increasing the proportion of unsaturated fatty acids in the diet can reduce blood cholesterol and TAG levels. Substitution of SFA with MUFA or PUFA has been found to lower LDL but not HDL cholesterol, even when total fat and energy intakes are maintained. MUFA are less susceptible than PUFA to oxidation, and high MUFA diets may decrease the susceptibility of the LDL particle to oxidation, reducing its atherogenicity.

- The long-chain *n*-3 PUFA of marine phyto-plankton and algae that are concentrated in the body oils of fish have well-documented inhibitory effects on the inflammatory arm of the immune system. They regulate the expression of genes responsible for cytokine production and modulate the type of eicosanoids produced by cells (type 3 prostaglandins and type 5 leukotrienes), which attenuates inflammation and regulates the propensity for blood clotting (thrombus formation). The pattern of eicosanoid production may explain the effect of these fatty acids on cancer development and progression because PGE2 is an angiogenic factor and new vascularisation is important for tumour growth. Long-chain *n*-3 PUFA also reduce plasma TAG concentrations significantly thereby attenuating another risk factor for CVD.

- Although it has been proposed that the unique antioxidant properties of the phenolic compounds present in olive oil may contribute to the beneficial effects of the Mediterranean diet, the evidence is insufficient to draw any conclusions.

- The effects of CLA and other conjugated fatty acids derived from plant linoleic and linolenic acids appear similar to those observed for *n*-3 PUFA. CLAs have also been shown to induce apoptosis in different types of human cancer cells by regulating pro- and anti-apoptotic oncogene expression. The same could also be the case for other plant-derived PUFA with conjugated double bonds in their structures.

- Data from animal studies demonstrating anti-cancer effects, reductions in body fat mass and improved lipid profiles have led to interest in the potential role that CLA might have for human health. However, with the exception of body fat reduction, the results of studies reported to date have been inconsistent. This is probably due to the different doses, the mix of isomers used and the characteristics of the subjects studied. There may also be synergism or antagonism between different CLA isomers.

- Sphingolipids are a structurally diverse class of complex, polar lipids present in all eukaryotic and some prokaryotic cell membranes. Consequently they are ubiquitous in human foods of both animal and plant origin. Sphingolipids are similar in structure to glycerophospholipids but utilise sphingosine as the 'backbone' of the diacyl ester rather than glycerol. Studies *in vitro* and animal models have shown that plant- and animal-derived sphingolipids such as sphingosine-1-phosphate regulate the function of cancer cells and endothelium, and so may be beneficial in preventing cancer, particularly bowel cancer, and also vascular disease.

- Refining of vegetable oils significantly reduces the content of sterols, and the potential to lower serum cholesterol through a normal diet.

- Plant sterol and stanol esters significantly reduce serum cholesterol levels by inhibiting cholesterol uptake and facilitating its elimination. With respect to cholesterol lowering, results suggest that a daily intake of up to 2 g/day of plant stanol or sterol esters is effective, and that higher doses may not increase their efficacy. Sterol and stanol esters appear to be equally effective.

11
Miscellaneous Foods

11.1 Chocolate (see also Chapter 9, Section 9.5 on cocoa)

11.1.1 Introduction

Cocoa comes from the tree *Theobroma cacao*, which originated in the tropical regions of South America. Although the Western world first came into contact with cocoa at the beginning of the 16th century when Cortez visited Montezuma's court in 1519, the tree had already been cultivated in Central America for over 2000 years. Cocoa was a major item of commerce for the Aztecs and their predecessors. It is thought that the wild cocoa tree originated in the upper regions of the Orinoco and Amazon river systems but here the crop was never valued as it was by the Aztecs (Young, 1994).

In the 18th century, France and Spain established cocoa plantations in the Caribbean and the Philippines, respectively. The English introduced cocoa into the Gold Coast colony in West Africa in the 1880s (Bloom, 1998) and subsequently into Nigeria and the Ivory Coast.

The chocolate that the Spanish found when they arrived in Mexico in the 16th century was a high-status product. Beans were both used as currency and processed into beverages (see Chapter 9). The roasted beans were also ground to a liquid and allowed to set. The resulting block could then be transported and eaten or used as a medicine. In 1828, the Dutch inventor Conrad van Houten invented a machine to press some of the fat out of cocoa beans. His process gave a powder that was easier to mix with water and a fat known

as cocoa butter. Combination of this fat with ground beans and sugar gave the first blocks of chocolate, but it was not until 1876 that milk chocolate was first made and sold by Daniel Peter of Vevey, Switzerland.

11.1.2 Cultivation and variety

The cocoa plant is now cultivated worldwide, the major producers being the Ivory Coast, Ghana, Nigeria, Indonesia, Brazil and Cameroon. Table 11.1 shows that now the Ivory Coast is the producer of nearly half the world's crop.

Theobroma cacao is demanding in its cultivation, requiring shade when young, protection from wind and frost and an even temperature and humidity. It is a very labour-intensive crop, a smallholder crop, and over 80% is produced by growers with less than 5 hectares. It is susceptible to a range of diseases including the so far untreat-

Table 11.1 Yearly production of the major cocoa-producing countries.

Country	Yearly production in 1997–8 (000s tonnes)
Ivory Coast	1105
Ghana	390
Indonesia	345
Brazil	162
Nigeria	155
Malaysia	95
World total	2673

Source: Lass (1999).

able witches broom. The main cultivated form is *T. cacao* var. *forastero*, which accounts for more than 90% of the world's usage. Other varieties such as *criollo* and *trinitario* are also grown and some regard these as providing better flavour qualities to cocoa-based products (Leung & Foster, 1996).

Theobroma cacao grows up to 15 m high but is usually pruned to allow easier harvesting of the pods, which are borne directly on the trunk and larger limbs. The tree bears 30–40 pods in a year, which yields in total about 2 kg of dried beans (see below). Within the pod, which is yellow–orange when ripe, the seeds (or beans) are surrounded by a sweet white mucilagenous pulp comprised mainly of sugars. It is thought that it was the pulp that first brought the fruit to the attention of the native Indians. Indeed, in some South American populations it is still the pulp that is consumed as a refreshing drink, while the beans are discarded.

11.1.3 Harvesting and production of cocoa

Ripe cocoa pods contain about 30–40 seeds. The pods are harvested and broken open and the pulp and seeds are formed into large mounds about 1 m high, covered with leaves and left to ferment for 6–8 days. During this period, sucrose is converted to glucose and fructose by invertase and the glucose is subsequently utilised in fermentation, yielding ethanol which is metabolised to acetic acid. As the tissues of the beans lose cellular integrity and die, storage proteins are hydrolysed to peptides and amino acids. The beans change colour from purple to brown and develop the flavour precursors that will become chocolate flavour on roasting. Polyphenol oxidase converts phenolic components to quinones, which polymerise yielding brown, highly insoluble compounds that give chocolate its characteristic colour (Haslam, 1998; Lass, 1999). Also, during this process, the simple polyphenols are complexed and careful control of fermentation is required if flavour is to be developed without significant loss of simple polyphenol content. After fermentation, the seeds are dried in the sun, reducing the moisture content from 55 to 7.5%.

The resulting cocoa beans are then packed for the wholesale trade and shipped worldwide. Cocoa beans are used extensively in the manufacture of chocolate and the beverage, cocoa (see Chapter 9). Cocoa powder is also used in products such as ice cream, cakes and biscuits.

Cocoa processing is full of its own terminology. Each bean is contained within a shell (hull) and the bean after separation from the shell is known as a 'nib'. Beans or nibs are roasted (depending on whether the shell is separated off before or after roasting) and then ground. After grinding, the product is known as cocoa mass or cocoa liquor. To produce the cocoa powder used in the beverage, the beans are roasted at 150°C and the shells and nibs are mechanically separated. The nibs, which contain about 55% cocoa butter, are then finely ground while hot to produce a liquid 'mass' or 'liquor'. This sets on cooling and is then pressed to express the 'butter' that is used in the manufacture of chocolate. The residual cake is ground up to produce cocoa powder (see Chapter 9).

An alkalisation process (known as the 'dutch process') is also often employed nowadays to modify the dispersibility, colour and flavour of cocoa powders which can have a range of colours from red through brown to black. This process can be carried out on nibs before or after roasting. The alkali is usually potassium carbonate but can also be calcium carbonate or sodium hydroxide (Bixler & Morgan, 1999).

11.1.4 Production of chocolate

To make plain or dark chocolate, the only ingredients are cocoa mass, cocoa butter, sugar and flavour, and perhaps lecithin. These are mixed together and the particle size of the mixture is reduced in a refiner before conching. This is a process that is basically little more than stirring, but it has a considerable effect on the flavour and texture of the chocolate, removing both moisture and volatiles while improving flow. The process is, even now, not well understood (Bixler & Morgan, 1999).

Milk chocolate can be made by a similar process using milk powder with the other ingredients

Table 11.2   Typical composition of European milk chocolate.

Component	% weight
Sugar	48.5
Cocoa mass	12
Whole milk powder	19
Cocoa butter	20
Lecithin and flavouring	0.5

Source: Jackson (1999).

but in the UK it is often made by the crumb process, where cocoa mass is added to full-cream sweetened condensed milk and the resultant paste dried in a vacuum oven. The material is ground to a powder and cocoa butter added before refining. The composition of typical European milk chocolate is shown in Table 11.2.

Block milk and plain chocolate is generally made from natural cocoa (not alkalised) but alkalised cocoa is sometimes added to darken the colour of plain chocolate. The level of cocoa solids in plain chocolate varies a great deal. The European Directive 2000/36 EC defines chocolate as containing not less than 35% cocoa solids including not less than 18% cocoa butter and not less than 14% non-fat cocoa solids. Some consumers prefer their chocolate to be bitter and the cocoa solids in retail products can be as high as 75%. Milk chocolate is also defined in the Directive, as is cocoa powder, which is to contain 20% cocoa butter while fat-reduced cocoa powder is to contain 10%. Drinking chocolate is made from natural cocoa (see Chapter 9) while instant chocolate drinks can be made from natural or alkalised cocoa, the latter tending to give a more rounded flavour and darker colour.

11.1.5   Composition of cocoa

(i)   Cocoa butter

The fermented bean consists of roughly 12% shell and 88% nib. The fat content of the cocoa bean depends mainly on the origin. Typically West African beans will contain 55–57% fat, South American can be as low as 51% and some Asia-Pacific beans can reach 60%. Cocoa butter consists mainly of triglycerides of stearic, oleic and palmitic acids with about 60% being saturated fatty acids (see below).

(ii)   Methylxanthines

Cocoa mass contains about 1.2% theobromine and 0.2% caffeine while cocoa powder contains 1.89–2.69% theobromine and 0.16–0.31% caffeine (Apgar & Tarka, 1999). There are few data on intake of methylxanthines from chocolate but from the above it would be expected that a cup of drinking chocolate would contain about 100–150 mg of theobromine and 10–15 mg of caffeine (see Chapter 9). The intake from chocolate bars will depend on the level of cocoa solids in the product.

(iii)   Polyphenols and phenolics

Polyphenols and phenolic acids comprise about 14% of dried unfermented cocoa beans (Jardine, 1999). The raw cocoa bean contains 12–18% flavonoids (Kim & Keeney, 1984) with at least 60% of these being procyanidin oligomers of epicatechin. As with tea (Chapter 9), the dominant polyphenols in cocoa appear to be flavan-3-ol derivatives. The principle components in fresh beans are (–)-epicatechin, the dimeric procyanidins B-2 and B-5 (Fig. 11.1), the trimer C-1 and higher oligomers. Other flavonoids include gallocatechin, epigallocatechin, epicatechin gallate, quercetin and quercetin glycosides. Caffeic, ferulic and 4-coumaric acids (Borchers *et al.*, 2000) have also been reported in cocoa beans, mass and powder.

During fermentation, these components are converted to the insoluble red–brown polymeric compounds of undetermined structure, and as a consequence the level of soluble polyphenols falls by about 90% (Haslam, 1998; Hammerstone *et al.*, 1999; Jardine, 1999; Würsch & Finot, 1999). The extent of the decrease in flavonoid content depends on the origin of the beans and on the processing, roasting and drying conditions (Kim & Keeney, 1984; Almeida *et al.*, 1998). Alkalisation

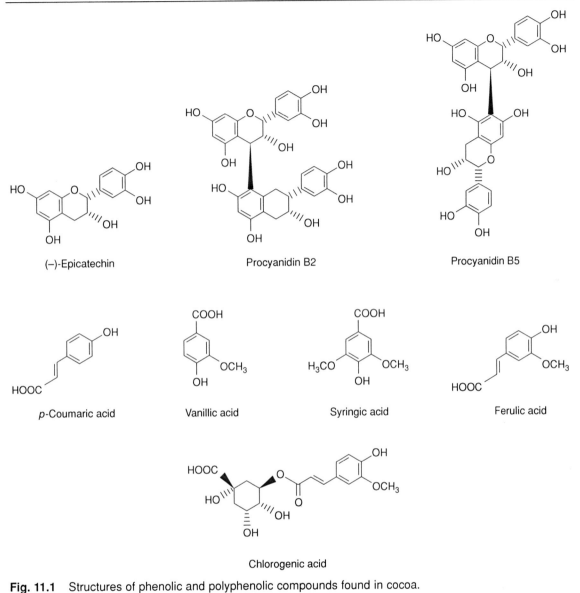

(−)-Epicatechin   Procyanidin B2   Procyanidin B5

p-Coumaric acid   Vanillic acid   Syringic acid   Ferulic acid

Chlorogenic acid

Fig. 11.1 Structures of phenolic and polyphenolic compounds found in cocoa.

reduces the flavonoid content still further, in some cases to zero (Meursing, 1994).

Among the flavonoids, procyanidin oligomers have been detected in apple, grape seed extract (Cheynier *et al.*, 1997) and cocoa. Compounds with degrees of polymerisation up to the decamer have been identified and quantified by HPLC/MS for some samples of cocoa mass and chocolates. It should be noted that although peaks can now be cleanly separated, they still represent a number of compounds with the same degree of polymerisation. The analysis shown in Table 11.3 is for a sample of Brazilian cocoa mass (Adamson *et al.*, 1999).

Levels of total procyanidin in plain (dark) chocolate have been determined in the range 1.7–15.8 mg/g, depending on the source of the cocoa and percentage of cocoa in the product

Table 11.3 Procyanidin oligomers in Brazilian cocoa mass (mg/g).

Monomers	4.9
Dimers	4.2
Trimers	2.8
Tetramers	2.2
Pentamers	1.7
Hexamers	1.4
Heptamers	0.7
Octamers	0.6
Nonamers	0.7
Decamers	0.3

Source: Adamson *et al.* (1999).

(Adamson *et al.*, 1999; Richelle *et al.*, 1999; Hammerstone *et al.*, 2000).

In addition, a considerable range of phenolic acids have been identified in cocoa, including vanillic acid, syringic acid, 4-coumaric acid, caffeic acid, ferulic acid and chlorogenic acid (Fig. 11.1). However, there is little information on how these phenolics are affected by the production process used to manufacture cocoa powder. For example, as a result of fermentation, some conjugated phenolics may be hydrolysed by galactosidases, liberating the aglycone.

11.1.6 Bioavailability of cocoa polyphenols

A number of studies have shown that epicatechin levels in blood increase after consumption of dark chocolate. Richelle *et al.* found plasma epicatechin levels of 0.7 µmol 2 h after consumption of 80 g of European dark chocolate (Richelle *et al.*, 1999). In a study using American dark chocolate, Rein *et al.* found levels of 0.257 µmol 2 h after consumption of 80 g of procyanidin-rich chocolate and 0.153 µmol after 6 h compared with a baseline of 0.022 µmol. The inter-individual variation in this trial was considerable, with a range of ±0.066 and ±0.069 µmol at the two time points (Rein *et al.*, 2000a). Wang *et al.* also demonstrated a positive relationship between amount of chocolate consumed and plasma epicatechin concentration and their experiment had smaller inter-individual variation (Wang *et al.*, 2000). Further studies are required to identify more of

the oligomers and metabolites present in plasma after eating chocolate

11.1.7 Health implications of cocoa and chocolate

(i) Methylxanthines

The physiological effects of caffeine are well known, including stimulation of the central nervous system, stimulation of cardiac muscle and diuretic effects. Theobromine has been less studied but those studies that have been carried out tend to show it having less physiological effect than caffeine. It has also been reported not to affect alertness in the same way as caffeine (see also Chapter 9).

(ii) Cholesterol

Saturated fatty acids, on average, have been shown to raise cholesterol levels and are thought thereby to contribute to atherosclerosis. However, there is evidence that both stearic acid and cocoa butter are neutral with respect to blood cholesterol levels (Kris-Etherton *et al.*, 1993; Kris-Etherton & Yu, 1997).

(iii) Cocoa polyphenols as antioxidants

Arts has shown that, in the Netherlands, chocolate may be a significant contributor to the total flavonoid content of the diet (Arts *et al.*, 1999). Recent studies have identified a number of ways in which procyanidins such as those present in chocolate may benefit human health. Because this is a new area of interest and many of these experiments have been carried out *in vitro*, more studies need to be carried out to confirm these initial findings (Schenker, 2000).

(iv) LDL oxidation

The oxidation of apolipoprotein B, the structural protein of LDL, is recognised as being a prerequisite step for the uptake and deposition of cholesterol in the arterial wall. It is hypothesised that reducing this oxidation will reduce deposition and hence the risk of cardiovascular disease. LDL in the bloodstream is oxidised by reactive oxygen species released by endothelial cells and it is thought that the antioxidants in plasma may inhibit this reaction by combining with the reactive species (see Chapter 4). The ability of antioxidants to do this is measured *in vitro* by an assay of antioxidant capacity. There are a number of different assays. In oxygen radical absorbance capacity (ORAC) assays the antioxidant capacity of a series of chocolate products correlated closely with the total polyphenol content; the antioxidant potential of cocoa was shown to be greater than that of green tea and much greater than that of blueberry, garlic or strawberry (Adamson *et al.*, 1999). In a later study, the inhibition of copper-induced LDL oxidation was shown to be dependent upon the degree of polymerisation of the oligomers with the hexamer being most efficient (Bearden *et al.*, 2000). A further study on the impact of consumption of a cocoa polyphenol-rich meal on the antioxidant capacity of plasma demonstrated a 36% reduction 2 h after consumption of 80 g of procyanidin-rich chocolate. The level returned to the baseline after 6 h but the level of thiobarbituric acid-reactive substances (TBARS) was reduced by 40% at 2 h and was still 30% below the baseline after 6 h (Rein *et al.*, 2000a). However, a subsequent study to determine a dose-dependent relationship between chocolate consumption and plasma antioxidant capacity failed to find such a relationship. This was believed to be due to differences in experimental method and illustrates the difficulties inherent in these studies (Wang *et al.*, 2000).

A recent novel approach has been to examine the use of cocoa bran in a breakfast cereal where it was found to increase faecal bulk and to decrease the LDL:HDL ratio (Jenkins *et al.*, 2000).

(v) Action against specific oxidants

A number of reactive oxygen species are generated in the cell during normal cell processes but excessive production can lead to damage of cell membranes and biological molecules, leading to disease. It is hypothesised that antioxidants in the bloodstream can reduce the levels of these reactive oxygen species and it has been shown that polyphenols extracted from cocoa mass inhibit the production of hydrogen peroxide and O_2^- by activated granulocytes and lymphocytes *in vitro* (Sanbongi *et al.*, 1997). Polyphenols have also been shown *in vitro* to have the ability to intercept peroxynitrite and its precursors, possibly by being oxidised or nitrated themselves (Kerry & Rice-Evans, 1998; Pannala *et al.*, 1998). It has been shown that the individual epicatechin oligomers present in cocoa inhibit the action of peroxynitrite *in vitro*. The extent of the inhibition depends on the degree of polymerisation with the tetramer, having a similar effect to epicatechin gallate (Arteel & Sies, 1999).

(vi) Cocoa polyphenols and platelet function

Platelets are found at the site of early atherosclerotic lesions and enhanced platelet reactivity has been associated with higher risk of coronary heart disease (see Chapter 4). The reactivity of platelets can be assessed *ex vivo* by measuring both expression of fibrinogen-binding conformation of platelet GPIIb–IIIa complex and the production of haemostatically active platelet microparticles. A number of studies have shown that flavonoids decrease platelet aggregation *in vitro* (Corvazier & Maclouf, 1985) and recent studies have demonstrated that the consumption of a cocoa beverage suppressed both unstimulated GPIIa–IIIb expression and epinephrine-induced activated GPIIa–IIIb expression at 2 and 6 h after ingestion. Consumption of the beverage also decreased microparticle production and prolonged closure time at both 2 and 6 h after consumption. These effects were attributed to the flavonoid components of the beverage because the consumption of both water and a caffeine solution did not have these effects (Rein *et al.*, 2000b).

(vii) Chocolate and vascular smooth muscle

It is hypothesised that one of the potential means by which red wine has a beneficial impact on cardiovascular disease is by inducing endothelium-dependent relaxation of aortic smooth muscle (see Chapters 4 and 9). This effect has been shown *in vitro* to be due to red wine flavonoids rather than alcohol. Recent studies have shown that some cocoa polyphenols also induce such relaxation but that the effect is limited to tetramers and higher oligomers (Karim *et al.*, 2000).

(viii) Chocolate and immune function

In addition to their studies on reactive oxygen species, Sanbongi *et al.* showed that cocoa polyphenols reduce the expression of interleukin-2 in human lymphocytes (Sanbongi *et al.*, 1997). In further studies, Mao *et al.* have shown that both a crude water-soluble cocoa extract and a purified procyanidin fraction reduced the expression of interleukin-2 by phytohaemagglutinin stimulated peripheral blood mononuclear cells (PBMC) by over 50% (Mao *et al.*, 1999). Examination of the effects of individual cocoa oligomers showed that the monomer had little effect while the pentamer, hexamer and heptamer caused 61–73% inhibition.

Mao *et al.* have also shown that cocoa fractions inhibit the expression of interleukin-1β by phytohaemagglutinin stimulated PBMC (Mao *et al.*, 2000b). In this case the crude water-soluble cocoa extract had no effect but the purified procyanidin fraction reduced expression by 30%. For the individual oligomers it was shown that the monomer tended to increase expression whereas the higher oligomers, particularly the hexamer, decreased expression. Similar results have been obtained in experiments on the secretion of interleukin-4 (Mao *et al.*, 2000a).

11.2 Herbs, spices and condiments

11.2.1 Introduction

Unlike the foods discussed elsewhere in this report, herbs, spices and condiments are not staples (such as cereals and pulses), nor are they consumed in quantitatively large amounts (such as fruits and vegetables, fats and beverages). The plants, or parts of plants, that are used to flavour, colour and add aroma to foods are consumed in very small amounts (see below). However, although such foods are eaten in small absolute amounts on a single occasion, in many cultures they are central to traditional recipes and so are consumed regularly; the cumulative intake of some of the bioactive compounds they contain may therefore be important.

Historically, many herbs and spices were rare and expensive and treated as a commodity in the same way as precious metals. The Romans carried herbs and spices to other parts of their Empire, and in the 15th century the Europeans' search for more direct trade routes to spice-producing countries led to great voyages of exploration and to also to wars. In Europe, herb and physicke gardens were common in monasteries and large estates. Herbals, detailed manuals describing the properties and uses of herbs and spices, and other plants, were produced from the 15th century. The vernacular names given to plants at that time give an indication of their properties and uses, *e.g.* 'selfheal', 'feverfew' and 'heartsease'. The Latin names given to plants by early herbalists also give an indication of their use. For example, those ending with *officinalis*, *culinaris*, *odorata* and *fragrans* were sold by apothecaries, used for cooking and have a sweet fragrance, respectively. Until the recent past, people had access only to those herbs and spices that were locally available; most plants used as herbs and spices originated in the Far East, the Indian subcontinent and Mediterranean areas. Today, herbs and spices are much more widely consumed as a result of the ease of travel and imports/exports around the world.

As discussed in Chapter 2, many secondary metabolites have a key role in protection against herbivores and microbial infection, including as attractants for pollinators and seed-dispersing animals, as allelopathic agents and UV protectants. Secondary metabolites are also of interest to humans because of their food use (*e.g.* as flavouring and colouring agents) and non-food use (*e.g.* in dyes, waxes, drugs and perfumes), and they are viewed as potential sources of new natural drugs, antibiotics, insecticides and herbicides (Croteau *et al.*, 2000). Because herbs and spices are plants or parts of plants they can contain the same classes of bioactive compounds, and for the same reasons, as the plant foods discussed in other Chapters (see Chapters 2, 7, 8 and 9). Carotenoids are ubiquitous in leaves and stems because they are an essential part of the photo-synthetic process and protect against photo-oxidative damage. Phenolic compounds are associated with the defence of the plant against browsing animals, insects, bacteria and fungi and with inhibiting the growth of competing plants. Flavonols in epidermal cells of leaves and the skins of fruit provide protection against the dam-aging effects of UVB irradiation, and they are also involved in fertilisation, by promoting the growth of pollen tubes in the style of flowers. Polyphenols and carotenoids provide colour to stems, leaves, flowers and fruits.

The presence of bioactive compounds in herbs and spices is more immediately obvious than in many other foods because as well as being colourful, many of the compounds – the essential oils and oleoresins – are volatile (see below). Characteristic aromas and flavours can be released simply by the plant (or part of plant) being brushed or lightly crushed. The bioactive compounds in herbs and spices are the reason why they have been used for centuries throughout the world to flavour, preserve and colour foods, and to disguise the appearance and taste of foods that have putrified or are otherwise 'past their best'. Herbs and spices are also used to flavour beverages (*e.g.* juniper in gin, anise in Pernod, oil of bergamot in Earl Grey tea, chamomile and mint 'teas', etc., ground chicory root to flavour coffee, elderflower cordials, and hops in beer) and confectionery (*e.g.* peppermint, spearmint, aniseed, liquorice).

Herbs and spices also have a long history of use as medicines, both ingested (as pills and potions) and applied topically (*e.g.* mustard poultices), perfumes (as essences, pot pourri, pomanders, nosegays, etc.), cosmetics, insect repellents and antiseptics. Many traditions and superstitions (*e.g.* the use of basil to ward off evil, bay to deflect lightning, which is why bay trees were often plant-ed outside houses) have built up around the use and properties of herbs and spices. Herbs have been used medicinally for thousands of years.

Many modern mass-produced drugs have their origins in plant extracts (*e.g.* salicin, an analogue of aspirin, found in many species of willow, *Salix*, and digitoxin, from foxglove, *Digitalis purpurea*). Salicylic acid (see Chapter 7 and Fig. 7.3) is pro-duced rapidly in some plants as a signal molecule that initiates defence responses following attack by insects, fungi, bacteria and virus. Methyl sali-cylate, the principal component of oil of winter-green (from *Gaultheria procumbens*), which has been used for pain relief for centuries, is derived from salicylic acid. Acetylsalicylic acid (aspirin) has been found in some herbs and spices, most notably cinnamon, oregano and rosemary (Venema *et al.*, 1996). 'Herbal medicine', as practised centuries ago in Europe and as still practised today in many other countries, is cur-rently an area of great interest and debate in lay, medical and nutrition arenas in many Western countries including the UK. When herbs (includ-ing the leaves, bark, stem and roots of the plants) are used as medicines, they are concentrated into powders, granules, tinctures, essences and gels (Readers Digest Association Ltd, 2000). They can have very potent, sometimes lethal effects, and can also interact adversely with conventional drugs. The use of herbal preparations for medici-nal purposes is outside the scope of this chapter; further information, including the legislation that governs their use as medicines, can be found in recent reviews (Craig, 1999; Arab, 2000; Wills *et al.*, 2000; Buttriss, 2001).

11.2.2 Definitions of herbs, spices and condiments

The common use of the terms 'herbs' and 'spices' makes culinary rather than botanical distinctions, although in general spices tend to originate from plants grown in semi-tropical climates, whereas herbs tend to originate from plants found in more temperate regions.

(i) Herbs

The *OED* defines a herb as *Plant of which the stem is not woody or persistent and which dies down to ground level after flowering; plant of which leaves are used for food, medicine, scent, flavour, etc. Benders' Dictionary of Nutrition and Food Technology* defines herbs as *Soft stemmed aromatic plants used fresh or dried to flavour and garnish dishes, and sometimes for medicinal effects. Not clearly distinguished from spices except that herbs are usually the leaves or the whole of the plant while spices are only part of the plant, commonly the seeds, or sometimes the roots or rhizomes* (Bender & Bender, 1999). In the *Handbook of Herbs and Spices*, herbs are defined as *The dried leaves of aromatic plants used to impart flavour and odour to foods with, sometimes, the addition of colour. The leaves are commonly traded separately from the plant stems and leaf stalks* (Peter, 2001).

(ii) Spices

The OED defines spice as *Aromatic or pungent vegetable substance used to flavour food* and *Benders' Dictionary* says *Spices are distinguished from herbs in that part, instead of the whole of the aromatic plant is used; root, stem or leaves* (Bender & Bender, 1999). In the *Handbook of Herbs and Spices*, spices are defined as *The dried parts of aromatic plants with the exception of the leaves. This definition is wide-ranging and covers virtually all parts of the plant* (Peter, 2001).

(iii) Condiments

A condiment *is a substance used to give relish to food, seasoning* (OED). Many condiments, *e.g.* vinegars, pickles and chutneys, tomato ketchup, horseradish sauce, mustard and soy sauce, are of plant origin.

The International Organisation for Standardisation (ISO) defines spices and condiments as *Vegetable products or mixtures thereof, free from extraneous matter, used for flavouring, seasoning and imparting aroma in foods.* As in Chapter 7 (fruits and vegetables), to avoid confusion, in this section foods will be classed according to their common usage. Examples of herbs and spices with their common and botanical names are given in Table 11.4.

11.2.3 Constituents of plants used as herbs and spices and in condiments

The culinary use of plants as herbs and spices, and in condiments, exploits all parts of a plant: leaves (*e.g.* sage, bay, basil), stems (*e.g.* ginger, angelica), bark (cinnamon), rhizomes (*e.g.* ginger, turmeric), roots (*e.g.* horseradish), stolons (*e.g* liquorice), flower buds (*e.g.* cloves), flowers (*e.g.* bergamot), stamens (saffron), seeds (*e.g.* aniseed, mustard, cumin), seed pods (*e.g.* vanilla), kernels (*e.g.* nutmeg), aril (*e.g.* mace) and fruits (*e.g.* peppers, juniper). In some cases more than one part of the same plant is utilised, *e.g.* the leaves and seeds of coriander and the stem and root of ginger. More examples of the parts of plants that are commonly used as herbs and spices are given in Table 11.4.

11.2.4 Essential oils and oleoresins

In many herbs and spices, the flavour and aroma are provided by the components of essential oils and oleoresins. Essential oils are the volatile materials present in plants. They can be obtained by distillation, are generally colourless or lightly coloured, low-viscosity liquids and are the concentrated essences of the spice or herb aroma. Because they do not contain the non-volatile components, the flavour may not be representative of the original spice or herb. Some essential oils have only a few main constituents, but it is the minor components that generally determine the characteristic aroma. The hydrocarbons in essential oils are made up of isoprene units (see below): terpenes, sesquiterpenes and diterpenes. They contribute little to aroma and flavour, even though they may be a major constituent of the oil. Furthermore, they are readily oxidised and polymerised. Some of these essential oils (*e.g.* in cloves, cinnamon and mustard) have a preservative effect (Fisher, 2002).

Many oils may contain aromatic and terpenoid components, but usually one group predominates. As with other bioactive compounds, the oil yields and the exact composition of any sample of oil will be variable depending on the particular plant material used in its preparation (Dewick,

Table 11.4 Plants or parts of plants used to flavour, colour, add aroma to foods and preserve foods.

Common name	Botanical name	Family	Part(s) of plant used
Allspice	*Pimenta officinalis*	Myrtaceae	Dried unripe berry
Aniseed or anise	*Pimpinella anisum*	Umbelliferae	Seeds (and oil)
Angelica	*Angelica officinalis*	Umbelliferae	Stalks
Basil	*Ocimum basilicum*	Labiate	Leaves
Bay	*Laurus noblis*	Lauraceae	Leaves
Bergamot	*Monarda didyma*		Peel, flower
Black pepper	*Piper nigrum*	Piperaceae	Unripe fruit
Borage	*Borago officinalis*	Boraginaceae	Leaves
Caraway	*Carvum carvi*	Umbelliferae	Seeds
Cardamom	*Eletaria cardamomum*	Zingiberaceae	Seeds
Cayenne pepper	Various spp. of *Capsicum frutescens*	Solanaceae	Dried and ground fruit
Chamomile	*Chamomilla recutita*	Compositae	Flower heads
Chervil	*Anthriscus cerifolium*	Umbelliferae	Leaves
Chicory	*Cichorium intybus*	Composite	Roots (coffee), leaves
Chilli powder	Various spp. of *Capsicum frutescens*	Solanaceae	Dried and ground fruit
Chives	*Allium schoenoprasum*	Alliaceae	Leaves
Cinnamon	*Cinnamon zeylanicum*	Lauraceae	Bark
Cloves	*Eugenia caryophyllata*	Myrtaceae	Dried flower buds
Coriander	*Coriandrum sativum*	Umbelliferae	Leaves and seeds
Cumin	*Cuminum cyminum*	Umbelliferae	Seeds
Dill	*Anethum graveolens*	Umbelliferae	Seeds and leaves
Elderberry	*Sambucus niger*	Honeysuckle	Flowers and berries
Fennel	*Foeniculum vulgare*	Umbelliferae	Seeds and leaves
Fenugreek	*Trigonella foenumgraecum*	Fabaceae	Seeds
Ginger	*Zingiber officinale*	Zingiberaceae	Roots and stems
Hops	*Humulus lupulus*	Cannabaceae	Flowers
Horseradish	*Armoracia rusticana*	Brassica	Root
Juniper	*Juniperus communis*	Cupressaceae	Fruit (berry)
Lemon balm	*Melissa officinalis*	Labiate	Leaves
Lemon grass	*Cymopogon citratus*	Graminae	Leaves
Liquorice	*Glycyrrhiza glabra*	Leguminosae	Rhizome and root
Mace	*Myristica fragrans*	Myristicaceae	Aril (husk) surrounding nutmeg
Marjoram	*Origanum marjorana*	Labiate	Leaves
Mints	*Mentha* spp.	Labiate	Leaves
Mustard	*Sinapsis alba, Brassica nigra, Brassica juncea*	Cruceriferae	Seeds
Nutmeg	*Myristica fragrans*	Myristicaceae	Kernel
Oregano	*Origanum vulgaris*	Labiate	Leaves
Paprika	Various spp. of *capsicum frutescens*	Solanaceae	Dried and ground fruit
Parsley	*Petroselinium crispum*	Umbelliferae	Leaves
Peppermint	*Mentha piperita*	Labiate	Leaves
Rosemary	*Rosmarinus officinalis*	Labiate	Leaves
Sage	*Salvia officinalis*	Labiate	Leaves
Saffron	*Crocus sativus*	Iridaceae	Styles of unopened flowers
Spearmint	*Mentha spicata*	Labiate	Leaves
Star anise	*Illicium verum*	Illiciaceae	Seeds
Tamarind	*Tamarindus indica*	Cesalpiniaceae	Pulp from the pods
Tarragon	*Artemisia dranunculus*	Composite	Leaves
Thyme	*Thymus vulgaris*	Labiate	Leaves
Turmeric	*Curcuma longa*	Zingiberaceae	Rhizome
Vanilla	*Vanilla planifolia*	Orchidaceae	Bean or pod, and seeds
White pepper	*Piper nigrum*	Piperaceae	Ripe fruit

Sources: Grey-Wilson (1987); Peter (2001); Aggarwal *et al.* (2002); Dewick (2002).

Table 11.5 Volatile oils containing principally aromatic compounds and which are derived by the shikimate pathway.

Oil	Oil content (%)	Major constituents with typical composition (%)
Aniseed (anise)	2–3	Anethole (80–90), estragole (1–6)
Star anise	5–8	Anethole (80–90), estragole (1–6)
Cinnamon	1–2	Cinnamaldehyde (70–90), eugenol (1–13), cinnamyl acetate (3–4)
Clove	15–20	Eugenol (75–90), eugenyl acetate (10–15), β-caryophyllene (3)
Fennel	2–5	Anethole (50–70), fenchone (10–20), estragole (3–20)
Nutmeg	5–16	Sabinene (17–28), α-pinene (14–22), β-pinene (9–15), terpinen-4-ol (6–9), myristicin (4–8), elemicin (2)

Source: Dewick (2002).

2002). Table 11.5 illustrates some examples of volatile oils containing principally aromatic compounds and which are derived by the shikimate pathway (see Chapter 2). Table 11.6 illustrates some examples of volatile oils containing principally terpenoid compounds and which are derived by the deoxyxylulose phosphate pathway (see Chapter 2).

Oleoresins are the solvent-extractable components of a botanical raw material. They are liquids, which can vary in consistency from that of a vegetable oil, to a semi-solid paste. Oleoresins contain the volatile and the non-volatile components of the herb or spice. For example, the non-volatile fraction may contain active flavour components such as the alkaloid piperine, which gives black pepper its pungency, and pigments such as carotenoids (Fisher, 2002).

11.2.5 Bioactive compounds found in herbs, spices and condiments

The major groups of secondary metabolites (see Chapter 2) can be found in the plants commonly used as herbs and spices and in condiments. In the following sections particular compounds and foods will be highlighted, but this should not be taken as an indication that these are the only ones associated with the foodstuff. Some bioactive compounds have been investigated in detail whereas others have received very little, if any, attention. For details of the physico-chemical

properties of specific compounds that have been isolated from a range of herbs and spices see the books by Dewick and Peter (Peter, 2001; Dewick, 2002). The former also contains a wealth of information about international quality specifications and regulatory issues and the methods of cultivating and processing herbs and spices.

(i) Nitrogen-containing alkaloids and sulphur-containing compounds

Glucosinolates are nitrogen- and sulphur-containing glucosides. As discussed elsewhere in this report (Chapters 2, 5 and 7), glucosinolates are found in members of the genus *Brassica* (in the family Cruciferae). The vegetables commonly consumed as foods in this family are discussed in detail in Chapter 7. Of relevance to this section is the fact that some *Brassica* species are central components of some condiments (mustard, horseradish sauce, pickles). The breakdown products (see Chapters 2, 5 and 7) of glucosinolates include isothiocyanates, hot and bitter compounds, commonly termed 'mustard oils', which are often volatile with an acrid smell (see Section 7.4.3). These are responsible for the spicy/hot flavour of, for example, mustard and horseradish (see Section 11.2.6). There is also evidence that glucosinolates have antifungal and antibacterial activities and their presence in the plant may contribute to resistance to infection by mildew and other fungi.

Table 11.6 Volatile oils containing principally terpenoid compounds and which are derived by the deoxyxylulose phosphate pathway.

Oil	Oil content (%)	Major constituents with typical composition (%)
Bergamot	0.5	Limonene (42), linalyl acetate (27), γ-terpenine (8), linalool (7)
Caraway	3–7	(+)-Carvone (50–70), limonene (47)
Cardamom	3–7	α-Terpenyl acetate (25–35), cineole (25–45), linalool (5)
Coriander	0.3–1.8	(+)-Linalool (60–75), γ-terpinene (5), α-pinene (5), camphor (5)
Dill	3–4	(+)-Carvone (40–65)
Ginger	1.5–3	Zingerberene (34), β-sesquiphellandrene (12), β-phellandrene (8), β-bisabolene (6)
Juniper	0.5–2	α-Pinene (45–80), myrcene (10–25), limonene (1–10), sabinene (0–15)
Lemon-grass	0.1–0.3	Citral (= geranial + neral) (50–85)
Peppermint	1–3	Menthol (30–50), menthone (15–32), menthyl acetate (2–10), menthofuran, (1-9), α-terpineol (65)
Rosemary	1–2	Cineole (15–45), α-pinene (10–25), camphor (10–25), β-pinene (8)
Sage	0.7–2.5	Thujone (40–60), camphor (5–22), cineole (5–14), β-caryophyllene (10), limonene (6)
Thyme	0.5–2.5	Thymol (40), *p*-cymene (30), linalool (7), carvacrol (1)

Source: Dewick (2002).

The sulphur-containing compounds *S*-alkylcysteine sulphoxide and *S*-methylcysteine sulphoxide (see Chapter 7, Fig. 7.7) are present in all members of the *Allium* genus (see Chapters 2 and 7), including chives (*Allium schoenoprasum*). The amino acid cysteine is the precursor of all these *S*-alkylcysteine sulphoxides (see Chapter 2, Fig. 2.28). The major compound found in chives is *S*-propylcysteine sulphoxide. The properties and breakdown products of the sulphur-containing compounds found in members of the *Allium* genus are discussed in detail in Chapter 7.

(ii) Terpenoids

The terpenoids comprise the largest group of natural plant products (see Chapters 2, 7 and 11). Members of the terpenoid family are diverse in structure and have an extremely wide range of actions. All terpenoids are derived chemically from the five-carbon isoprenoid precursor isopentenyl diphosphate (IPP, a hemiterpene) (see Chapter 2, Fig. 2.15), and thus are also known as isoprenoids (see Chapter 2). Terpenoids are classified according to the number of C_5 isoprenoid units that they contain. The biosynthesis and classification of these compounds are discussed in detail in Chapter 2. Many monoterpenes (C_{10}), sesquiterpenes (C_{15}), triterpenes (C_{30}) and tetraterpenes (C_{40}) are responsible for the flavouring, aromas and other properties of plants commonly referred to as herbs and spices.

(a) Monoterpenes (C_{10})

A number of monoterpenes are components of volatile oils used as flavourings (see Chapter 2 and Table 11.6). Examples include geranial found in lemon grass, β-myrcene (found in hops and juniper), linalool (found in bergamot, cardamom, coriander and thyme), (−)-methol (found in peppermint), and (+)-limonene and (−)-limonene which have the fragrance of oranges and lemons, respectively. Limonene is found in bergamot, juniper, caraway and sage. Limonene is the precursor of carvone; (+)-carvone provides the characteristic odour of caraway and is also found in dill; (−)-carvone smells of spearmint. Thyme contains *p*-cymene, thymol and carvacrol (see Chapter 2, Fig. 2.17).

(b) Sesquiterpenes (C₁₅)

Sesquiterpenes (see Chapter 2, Fig. 2.18) include bisabolene, which contributes to the aroma of ginger (*Zingiber officinale*). Other C_{15} compounds include α-cadinene, which is one of many terpenoids found in juniper berries (*Juniperus communis*) used in making gin.

(c) Triterpenoids (C₃₀)

C_{30} derivatives include triterpenoid saponins, such as glycyrrhetic acid, which is found as a diglucuronide conjugate, glycyrrhizic acid in liquorice root (*Glycyrrhiza glabra*).

(d) Tetraterpenoids (C₄₀)

Carotenoids (see Chapters 2, 6 and 7) are the sole tetraterpenoid group although numerous variations on the basic structure occur in nature. Carotenoids include lycopene, the precursor of both β- and α-carotene, which occurs widely in plants and is a significant dietary component because of its presence as the red colorant in tomatoes and tomato-based products, such as tomato ketchup and tomato purée (see Section 11.2.6). Capsanthin (see Chapter 7, Fig. 7.17), the bright red pigment of peppers (*Capsicum annuum*), is a metabolite of violaxanthin, an oxidation product of β-carotene. When fresh red pepper is processed to paprika, rapid drying leads to the destruction of carotenoids, but slow drying induces an increase in carotenoid concentration (see Chapter 12). There are many varieties of smaller and much hotter chilli peppers. Capsaicin (see Chapter 7, Fig. 7.17) has been identified as the chemical that gives the heat to chilli peppers.

11.2.6 Quantification of bioactive substances in herbs and spices

There is very little information about the amounts of bioactive substances present in different plants. As discussed elsewhere in this report,

the levels of bioactive compounds present in plant foods also depend on the variety, the conditions under which the plant is grown, harvested, processed and stored and the period of storage before consumption (see Section 7.3.2). The levels of plant bioactive compounds recorded have to be considered in context and no single figure can be regarded as representative of a plant species. Many oils may contain aromatic and terpenoid components, but usually one group predominates (see Tables 11.5 and 11.6). The oil yields and the exact composition of any sample of oil will be variable depending on the particular plant material used in its preparation. As discussed in Chapters 2 and 7, with some significant exceptions, plant bioactive compounds are present in relatively small amounts. Two other issues pertain particularly to herbs and spices. First, because many of the compounds are aromatic, the amounts can decline rapidly (this is why in many instances the particular plant, or part of plant, is not picked, ground or crushed until it is actually needed in a recipe). Second, the amounts of herbs and spices required to achieve the desired culinary effect are extremely small. This is because the colours are very intense, and because the aromatic compounds are very potent/pungent. Hence serving sizes rarely approach even gram quantities (except in the case of fresh parsley or basil used in pesto) and are mostly at milligram levels. Even if values are expressed as mg/kg, the actual amounts consumed are orders of magnitude lower than this. Typically, quantities are described in terms of a 'pinch' or 'sprinkle', or 'to taste'. Dried herbs weigh less than fresh herbs, but may have a higher concentration of bioactive compounds.

11.2.7 Potential protective effects of herbs and spices

Because they contain many of the same bioactive compounds as fruits and vegetables and other plant foods, many of these compounds are of interest for their potential protective effects against CVD and cancer. In particular, extracts of the essential oils have been found to possess antioxidant and other properties in *in vitro* studies and in animal models, for example inhibiting the growth of tumours (Craig, 1999, 2001; Aggarwal *et al.*, 2002). However, the compounds used are often very concentrated and given in isolation. Hence, their use in this manner is more medicinal than culinary.

11.2.8 Condiments

Many condiments, *e.g.* vinegars, pickles, chutneys, mustards and sauces, are of plant origin.

(i) Mustard

The breakdown products (see Chapters 2, 5 and 7) of glucosinolates include isothiocyanates, hot and bitter compounds, commonly termed 'mustard oils', which are often volatile with an acrid smell (see Section 7.4.3). These are responsible for the spicy/hot flavour of mustard. English mustard contains mostly white mustard seed (*Sinapsis alba*), whereas French and German mustards contain small amounts of black mustard seeds (*Brassica nigra* and *Brassica juncea*). The glucosinolate sinalbin accumulates in white mustard seed and when moistened and crushed the glucose moiety is cleaved by myrosinase to form acrinyl isothiocyanate (see Figs. 2.26 and 7.10) which is responsible for the hot pungent taste. Black mustard seeds contain sinigrin which is similarly hydrolysed to allyl thiocyanate (see Figs 2.26 and 7.10), which is considerably more volatile than acrinyl isothiocyanate, and which gives black mustard powder a pungent aroma as well as a hot spicy taste.

(ii) Horseradish sauce

The breakdown products (see Chapters 2, 5 and 7) of glucosinolates include isothiocyanates, hot and bitter compounds, commonly termed 'mustard oils', which are often volatile with an acrid smell (see Section 7.4.3). These are responsible for the spicy/hot flavour of, for example, horseradish. The indole glucosinolate glucobrassicin (see Chapters 2 and 7) is found in a number of Brassica species including horseradish (*Armoracia rusticana*).

(iii) Tomato ketchup, tomato purée and tomato-based sauces

As discussed elsewhere in this report, food processing enhances the bioavailability of some carotenoids. When fat or oil is added to vegetables during blanching and cooking, the retention of carotenoids improves considerably (see Chapter 12). The bioavailability of lycopene (see Section 6.5.1 and Fig. 2.21) is known to increase when processing occurs in the presence of a small amount of oil/fat. This is because heating tomato-based foods in the presence of oil enhances the conversion of lycopene from the *trans* to the *cis* form, which is more easily absorbed. Thus tomato ketchup (widely used as a relish), tomato purée and tomato-based sauces (widely used in composite dishes such as casseroles and stews and on pasta and pizzas) is a good source of bioavailable lycopene. Several case-control and large prospective studies have suggested that the intake of tomatoes and tomato products may be associated with a lower risk of prostate cancer. It has been hypothesised that lycopene is one of the compounds in raw and processed tomatoes that may contribute to this lower risk (Cohen, 2002; Giovannucci *et al.*, 2002; Vogt *et al.*, 2002), but this remains to be investigated further (Miller *et al.*, 2002). Preliminary results from the EPIC study found no link between tomatoes/tomato products and prostate cancer; the final results are awaited. Other carotenoids and other bioactive compounds may also contribute to these proposed benefits. In the meantime, the reported correlations or associations between the consumption of tomato products and prostate cancer should not be interpreted as causal until additional data are available from a variety of studies in different populations (Miller *et al.*, 2002).

(iv) Soy sauce

The level of isoflavones in a typical portion of soy sauce is negligible (see Chapter 8, Table 8.3).

(v) Vinegar

Vinegar is formed as a result of *Acetobacter* spp. of bacteria fermenting alcohol to acetic acid. There are a number of different types of vinegar, which is basically a solution of acetic acid. In most countries vinegar is made from grape juice. Balsamic vinegar is also made from grape juice, but is produced by a very slow fermentation process in only one area of Italy (Modena). Wine vinegar may be made from red, white or rosé wine. Malt vinegar is made from malted barley, cider vinegar (known simply as 'vinegar' in the USA) from apple juice and rice vinegar from sake. Many vinegars are also flavoured with herbs (Bender & Bender, 1999). Although there are many anecdotes about the healthy attributes of vinegars, particularly cider vinegars, no large-scale scientific studies have been conducted. Vinegars might be expected to contain the same classes of bioactive compounds as the alcohol from which they are derived. However, in the vinegar industry, polyphenols are mainly regarded as 'likely haze formers'. It is likely that polyphenols are found at a lower level in vinegars than in wines because they are less soluble at a lower pH, and so tend to precipitate over a period of time. It is partly for this reason that vinegars are stored for 2 or more months to allow for sedimentation. Some years ago vinegars were left in storage for approximately 12 months before being filtered and used. This gave a very stable product free from haze-forming products such as polyphenols and tannins (W.H. Grierson, personal communication).

11.3 Research recommendations

- As with flavonoids in other foods, further research is needed with respect to chocolate. The molecular weight range of flavonoids that can be absorbed from the gut into the plasma is unknown, as is the lifetime of the molecules in the plasma, whether they can be taken up by the tissues of interest, and the nature and activity of their metabolites

- Whilst the bioavailability is readily apparent because of their use as medicines, the properties, bioactivity and possible effects *in vivo* of the bioactive compounds found in herbs and spices remain to be established for the very small amounts required for culinary purposes.

11.4 Key points

- Chocolate is derived from the cocoa plant, which is a source of theobromine, caffeine and a range of other bioactive substances. In particular, polyphenolics and phenolic acids comprise about 14% of the weight of the dried cocoa bean, with at least 60% of these being procyanidin oligomers of epicatechin (a flavan-3-ol). The hydroxycinnamates caffeic, ferulic and 4-coumaric acids are also present in the unfermented cocoa bean.
- Procyanidin levels have generally been shown to be higher in dark (plain) chocolate and epicatechin levels in blood have been shown to rise after dark chocolate consumption.
- There is an increasing body of largely *in vitro* evidence that the consumption of cocoa derivatives has the potential to increase the antioxidant capacity of the plasma and the potential to modify beneficially a number of processes thought to be associated with cardiovascular disease, *e.g.* LDL oxidation, inhibition of peroxynitrite and inhibition of platelet activity.
- It should be noted that much of this work has been conducted *in vitro* and needs to be corroborated in *ex vivo* or *in vivo* human studies.
- It should also be remembered that any potential benefits have to be considered in context. Chocolate, and products containing it, are often energy-dense and contain relatively high amounts of fat and sugar, and thus should be eaten in moderation (see Balance of Good Health in Chapter 13).
- Herbs and spices have been used for culinary purposes all over the world for thousands of years, for flavouring, preserving and colouring foods.
- The culinary use of plants as herbs and spices utilises all parts of the plant – leaves, stems, roots, seeds, seed pods and flowers. Thus a range of bioactive substances present in plants will be consumed in this way.

- Herbs and spices also have a long history of use as medicines, perfumes, cosmetics, insect repellents and antiseptics. Many 'modern' mass-produced drugs have their origins in plant extracts and are based on knowledge gained over centuries of traditional use.
- In Western societies there is a resurgence of interest in the properties of herbs and spices, particularly in their use as medicines.
- The use of herbs and spices for medicinal purposes, and more recently in *in vitro* and *in vivo* studies for potentially beneficial effects on CVD and cancer, usually requires tinctures or essences or very concentrated extracts in the form of powders, granules and gels to be used. Thus intakes or 'doses' are much higher than would be from culinary use.
- The bioactive compounds contained in plants used as herbs and spices (and condiments such as horseradish sauce and mustards) are more immediately obvious than many other bioactive compounds, because many of them are aromatic, and released by the plant simply by being brushed or crushed.
- The bioactive compounds found in herbs and spices are mostly terpenoids and it is these oils that are responsible for flavours, taste and aromas.
- The bioavailability of bioactive compounds in herbs and spices is readily apparent because of their use as medicines. However their properties, bioactivity and possible effects *in vivo* when used in very small amounts required for culinary purposes, and as part of typical recipes, remain to be established.
- Although herbs and spices are eaten in very small amounts on an absolute basis, in many cultures they are essential to traditional recipes, and so are consumed regularly; the cumulative intake may therefore be important. Furthermore, until recently people would have used only those herbs and spices that were locally grown and available. Today they are much more widely consumed by

12
The Effect of Agronomy, Storage, Processing and Cooking on Bioactive Substances in Food

12.1 Introduction

The purpose of food processing and cooking is to convert raw plant and animal ingredients into safe and edible foods. Because of different food processing techniques, we are able to enjoy a variety of foods that otherwise would not be edible or available for consumption. Increased stability of processed foods allows us to consume perishable foods outside their growing season, widening the choice of foods that provide a varied, healthy and balanced diet all year round.

The chemical and physical changes that occur as a result of food processing and cooking can be desirable or undesirable. Food processing, especially heat treatment, is recognised to cause a reduction in anti-nutritional factors present in raw materials and a release of nutrients and other bioactive substances from the food matrix to which they are bound, improving the digestibility and bioavailability of the beneficial components. Some food processing techniques, *e.g.* fermentation, are known to lead to the formation of beneficial components.

Despite many favourable attributes associated with food processing, there can also be losses of chemically sensitive compounds, including those discussed throughout this report. In developing countries, for example, significant losses occur because of inadequate storage facilities and long storage times. The extent of the losses depends on the nature of the compound and its sensitivity to different processing conditions. Factors that contribute to losses include exposure to heat, air (oxygen) and light, pH, water content and the presence of natural biological enzyme systems in the plants. The impact of the losses of potentially beneficial components resulting from storage, processing and cooking needs to be evaluated in the context of that food's role as a source of the compound of interest. The other advantageous effects that food processing offers by providing a varied, healthy and balanced diet to urbanised communities also has to be considered. It should also be noted that the same chemical and physical principles apply in domestic kitchens and in commercial food production. Hence it could be that the biggest losses of bioactive compounds due to storage, processing and cooking can occur in the kitchen.

It is also important to appreciate that the effects of storage, processing and cooking on the content of bioactive compounds in plant foods are only a part of the equation. Pre-harvest conditions and factors may play an even bigger role. The content in fruits and vegetables has been shown to depend on the species, and it can vary greatly between sub-species and varieties (see Chapter 7). Environmental factors such as temperature and humidity, the quality of land and its geographical location are also known to influence the accumulation of bioactive compounds in plant crops, as are cultivation practices such as the use of fertilisers, herbicides and pesticides. The state of maturity at harvest also influences the content of bioactive compounds in fruit and vegetables. For example, if the colour of ripe fruit is due to pigments other than carotenoids, the carotenoid concentration decreases during ripening. In fruits where carotenoids are the main pigments, their concentration increases with maturation. The content of bioactive compounds has been shown to vary in different parts of the plant; for example, according to one report the outer dark-green leaves of Savoy cabbage contain up to 150-fold more lutein and 200-fold more carotene than the paler inner leaves (van den Berg *et al.*, 2000).

In this chapter, some of the studies that have looked at the effect of storage, processing and cooking on the content of bioactive compounds in plant foods will be reviewed. As discussed elsewhere in this report, there are thousands of different compounds in plants, whose distribution and potential role in human health are not yet fully understood. Therefore, only limited data are available on the effects of storage, processing and cooking on these some of these compounds. Furthermore, the majority of the research has been conducted on rarer plant foods in small-scale studies and many of these plants are not consumed in developed countries. The priority is to determine the distribution of the bioactive compounds and their role in human health first. Once this has been achieved, the effects of storage, processing and cooking can also be more precisely investigated in more commonly consumed plants. However, the existing data show that the retention of a compound depends on its chemical and physical properties, the type of food in which it is present and the processes used.

Definitions of the different types of storage, processing and cooking techniques referred to in this chapter can be found in the Appendix. Table 12.1 summarises the effects of different types of processing on some plant bioactive compounds.

12.2 Terpenoids

The terpenoids comprise the largest group of natural plant products, and over 20 000 from plant sources have been described (see Chapters 2, 7 and 11). This category of substances includes the carotenoids (see Section 12.4) and examples of other typical plant terpenoids are camphor, limonene, abscisic acid, aucubin, gossypol and gibberellic acid. They are derived chemically from the five-carbon precursor isoprene and hence are also known as isoprenoids (see Chapter 2). A limited amount of information is available on the effects of storage, processing and cooking on terpenoids. Howard & Dewi found that terpenoid concentrations in peeled carrots declined by 72% after 17 days of storage at 2°C for 14 days and then at 10°C for an additional 3 days (Howard & Dewi, 1996). Terpenoid levels have also been found to be reduced when air is removed (Talcott *et al.*, 2000).

12.2.1 Saponins

Saponins are triterpenoid compounds (see Chapter 2 and Fig. 2.25). They are glycosides with the surfactant property of forming a durable foam when shaken in solution. In addition to genetic, environmental and agronomic factors, storage, cooking and industrial processing affect the saponin content of food. The solubility of saponins in water, their ability to bind to other components of the plant matrix and their susceptibility to partial or complete hydrolysis may all be factors causing changes in levels during processing.

Mechanical removal of the outer layer of soya beans by acidic hydrolysis, fermentation and other procedures such as the removal of insoluble material from, and defoaming of, soya 'milk', have been shown to reduce saponin levels in traditional Japanese soya bean products (Davidek, 1995) (see also Chapter 8).

Cooking and canning have a small effect on the saponin content of broad beans and navy beans, but soaking prior to cooking and canning has resulted in significant losses (Drumm *et al.*, 1990). The loss of saponins during cooking has been attributed to the leaching into the soaking medium through simple diffusion, but losses during cooking indicate the thermolability of saponins. Cooking significantly decreases the saponin content of chickpeas (Jood *et al.*, 1986).

12.2.2 Carotenoids

Carotenoids belong to the terpenoids family and are fat-soluble, highly unsaturated hydrocarbons found in plant cells. Chemically, carotenoids can

Table 12.1 Stability of phytochemicals under different conditions.

Bioactive compound / Main food sources	Storage					Cooking		Processing	
	Air	MAP	Chilled	Room temperature	Frozen	Microwave	Traditional	Canning	Drying
Terpenoids (other than carotenoids)									
Oil in citrus peel, olive oil			U						
Saponins									
Soya bean, ginseng, liquorice							U	U	
Carotenoids									
Carrots, oranges, unrefined palm oil	U	S	S	S	S	S/U	S/U	S/U	U
Phytosterols									
Vegetable oils	U					S			U
Flavonols									
Endive, onions, spinach	U	U	U	U		S/U	S/U		
Anthocyanins									
Berries, cherries, grapes	S	S	S	U		S	S/U		S
Flavan-3-ols									
Tea							S/U		S
Isoflavones									
Soya bean							U	U	
Lignans									
Wholegrain products, seeds									
Glucosinolates									
Brussels sprouts, cabbage, broccoli			U		U				
Sulphides			U						
Protease inhibitors									
Apples, cabbage, barley							U	U	
Coumarins									
Cassava, citrus fruit									
Vitamin E									
Beans, asparagus, cabbage	U		U	U	U	U	U	U	U
Vitamin C									
Oranges, strawberries, blueberries	S	S	U	U	S	U	U	U	U
Folate									
Green leafy vegetables	U	S	U	U	S	U	U	U	U

U, unstable under the conditions specified; S, stable under the conditions specified.

be divided into two sub-classes. The first includes carotenes and lycopene, which contain no oxygen and are usually orange or red in colour (see Chapters 2, 7, 9 and 11). Carotenes have a cyclic structure at the end of the hydrocarbon chain, whereas lycopene has no cyclic structure. Nutritionally, the most important carotenes are α- and β-carotenes, found in orange fruit and vegetables, green leafy vegetables and unrefined red palm oil (see Chapter 1). Lycopene is the main carotenoid in tomatoes, and is also found in watermelon, guava, rosehip, papaya and pink grapefruit (see Section 7.5.5). The other sub-class of carotenoids is xanthophylls, which contain one or more oxygen atoms in their cyclic structure. Of these, spinach and other greens are good sources of lutein, and cryptoxanthin is found in mango and pawpaw (Ainsworth, 1994). Further information can be found in Section 6.5.

Storage, processing and cooking change the chemical composition and content of carotenoids and their bioavailability. During food processing the stability of carotenoids depends both on the individual carotenoid *per se* and the type of fruit or vegetable in which it is found. As highly unsaturated compounds, carotenoids are susceptible to oxidative damage. The structural integrity of the plant and optimal storage conditions in relation to light, oxygen, moisture content and temperature are important determinants of the maximal retention. Storage of fruit and vegetables at low temperatures, protected from light and oxygen, ensures the best retention.

Although temperature is the most important factor in relation to biochemical reactions, carotenoids are relatively stable at different storage temperatures. When the β-carotene content of spinach and amaranth leaves was determined after storage in polyethylene bags for 24 and 48 h at either 5 or 30°C, the losses were only in the region of 1% at both temperatures (Kala-Yadav & Sehgal, 1995). During cold storage the effect of light on carotenoid retention has been found to depend on the vegetable in question. Storing raw spinach in the dark for 8 days caused a reduction only in the concentration of β-carotene, by 18%, whereas exposure to light reduced the concentration of all carotenoids ranging from 22% for lutein to 60% for violaxanthin. Exposing carrots to light did not have any significant effect on major carotenoids (Kopas-Lane & Warthesen, 1995). The damaging effect of atmospheric oxygen on carotenoid retention was demonstrated in a study in which fresh broccoli florets had been stored for 6 days at 5°C in different atmospheric conditions. Florets stored in a modified atmosphere retained total carotenoids well, whereas losses in other conditions (ventpackaging and automatic misting) ranged from 42 to 57% (Barth & Hong, 1996). In another study the effect of modified atmosphere on carotenoid retention of jalapeno pepper rings (structural integrity of the plant broken) was investigated. After 12 days at 4.4°C followed by 3 days at 13°C, losses under modified atmospheric packaging were smaller (32–72%) than those in control samples (44–100%). Losses of β-cryptoxanthin and α-carotene were greater than the losses of β-carotene (Hernandez & Howard, 1996).

The effect of irradiation on carotenoid retention has been studied in sweet potatoes. In non-irradiated sweet potatoes, the content of carotenoids was shown to decrease at storage temperatures of 15 and 20°C, but to increase at 4 and 25–30°C. Irradiation of sweet potatoes caused a reduction in total carotenoid concentration at all temperatures (Bhushan & Thomas, 1990). As with lycopene, the bioavailability of these carotenoids increases in the presence of fat and oil.

The effect of heat treatment on carotenoid retention during the processing of carrot juice has also been investigated (Chen *et al.*, 1983). Pasteurisation (105°C for 25 s) had a minimal effect on total carotenoid concentration. Heating the carrot juice at 110°C for 30 s caused reductions in concentration of 45% for β-carotene and 30% for lutein; 48% of β-carotene was degraded after heating at 120°C for 30 s. Under canning conditions (121°C for 30 min), the β-carotene content of carrot juice was increased, but the α-carotene and lutein concentrations decreased by 60 and 50%, respectively. When fat or oil is added during blanching and cooking, carotenoid retention improves considerably (Kala-Yadav &

Sehgal, 1995). The bioavailability of lycopene (see Section 6.5.1) is also known to increase when processing occurs in the presence of a small amount of oil/fat. This is because heating tomato-based foods in the presence of oil enhances the conversion of lycopene from the *trans* to the *cis* form, and as a consequence absorption is increased (Shi & Le Maguer, 2000).

During heat treatment, the stability of lycopene shows similar trends to those seen with other carotenoids. Heating tomato juice for 7 min at 90 and 100 °C caused a decrease in lycopene content of less than 2%. Greater losses were observed at higher temperatures with longer holding times, *e.g.* at 130 °C a loss of 17.1%. In the presence of an oxidising agent, *e.g.* copper, the losses increase markedly to 60 and 90% at 65 and 100 °C, respectively. The exposure to oxygen during thermal treatment has a considerable impact on lycopene degradation; more than 30% is degraded when heated at 100 °C in the presence of oxygen, whereas only 5% is lost in the presence of carbon dioxide (Shi & Le Maguer 2000).

In some studies, thermal processing has been shown to increase the carotenoid content of processed vegetables. This might be due to unaccounted losses of moisture and soluble solids that concentrate the sample per unit weight, or because thermal and mechanical disruption of plant cells makes carotenoids easier to extract from the food matrix. The bioavailability (see Section 6.5) of different carotenoids varies depending on the vegetable; the bioavailability of lutein from spinach is higher than that of β-carotene, 67 and 14%, respectively. Enzymic disruption of the cell wall structure has been shown to enhance the bioavailability of β-carotene from whole leaf and minced spinach, but has no effect on the bioavailability of lutein (Erdman, 1999). Generally, the bioavailability of carotenes from raw vegetables is low (3–4%), but is markedly increased by cooking and puréeing processes, by up to 4–5 fold (Rock *et al.*, 1998). Heat processing of vegetables promotes isomerisation of the carotenoids, the degree of which is dependent on the type of vegetables and the processing conditions. The *cis* isomers of lycopene from heat-processed tomato juice are more bioavailable

than *trans* isomers from unprocessed juice (van den Berg *et al.*, 2000).

Traditional sun-drying of fruit and vegetables causes a significant reduction in carotenoid content. Air-drying of carrots at 60–70 °C led to significant losses of the α- and β-carotene in fresh product, 18 and 28%, respectively. The use of sulphite, sodium metabisulphite and lower temperature (40 °C) is associated with improved carotene retention during drying (van den Berg *et al.*, 2000). When fresh pepper is processed to paprika, fast drying causes carotenoid destruction, but slow drying induces an increase in carotenoid concentration. Nitrogen flushing and high water activity have also been shown to increase the carotenoid retention in dried red peppers (Minguez-Mosquera *et al.*, 1993). Drying of tomatoes at low temperature and in osmotic conditions, instead of air or vacuum drying, has been shown to maximise the retention of lycopene (Shi & Le Maguer, 2000).

12.2.3 Plant sterols

Like saponins, plant sterols are also triterpenoid derivatives. As discussed in Chapter 10, plant sterols are an essential component of the membranes of all plants. The commonly consumed plant sterols are sitosterol, stigmasterol and campesterol, predominantly supplied by vegetable oils. These oils are also a rich source of sterol esters. Less important sources of sterols are cereals, nuts and vegetables. The effect of oil refining on plant sterols has been extensively studied. However, only a few studies concerning other processes, either industrial processes or different food preparation methods at home, have been published.

Plant sterol contents may change as a result of different processes because of the removal of sterols, or chemical reactions. A significant quantity of sterols in plant materials may be lost by removal of the sterol-rich parts such as the peel or seeds. Sterols are also removed when the oil is refined (see Section 10.9.3). Reactions leading to a decrease in sterol content, changes in sterol composition or reaction products of sterols include oxidation reactions, hydrolysis, isomerisation and other intramolecular transformations (Piironen *et al.*, 2000). Significant sterol losses may occur at temperatures reached during deep-frying.

Limited data are available on the stability of plant sterols according to different food preparation procedures used in the home. Normén *et al.* investigated sterol losses, resulting from cooking in 13 types of vegetables and fruits (Normén *et al.*, 1999). They concluded that there was no significant difference between raw and cooked samples at a group level. There are also no significant differences in the sterol content of untreated and treated oils when foods are microwaved (Albi *et al.*, 1997). Very few studies have looked at stability during storage; however no significant changes in total sterol contents are likely to take place in most practical situations. After prolonged storage, some oxidation products may be found.

12.3 Phenolic compounds

Plant phenolics (see Section 2.2) contribute to the colour and flavour of fruit and vegetables (see Section 7.2). During storage and processing, the reactivity of phenolic compounds and the activity of polyphenol oxidases can cause changes in colour, taste and nutritional value of the product.

12.3.1 Flavonoids

Flavonoids are water-soluble, bioactive secondary metabolites in plants (see Section 2.2.1). Structurally they are diphenylpyrans (C6–C3–C6) comprising two benzene rings, A and B, linked through a heterocyclic pyran or pyrone ring C. Flavonoids are classified in sub-classes according to the structure of the joining heterocyclic ring C. The most common classes are flavonols, flavones, flavanones, flavan-3-ols, anthocyanins and isoflavones. It is assumed that each family of plants has a characteristic pattern of flavonoids; most flavonoids have very restricted distribution within the plant kingdom and may occur in only one genus or even species. Flavonoids exist in plants almost entirely as glycosides, and a flavonoid can have many different glycosides (see

Chapters 2 and 6). Flavonoids are basically thermostable, but cooking can cause them to leach into the cooking liquor, resulting in altered chemical structures. The main sources of flavonoids in the UK diet are tea, onions, wine and apples (Peterson & Dwyer 1998a,b) (see Chapters 1, 6, 7 and 9).

(i) Flavonols

DuPont *et al.* have studied the effect of processing and storage on the flavonol content (mainly quercetin) and composition in eight varieties of lettuce and three varieties of endives (mainly kaemferol) (DuPont *et al.*, 2000). Shredding and subsequent exposure to light caused significant losses (6–94%) in the total flavonol content in these salad leaves. Seven-day refrigerated storage also resulted in a marked loss (7–46%) of flavonol glycosides. Among the individual glycosides, malonated conjugates decreased the most, but there was no evidence of formation of respective aglycones or an increase in other conjugates. Further studies in lettuce suggest that peroxidase, polyphenol oxidase and phenolase might be responsible for the rapid degradation of the flavonol aglycone moiety to phenolic acids and production of brown pigments on oxidation.

Modified atmosphere storage does not appear to have an important role in the retention of flavonols in leafy vegetables. Gil *et al.* have shown that the total flavonol content of minimally processed Swiss chard after 8 days of storage remained constant, although increased extraction was noticed during boiling in water (Gil *et al.*, 1998). Likewise, the total flavonol content of fresh-cut spinach was very similar whether stored in air or under a modified atmosphere (Gil *et al.*, 1999).

The main effect of heat on the flavonol (quercetin and kaempferol) content of vegetables seems to be in the leaching into the cooking medium, rather than chemical degradation. Boiling broccoli florets in water for 15 min resulted in only 14–28% of the individual glycosides being retained, the rest being leached into the cooking water (Price *et al.*, 1998a). When the different heating methods (blanching, boiling, microwaving and frying) used to process onions, green beans and peas were compared, it was noted that frying and blanching were less damaging than the other methods. However, for onions the major losses were associated with peeling off the outer flavonol-rich layers (Ewald *et al.*, 1999). The cooking losses of quercetin in tomatoes and onions have been shown to be greater during microwaving and boiling than after frying (Crozier *et al.*, 1997). On the other hand, canning has not been reported to cause chemical degradation of flavonols in green beans (Price *et al.*, 1998b).

(ii) Anthocyanins

Anthocyanins (see Section 2.2.1*iv*) are the most common group of flavonoids present in berries, cherries and grapes, and give them their specific colours (see Sections 7.6.1 and 7.6.2). The colour of anthocyanins is strongly dependent on pH; they are usually red in acid, purple or colourless in neutral and blue in alkaline conditions. Following oxidation of the benzene rings (A and B) their colour turns to brown. At a low pH, the anthocyanins are relatively stable and can withstand most food processing conditions (Ainsworth, 1994).

The effect of different cooking methods (steaming, boiling and frying) on anthocyanin levels has been studied in purple-fleshed potatoes. Anthocyanins in these potatoes are thermally stable. During frying and steaming they are relatively well retained, whereas during boiling, a substantially greater amount of the pigments is lost through leaching (Lewis *et al.*, 1996). Despite their apparent thermostability, the retention of anthocyanins in freeze-dried strawberry juice is dependent on storage temperature; their concentration decreases with increasing temperature (Irzyniec *et al.*, 1993).

In wine production (see Section 9.6), anthocyanins are degraded during fermentation (Rommel *et al.*, 1990). The choice of starting material in wine production also affects the stability of anthocyanins during storage. Wine made from flash-pasteurised, depectinised juice retains more anthocyanins than fermented fruit pulp or depectinised juice after both 6 months of storage

at 20 °C and 3 months at 2 °C. Addition of sulphur dioxide increases the retention of these pigments (Withy *et al.*, 1993).

(iii) Flavan-3-ols

Tea is a particularly rich source of flavonoids (see Section 9.3.3). Fresh tea-leaves can contain up to 30% of flavonoids on a dry weight basis. In the production of green tea, the leaves are picked, heated and dried. The main flavan-3-ols in green tea are catechins (see Section 2.2.1*iii*). Komatsu *et al.* studied the effect of pH on the degradation of catechins in green tea infusions and showed that the degradation of epicatechin is dependent on pH (Komatsu *et al.*, 1993). pH values greater than 6.0 increased the degradation, but catechins were stable under acidic conditions, although they tended to isomerise.

In black tea production (see Section 9.3) the leaves are fermented (enzymically oxidised). During this process, a substantial amount of catechins present in green tea are transformed to the polymerised forms, theaflavins and thearubigins (Poulter, 1998; Clifford, 2000c).

In lentils, different processing methods (soaking, cooking and germination) have been shown to increase the content of catechins and tannins (Vidal-Valverde *et al.*, 1994).

(iv) Isoflavones

The main chemical forms of isoflavones in soya beans are the malonylglucoside conjugates (see Section 8.6.2). Cooking and processing will change the content and the composition of the isoflavones in soya beans. Most soya foods contain a mixture of aglucones, and three different glucosides, malonyl-β-glucoside, β-glucoside and acetyl-β-glucoside of isoflavones. Minimally processed soya products, such as defatted soya flour (produced by grinding and fat extraction with hexane), have an isoflavone concentration and profile comparable to that of intact soya beans (Huei, 1995).

The processing of soya beans to produce tempeh, soya 'milk', tofu and soya protein isolate causes variable changes in the content and profile of isoflavones. Soaking removes 12% of isoflavones in soya beans, probably through increased β-glucosidase activity (Budi-Santosa & Wei, 1996). In the production of tempeh, cooking can cause up to a 50% decrease in isoflavones; heat treatment induces decarboxylation of malonyl conjugates to form acetyl conjugates and further degradation to minor constituents. During protein coagulation in tofu making, 44% of isoflavones are lost (Huei & Murphy, 1996). Fermentation increases the concentration of aglycones, especially the polyhydroxylated forms (Klus & Barz, 1998); fungal enzymic hydrolysis and the aglycones of isoflavones are more prevalent in miso and tempeh than non-fermented products (Huei, 1995). The bioavailability (see Section 6.4) of isoflavones from fermented soya products is greater than from non-fermented products because aglucones are absorbed faster and in greater amounts than their glucosides (Izumi *et al.*, 2000).

In the production of soya protein isolate, alkaline extraction results in the formation of aglycones and large losses of isoflavone components. Only 26% of the original isoflavone concentration is found in soya protein isolate (Wang *et al.*, 1998). However, it has been shown that the retention of isoflavones depends on the extraction method used. Acid and hot water extraction cause retentions of nearly 80 and 75% of the original genistin and genistein content, respectively, whereas alcohol extraction results in over 90% losses of these isoflavones (Pandjaitan *et al.*, 2000b). The bioavailability (see Sections 6.4 and 8.6.2) of genistein from soya protein concentrate can be increased by the addition of a hydrolysing enzyme, β-glucosidase (Pandjaitan *et al.*, 2000a).

Extrusion cooking has been shown to cause a decrease in malonylglucosides because of the high temperature required. Total isoflavones are reduced when extracted with 80% aqueous methanol. Hydration of the soya beans before extraction can prevent the losses of isoflavones in extruded soya beans, simultaneously increasing the proportion of aglycone forms of isoflavones (Mahungu *et al.*, 1999). Isoflavones present in soya foods are stable for domestic cooking processes; boiling and baking do not alter the levels (Coward *et al.*, 1993).

(v) Flavanones

The only type of processing to be investigated is the effect of irradiation on flavanones, which has been shown to stimulate the synthesis of phenolic compounds in citrus fruit. When Moroccan clementines were irradiated with a mean dose of 0.3 kGy before storing them for 49 days at 3°C, an enhanced formation of the major flavanone hesperidin and the flavones nobiletin and heptamethoxyflavone was recorded. This was thought to be related to an improved resistance to pathogens (Oufedjikh *et al.*, 2000).

(vi) Lignans

Lignans are chemically related to the polymeric lignins of the plant cell wall and are found mainly in woody tissues (see Section 8.6.3). Lignans present in linseed were found to be stable under normal baking temperatures. Levels of the precursor secoisolariciresinol (seco) in baked goods were found to be similar to the estimates of seco added to the dough (Muir & Westcott, 2000).

(vii) Coumarins

The 700 or more plant coumarins can all be derived from the parent compound coumarin, which has a characteristic odour of new-mown hay. Coumarins occur widely (see Section 2.3*ii*), usually in a bound form. They are widely distributed in natural flavourings such as Tonkin beans, usually as the result of a fungal attack, and are also present in essential oils. For mammals, including humans, the most dangerous coumarins are the aflatoxins, which are fungal metabolites and hepatotoxic, and dicoumarol, which is a blood anticoagulant. They occur widely, but are extensively tested for, and the levels permitted in foods are extremely low.

There are limited data on the effects of processing on coumarins. The levels of five coumarins present in grapefruit juice were reduced by 50% by centrifugation (Berry & Tatum, 1986). Another successful method is the removal of coumarins and flavonoids from orange and grapefruit juices by treatment with β-cyclodextrin polymer (Shaw & Wilson, 1983). Coumarins are removed from mechanically treated citrus oils by winterising (Johnson *et al.*, 1978). During storage of cassava roots, coumarins and phenols are produced (Uritani *et al.*, 1984).

12.4 Sulphur-containing compounds

The glucosinolates are a large group of sulphur-containing compounds that occur in all the economically important varieties of Brassica vegetables (see Sections 2.5*ii*, 5.4.3 and 7.5.3). All the glucosinolates possess a common structure comprising a β-D-thioglucose group, a sulphonated oxime moiety and a variable side-chain derived from methionine, tryptophan, phenylalanine and some branched-chain amino acids (Fenwick *et al.*, 1983).

When the plant tissue is damaged by food preparation or chewing, glucosinolates are brought into contact with and hydrolysed by the endogenous enzyme myrosinase, releasing a complex variety of breakdown products including isothiocyanates. These hot and bitter compounds, commonly termed 'mustard oils', are often volatile with an acrid smell (see Section 7.4.3). Cutting the fresh plant tissue creates optimal conditions for myrosinase so that a high degree of glucosinolate hydrolysis can be expected. The effect of cooking on glucosinolates has received a relatively large amount of attention. Cooking reduces glucosinolate levels by approximately 30–60% depending on the method, cooking intensity and on the type of compound. Thermal degradation and washout also occur, leading to large losses of intact glucosinolates (Mithen *et al.*, 2000). Breakdown products of glucosinolates are apparently hardly detectable after prolonged cooking, with the exception of the thiocyanate ion and ascorbigen (MacLeod & MacLeod, 1968).

During the fermentation of white cabbage to produce sauerkraut, all glucosinolates were found to be hydrolysed within 2 weeks (Daxenbichler *et al.*, 1980). Blanching also causes a loss in glucosinolates. Goodrich *et al.* compared different blanching conditions for broccoli and Brussels sprouts. Large glucosinolate losses occurred in the former, but not the latter (Goodrich *et al.*, 1989).

Low-temperature storage conditions such as freezing and refrigerating can alter the metabolism of glucosinolates. Freezing without previous inactivation of myrosinase results in almost complete decomposition of glucosinolates after thawing (Quinsac *et al.*, 1994). On the other hand, storage of chopped cabbage at room temperature for 48 h leads to substantial increases in the levels of some indolyl glucosinolates (Verkerk *et al.*, 2001). In general, there is still little information about the influence of storage on total or individual glucosinolate content of Brassica vegetables. However, a predictive modelling approach to this problem has recently been reported (Verkerk, 2002).

12.5 Protease inhibitors

Protease inhibitors are widely distributed in plants, and cereals and pulses are particularly rich sources (see Section 8.3). Soya beans, kidney beans, chick peas and other pulses contain protease inhibitors, some of which survive canning and processing including that involved in making tofu. Plant breeding to eliminate protease inhibitor activity can, and is, being achieved. Moist heat treatment in the form of home cooking or industrial food processing is an effective method for decreasing protease inhibitor activity and improving the nutritional quality of the plant protein.

Normal cooking procedures significantly decrease the trypsin inhibitor activity of broad beans, cabbage and potatoes (Doell *et al.*, 1981). In addition, autoclaving almost completely eliminates the trypsin inhibitor content of faba beans (Sharma & Sehgal, 1992) and the activity of tofu and cooked tofu is 19 and 11%, respectively, of that in raw soya beans (Doell *et al.*, 1981).

Heat treatments including spray drying or canning and sterilisation, which are used to manufacture soya-based infant formulas from soya protein isolates, decrease the trypsin inhibitor activity effectively so that the final level is approximately 3% of that in raw soya flour (Churella *et al.*, 1976).

12.6 Vitamin C

Vitamin C is a water-soluble antioxidant (see Section 1.4.3, and Chapter 7). It is the most vulnerable of vitamins, and losses during storage and food processing can be substantial and nutritionally significant. However, the bioavailability of vitamin C is generally very high, similar to that of supplements. The vitamin C content of fruits and vegetables varies greatly and is affected by agronomic conditions and the maturity of plants at harvest (see Chapter 7). The use of increasing amounts of nitrogen fertiliser has been reported to decrease the vitamin C content of cauliflower (Lisiewska & Kmiecik, 1996), but climatic conditions were reported to have a greater impact on the vitamin C content of broccoli than the use of nitrogen fertiliser (Toivonen *et al.*, 1994). In sweet pepper cultivars, vitamin C was shown to increase with maturity (Howard *et al.*, 1994), whereas in potatoes there is an increase in vitamin activity up to 11 weeks after planting, followed by a decrease in activity (Mondy & Munshi, 1993).

Once fruits and vegetables have been harvested, the concentration of vitamin C immediately starts to decline. During fresh storage, vitamin C is lost through ascorbic acid oxidase-catalysed oxidation. The decease in vitamin C concentration is also influenced by the surface area of the plant, storage temperature, atmospheric oxygen, pH, light exposure and the presence of other oxygen scavengers in the plant (Shewfelt, 1990). In citrus fruits, because of the low pH, vitamin C is relatively stable, but in soft fruits vitamin C activity decreases more rapidly. Green leafy vegetables, peas and green beans are particularly vulnerable, whereas root vegetables (potatoes) can retain their vitamin C content for months (Favell, 1998). During storage, cruciferous vegetables retain vitamin C levels better than non-cruciferous vegetables. After 3 weeks of storage at 2 °C, Savoy cabbage had retained 75% and broccoli 98% of their initial vitamin C activity, whereas green beans retained only 16% over the same period (Albrecht *et al.*, 1990). Storage temperature is a critical factor in retention of vitamin C activity. For example, when fresh spinach and amaranth leaves were stored at 5 °C, the losses were in the range 1–6%, but at 30 °C the losses ranged from 55 to 66% (Kala-Yadav & Sehgal, 1995). Modified atmosphere packaging has been shown to improve vitamin C retention in blanched sweet green peppers (Petersen & Berends, 1993), broccoli florets (Barth & Hong, 1996) and lettuce (Serafini *et al.*, 2002). Reports of the effects of irradiation of potatoes are contradictory as some claim improved retention (Joshi *et al.*, 1990) and others increased losses of vitamin C activity (Shirsat & Thomas, 1998).

Vitamin C retention during frozen storage is dependent on the treatment before freezing. Blanching inactivates oxidative enzymes and improves the long-term storage retention of vitamin C, despite initial losses that are typically in the range of 20–25% of total vitamin activity for beans, peas, sprouts and cauliflower. In blanched vegetables, vitamin C retention can be in the region of 90% after 12 months at 25 °C, but if vegetables are frozen unblanched, then major nutrient losses can occur during storage (Favell, 1998).

During cooking, vitamin C is lost mainly through leaching and heat-induced degradation. When the effects of conventional cooking methods on vitamin C retention were studied, the shortest possible cooking time with the minimal amount of water retained the highest amount of vitamin C activity (Pither & Edwards, 1995). For example, during the application of conventional cooking processes to different vegetables (cauliflower, white cabbage, Brussels sprouts, French beans and potatoes), average losses ranged from 14% for microwave cooking to 53% for boiling (beginning with cold water). If the water was boiling before vegetables were added, losses were reduced to 38% (Ilow *et al.*, 1995). With green beans it has been demonstrated that vitamin C losses during cooking are lowest for steaming, followed by pressure cooking, then microwaving and boiling (De la Cruz-Carcia *et al.*, 2000). Washing vegetables before cutting and using a saucepan lid also minimise vitamin C losses (Tapadia *et al.*, 1995).

Canning, extrusion cooking and drying cause the biggest losses of vitamin C because these conditions are so extreme. During canning, losses of vitamin C are typically greater than 50% (Edwards *et al.*, 1990). In some acidic fruits, losses of vitamin C could be lower because of their low pH (Ang & Livingstone, 1974).

12.7 Vitamin E

Cereal grains and their products are important sources of vitamin E (see Section 8.2) and losses that occur during storage are of considerable practical importance. Vitamin E losses in intact grains stored under good commercial conditions are small, but losses are accelerated under adverse storage conditions and as a result of insect infestation (Pomeranz, 1992). Considerable losses in vitamin E have been observed during the storage of vegetable oils.

One of the most important industrial processes that impacts on the stability of tocopherols and tocotrienols is that of plant oil processing. Losses of tocopherols reported in refined oils were 15% in olive oil, 25% in soya bean and rapeseed oils, 32% in corn oil and 35–40% in cotton seed, sunflower and peanut oil (Kanematsu *et al.*, 1983). Substantial losses of tocopherols have also been observed during commercial frying operations, About 32% of the initial tocopherol in peanut oil was destroyed by heating for 30 min at 175 °C but losses were reduced by the addition of synergists (Bauernfeind, 1980). Losses of α-tocopherol in olive oils during a 6 month storage test at room temperature in the dark ranged from 14 to 32% (Manzi *et al.*, 1998).

Vitamin E is unstable in light, heat and air, so almost any processing method will adversely affect its concentration. Milling and industrial-scale bread-making cause significant losses of tocopherols and tocotrienols. The α-tocopherol content of some varieties of green olives is reduced during the debittering and fermentation process. It is assumed that because tocopherols and tocotrienols are fat-soluble, they are not as severely affected by home cooking for immediate consumption as the water-soluble vitamins. However, Wyate *et al.* measured the α- and γ-tocopherol contents of a range of cereals and legumes (see Chapter 8) before and after conventional cooking. They observed losses of vitamin E activity of 22–55% in cereals and 10–60% in legumes (Wyate *et al.*, 1998). This suggests that vitamin E losses during home cooking may be more substantial than have previously been considered.

12.8 Folate

Plant foods are a major source of dietary folate, a B vitamin required in one-carbon transfer reactions (see Section 1.4.4). The term folate refers to the multiple forms of folic acid (pteroyl-L-glutamic acid) present in the plant kingdom. The most common forms of naturally occurring folates are 5-methyltetrahydrofolate, tetrahydrofolate and 5-formyltetrahydrofolate, which are reduced forms (their oxidation state is lower than that of folic acid) and more reactive than the folic acid itself. Normally, one or more glutamyl residues are attached to the *p*-aminobenzoic group of the folic acid forming mono- or poly-glutamates. Different forms of folates exist in different plants (Witthoft *et al.*, 1999).

Because of their chemical reactivity and solubility, folates are easily lost during storage, processing and cooking. During fresh storage, temperature is a crucial factor in relation to retention. In spinach stored at ambient temperature for 10 h, the concentration of total folates was reduced by 7%. Keeping the spinach chilled improved folate retention; after 7 days of storage 64% of folates were retained. Although the total folate content of fresh vegetables declines significantly during storage, there is a proportional increase in free total folate due to the endogenous conjugase (Chen *et al.*, 1983). Blanching, as an enzyme inactivation process, minimises folate losses during frozen storage. In Brussels sprouts blanched before freezing, no further losses were noted during 6 months of storage, whereas un-blanched Brussels sprouts lost 48% of their folate content (Malin, 1977).

During cooking processes, folate is mainly lost through leaching. The losses increase with increasing temperature and time, and with the amount of water used. Blanching spinach in a microwave oven without added water caused a loss of 14% of total folates, whereas water blanching resulted in twice as much folate leaching into the cooking water (Chen *et al.*, 1983). The significance of leaching as a mechanism of folate loss has also been demonstrated (DeSouza & Eitenmiller, 1986). It was found that 40 and 68% of folate was lost from spinach and broccoli, respectively, during water blanching, compared with nominal folate losses of 1 and 4% during steam blanching. Identical boiling conditions (10 min) used for a selection of vegetables (asparagus, broccoli, Brussels sprouts, cabbage, cauliflower and spinach) resulted in folate losses ranging from 22% for asparagus to 84% for cauliflower. This indicates the existence of different forms of folate in different vegetables and the possible role of the food matrix in retention (Leichter *et al.*, 1978).

In legumes, pre-soaking prior to cooking facilitates folate losses. During 20 min of cooking, unsoaked legumes lost 40% of the folate content. Folate losses were increased to 65% if legumes were soaked in cold water for 16 h, and to 80% after quick soaking (boiled for 2 min and then left soaking for 1 h). When the cooking time was increased to 150 min, the differences in folate retention due to pretreatment disappeared; long cooking times resulting in high losses of folates in all cases (Hoppner & Lampi, 1993).

Irradiation has also been demonstrated to cause a reduction in vegetable folate content. When spinach, cabbage and Brussels sprouts were irradiated (2.5–10 kGy), up to 30% folate losses were recorded. Polyglutamate forms of folate were lost at a greater rate than monoglutamate forms, resulting in an increase in the bioavailability of retained folates (Mueller & Diehl, 1996).

12.9 Research recommendations

- There is a need for better information about the effects of storage, processing and cooking on the bioactive plant compounds found in commonly eaten foods. Such data should be collected using a large and representative sample of plant-based foods.
- These studies need to examine the effect of storage, processing and cooking conditions that are relevant to those undertaken both in a typical kitchen and during industrial-scale food production.
- The results of these studies then need to be translated into simple and practical advice for the consumer.

12.10 Key points

- Research on bioactive substances in foods is constantly expanding and developing. The emphasis has been on discovering and classifying their function in plants and their importance for human nutrition. In many cases, knowledge of the effects of storage, processing and cooking is very limited.
- The processing of plant crops has resulted in a wider choice of nutritious, good-quality produce being available all year round in a convenient form for the consumer.
- Retention of bioactive substances depends on their chemical and physical properties, the type of food in which they are found and the storage conditions and the processes used. As a rule, the higher the processing/cooking temperature, the longer is the holding time, and the greater the exposure to oxygen, the more detrimental is the effect on the content of fruit and vegetables.
- Bioactive substances can be classified as water-soluble (flavonoids, vitamin C and folate) or fat-soluble (carotenoids, other terpenoids and sterols). The main method of losing water-soluble substances is by leaching into the cooking medium, whereas fat-soluble substances are lost through oxidative degradation.
- Careful harvesting and keeping fresh plant foods at chilled temperatures and protected from exposure to air during storage minimise the losses of bioactive substances. Blanching

the plant products before freezing greatly improves the retention during frozen storage.

- During processing and cooking, the retention of water-soluble substances can be maximised by using the minimum amount of water, starting cooking with boiling water and cooking for a minimum amount of time. Losses are lower with steaming, frying or microwaving than with traditional boiling. In canning, a high proportion of water-soluble components is usually lost.

- Fat-soluble bioactive substances are basically stable during heat treatments, but rearrangements in their structure may occur. Addition of oil during cooking increases the retention and bioavailability of some of these compounds.

- Plant breeding may have an important role in developing plants with modified levels of bioactive compounds, and information about the optimal levels required for plant protection and human health will require further research.

Appendix: definitions of different types of storage, processing and cooking techniques

(a) Factors determining the shelf-life of a product

Storage stability and therefore shelf-life of fruit and vegetables are characterised by physical, chemical, enzymatic and microbiological reactions. These processes are influenced by the exposure to heat, air, light, pH and the water content of the plant.

(b) Storage

Storage is defined as the time between harvesting and consumption. Fruit and vegetables can be stored either fresh or processed. Processed products will have no active microbial population and minimal enzymatic activity before storage, whereas fresh vegetables will have an active microbial population and enzyme activity.

(c) Fresh storage

In fresh fruit and vegetables, respiration and other biochemical reactions continue during storage. As the rate of biological reactions is highly dependent on the temperature, the storage temperature is an important determinant of the shelf-life of fresh products.

(d) Modified atmosphere storage/packaging

The modification of the atmosphere in which foods are packaged, by decreasing the oxygen content and increasing the concentrations of nitrogen, an inert gas, and/or carbon dioxide, which together inhibit growth of bacteria.

(e) Processing techniques

(i) Freezing

Freezing is a cooling process in which the temperature of food products is rapidly reduced to around −20 °C and then stored frozen. Fruit and vegetables are often blanched (short heat treatment) prior to freezing in order to inactivate enzymes with deteriorative effects.

(ii) Canning

In canning, a vigorous heat treatment (115 °C, 25–100 min) is used to sterilise the product to give it indefinite storage life. Oxygen is also excluded.

(iii) Drying

In drying, the water content of plant foods is reduced to the level where biological reactions are inhibited.

(iv) Fermentation

In fermentation, available carbohydrates are used by natural or inoculated microbial populations to induce chemical and physical changes, forming a product that can be stored for extended periods.

(v) Milling

Milling is the process of separating endosperm from bran and germ, and then grinding down the endosperm into flour-sized particles.

(vi) Oil refining

The chemical modification of crude seed oils through neutralisation, bleaching and deodorisation results in a bland, stable oil. The characteristics of the oil are also affected by the raw material and the addition of antioxidants and heavy metal chelators after deodorisation.

(vii) Irradiation

High-energy ionising radiation is used in irradiation to control and disrupt biological processes in order to extend the shelf-life of fresh products. Currently, its use in the UK is limited to spices.

(viii) Cooking

In cooking, the temperature of the food is raised. Traditional wet cooking methods include blanching, boiling, steaming, pressure cooking, stewing and poaching. Dry cooking methods comprise frying, baking, roasting, barbecuing and griddling. Heat can also be applied to the food by electromagnetic radiation; short wavelengths are used in grilling and longer wavelengths provide the energy in microwave ovens.

13
Implications for Public Health

13.1 Introduction

Nutrition is a fundamental determinant of the health experience of communities. The patterns of chronic disease in developed countries are as much a product of nutritional exposures over life as is malnutrition in developing countries. Which individuals within those communities are most vulnerable to particular exposures may be determined by constitutional factors such as genetic predisposition, but the population's experience is rarely so. There are several definitions of what constitutes the discipline of public health. A particularly useful one is 'the science and art of preventing disease, prolonging life and promoting health through organised efforts of society' (Department of Health, 1988). Public health nutrition applies these principles to 'a focus on the promotion of good health through nutrition and the primary prevention of diet-related illness in the population' (www.nutsoc.org.uk) and in practice this requires appropriately trained professionals to execute the necessary roles (Landman et al., 1998). Specifically, skills are needed in the identification of nutrition related problems in the community; assessment of diet and of nutrition status; in the interpretation of information pertaining to nutrition status both in individuals and in populations; in the analysis of evidence relating to the impact of interventions on nutrition status at the individual, group or community level; and in the development and evaluation of appropriate and practical interventions based on evidence.

Within the UK it is recognised that there would be advantage if the balance of people's diets, in general, were shifted more toward vegetable and fruit consumption, as well as towards starchy foods. The evidence for likely and possible benefits of such plant foods is summarised in earlier chapters, but is also a cornerstone of the reports of national and international expert groups that have examined the issue (World Cancer Research Fund, 1997; Department of Health, 1998b), and of government programmes (World Health Organisation, 1990, 2003; Acheson, 1998; Department of Health, 2000b–d; Potter et al., 2000). The postulated benefits of greater inclusion of plant foods in the diet include reduced risks of cardiovascular diseases and of some cancers, and possible benefits in other conditions including diabetes, lung function and eye health (see Section 3.2). Cardiovascular diseases and cancer comprise around three quarters of deaths in the UK, so that any reduction in morbidity and premature death from these causes would have an important impact on public health. There are also likely to be benefits in relation to obesity, given that plant foods tend to be relatively low in energy content and hence their inclusion in the diet might help to maintain a healthy weight.

13.1.1 Approaches to changing eating behaviour

There are several different approaches that could be taken to influence population eating behaviours. They are not mutually exclusive, and in some situations may be complementary.

A primary distinction is whether to target individual behaviour within a population or to take actions that influence behaviour at the population level. Which of these to choose depends on a number of factors – the nature of the problem, the feasibility of the intervention and, crucially, the political environment in which the decision is to be taken. Population-based approaches are often seen as restrictive of individual freedoms, and therefore undesirable, while individual-based approaches are regarded as giving choice to consumers.

In fact, population-based approaches that restrict individual choice in the interests of public health are widespread – there is legislation controlling the addition of nutrients to flour and to margarines (see Section 13.7.1); there are laws relating to the information which may be provided on or about foods; and, although not a nutritional issue, there is legislation regarding wearing of seat belts. Other approaches at this level might include fiscal measures such as taxation (as already exists for tobacco and alcohol), or agricultural or import controls to influence the broad national food supply. Although not intended as a health policy – and controversial regarding its precise health impact – the Common Agricultural Policy has had a clear impact on the macro-economics of the food supply within Europe, distorting the usual relationships between prices, supply and demand.

Individual-based approaches seek to target people's choices more directly, by influencing their knowledge, attitudes or beliefs. At the simplest level, simply providing information can be regarded as a policy in its own right. Where nutrition information is provided on a food label, it must be provided in a standard, prescribed format. It can be argued that this then allows consumers to exercise choice in their selection of foods. Educational leaflets or campaigns may improve consumers' ability to utilise such information. Health promotion activity within a healthcare setting can target information, education and encouragement to change consumers on a one-to-one basis. Other factors that impact on consumers' ability to choose include their affluence and access to the foods.

In practice, it has proved difficult to manipulate overall dietary behaviour. In spite of evidence that over time the national diet has proved very variable, identifying, harnessing and directing the relevant pressures have not been possible. Consumers appear generally to be well informed about the essentials of healthy eating – but so-called optimistic bias means that they tend to perceive their behaviour as closer to desirable than it actually is (Shepherd, 1999). This naturally tends to minimise their response to targeted campaigns for changing behaviour. In addition, understanding of the healthy eating messages may not be deep (Buttriss, 1997), as education in schools and elsewhere about nutrition is not a priority, and conflicting messages delivered through a variety of channels including the media (radio, press and television) and the internet can confuse. Although one-to-one counselling can impact on individuals' behaviour, the effects are small (Langham *et al.*, 1996) and are resource intensive. It is difficult for people to maintain a pattern of eating that is substantively different from that of their family, peer group or community.

A number of health plans aim to diminish socio-economic variations in health through related behaviours (see Section 13.4), such as fruit and vegetable consumption. One means of doing this is to improve access (both economic and physical) to the components of a healthy diet. Food deserts projects are helping to inform about this process (Warm *et al.*, 2002). Information and education campaigns intended to achieve this are paradoxically most effective in the better off, who have less need to change. The outcome is often a widening of the inequality.

The centrality of food to social functioning means that efforts to alter behaviour out of context are likely to fail. Consequently, strategies most likely to succeed are those which combine individual-based approaches within a broader population strategy. The selection of policies which are effective and acceptable is often a matter of political or ethical concern, as much as a scientific or health issue.

Recent policies in England include the provision of fruit for primary school children in the NHS Plan (Department of Health, 2000c), emphasis on vegetables and fruit in statutory requirements for school lunches (Department for Education and Employment, 2000) and a general

Table 13.1 UK initiatives that focus on plant foods, particularly fruits and vegetables.

Initiative	Responsibility	Key aspects	References and websites
School fruit scheme	Department of Health	All 4–6 year olds at school in England; pilots began in 2000 and the scheme is to be fully operational by 2004. The pilots are focusing on three separate phases: 'farm to school gate', 'school gate to child's hand' and 'hand to mouth'. Complementary schemes that are not currently government-funded have been piloted in parts of Scotland and Wales	Department of Health (2000e) www.doh.gov.uk www.scotland.gov.uk www.wales.gov.uk www.northernireland.gov.uk
5-a-day programme	Department of Health	National campaign in England; pilots were completed in five areas of England in August 2001, and targeted a million people. The key issues being addressed are access, availability and affordability; awareness; acceptability. To increase provision and access, particularly in deprived communities, schools and hospitals, the government intends working with producers, retailers and other key stakeholders	Department of Health (2000e) www.doh.gov.uk/fiveaday
National standards for school lunches	Department for Education and Employment (now Department for Education and Skills)	Compulsory nutritional standards for lunches served in nursery, primary and secondary schools, in England and Wales came into force in April 2001. To meet the new standards, fruit and vegetables will have to be on offer every day as part of the school lunch. In Scotland, nutritional standards for school meals, developed by a joint Social Justice, Education and Health initiative were launched in February 2003, and will be in place by 2006.	Department of Education and Employment (2000) www.dfes.gov.uk www.scotland.gov.uk www.wales.gov.uk www.deni.gov.uk/schools/meals/index.htm
Healthy schools standard	Department for Education and Employment (now Department for Education and Skills)	This encourages schools in England to consider diet and nutrition issues in all aspects of school life, and is part of the Healthy Schools Programme, led by the Department for Education and Skills and Department of Health. Its overall aim is to help schools become healthier through the development and improvement of local schools programmes. Initiatives to support the Healthy Schools Programme include *Wired for Health*, a website (www.wiredforhealth.gov.uk) providing reliable information for teachers for each of the four National Curriculum Key Stages	

Table 13.1 (Cont'd)

Initiative	Responsibility	Key aspects	References and websites
Catering for health	Food Standards Agency & Department of Health	Practical guidelines for nutrition for use in the training of chefs and caterers, developed by the British Nutrition Foundation in 2000–1. Separate versions for use in Scotland and Wales were launched in May 2002	Food Standards Agency and Department of Health (2001) www.food.gov.uk www.scotland.gov.uk www.wales.gov.uk
Targets and activities in Wales	FSA Wales (Nutrition Strategy)	Targets are to increase intake of fruit and vegetables, particularly among infants, children, young people, low-income and vulnerable groups, women of childbearing age and middle-aged men. The target in the strategy, launched in February 2003, is to increase fruit and vegetable intake by 10% by 2010.	FSA Wales Food & Wellbeing 2003 www.food.gov.uk/wales/ nutritionstrategy
Targets and activities in Scotland	Scottish Executive	A Scottish Food and Health Co-ordinator has been appointed. A variety of activities are under way, some of which target fruit and vegetable consumption. The Scottish Community Diet project (developed by the Scottish Consumer Council) is working with low-income communities. Grants are being provided for a range of projects including garden/allotment schemes, and a Breakfast Clubs tool kit has been produced. Health Improvement Fund monies (derived from tobacco taxation) are being used to improve Scotland's health. Priority areas include provision of fruit in pre-school settings, fruit and breakfast clubs in schools, and a theatre production for primary schools on fruit and vegetables	www.scotland.gov.uk
Targets and activities in Northern Ireland		The Food and Nutrition Strategy is due to be reviewed in 2002. The first North/South Ireland Food Consumption Survey was completed in 2001 giving accurate information about fruit and vegetable consumption in the island of Ireland	www.healthpromotionagency. org.uk

recognition of the need for local health policies to focus on diet in *Our Healthier Nation* (Department of Health, 1999b). There are counterpart strategy documents from other countries within the UK, *e.g.* in Scotland and Wales (The Scottish Office Department of Health, 1996; FSA Wales, 2003) (see Table 13.1).

In addition, enhancement of fruit and vegetable intake is an inevitable part of a range of more general policies, which emphasise the benefits to health of a balanced and varied diet, and which focus on health inequalities, given that fruit and vegetable intake is one of the aspects of diet most affected (see Section 1.3.4). Examples of such policies are the NHS Plans (Department of Health, 2000c), Cancer Plan (Department of Health, 2000b) and the National Service Frameworks for coronary heart disease (Department of Health, 2000d; Welsh Assembly, 2001b) and diabetes (Department of Health, 2001b; Welsh Assembly, 2001a). The NHS Plan stated that eating at least five portions of fruit and vegetables a day could lead to estimated reductions of up to 20% in overall deaths from chronic diseases, such as heart disease, stroke and cancer.

A number of national programmes of locally based projects are under way, as indicated in Table 13.1, and details of some of these can be found in Section 13.4.2. In addition, many local health alliances have engaged in smaller projects such as fruit tuck shops in schools, community cafes, food co-ops and healthy cookery classes, which generally have a fruit and vegetable component. Examples of these are given in Section 13.4.3. The Health Development Agency (HDA) in England has assessed such projects to identify effective interventions; the results can be found on its website (www.hda-online.org.uk). A toolkit is also under development by the HDA, see website for details.

Similarly, in other parts of Europe and in North America, there has been an emphasis on increasing fruit and vegetable consumption. Examples can be found in Section 13.4.1.

13.2 What is the target intake?

The question arises as to whether it is possible to establish an absolute intake of plant foods, in general or specific terms, which could be reliably taken to improve health.

A key message of this Task Force is the need for a varied diet given that the substances of interest are found in every food group and a broad selection of foods within each group, including herbs and condiments through to tea and wine. Certainly it is not possible, as yet, to tease out particular compounds as more important than others.

Despite widespread acceptance that eating fruit and vegetables is a health-promoting strategy, reviews suggest that formal evidence is relatively sparse for cardiovascular disease (Ness *et al.*, 1999; van't Veer *et al.*, 2000), although it is more abundant for some types of cancer (van't Veer *et al.*, 2000) (see Section 3.3 for more details). It needs to be recognised that higher fruit and vegetable intakes tend to go hand in hand with other lifestyle habits that are thought to be healthy (*e.g.* not smoking, being physically active), and when account is taken of these, the risk reduction is attenuated. For example, a recent meta-analysis of studies on fruit and vegetable consumption and cardiovascular disease suggested a reduction in risk of just 15% once such factors were taken into consideration (Law & Morris, 1998), and in some individual studies findings ceased to be statistically significant once account was taken of such factors (Liu *et al.*, 2000).

Apparent cardiovascular benefits are not restricted to fruits and vegetables. Other plant products including whole grains and nuts have also been reported to be of value (Hu & Stampfer, 1999; Jacobs *et al.*, 1999; Liu *et al.*, 1999). Evidence of this nature, uncertainty about the mechanisms involved and the precise dose–response relationships, together with the importance of other dietary and nutritional factors, serve to emphasise the importance of focusing on dietary patterns rather than individual nutrients (Jacobs & Murtaugh, 2000), and many countries now have food group-based dietary recommendations such as the UK's *Balance of Good Health* and the American *Food Guide Pyramid*. All such guides emphasise the role of fruit and vegetables in a balanced diet and typically recommend that about one third of food intake should come from this food group. How well the UK diet matches up to such recommendations can be found in Section 13.3.

Advice from the COMA Working Group on Nutritional Aspects of Cardiovascular Disease (Department of Health, 1994) to increase fruit and vegetable consumption by 50%, from an average of three portions to at least five portions per person per day on average, is a potentially achievable goal and is likely to be conducive to better health in general and a lower risk of some types of chronic disease in particular. The COMA Working Group considered that any increase in fruit and vegetable consumption would be expected to confer benefit.

With regard to cancer, the COMA Working Group (Department of Health, 1998b) concluded that there is insufficient evidence to quantify the optimum level of fruit and vegetable consumption associated with the lowest cancer risk, although they did recommend that intake is increased in the UK as previously recommended in 1994. There is some suggestion from observational studies that there might be a level of consumption above which no further benefit is seen, but this is well above the current average consumption in the UK.

In relation to cancer protection on a global scale, the WCRF (World Cancer Research Fund, 1997) recommended a year-round consumption of a variety of vegetables and fruit together providing 7% or more of total energy intake. They calculated that this would correspond to 400–800 g, or five or more servings, per day. They also recommended consumption of a variety of starchy or protein-rich foods of plant origin, to provide a further 45–60% of total energy intake. They suggest that this amounts to 600–800 g, or more than seven servings per day of cereals, grains, pulses, roots, tubers and plantains. The combined WCRF goal would be difficult to achieve in the short to medium term for most Western societies, given the large discrepancy with current dietary patterns.

Current policies are based on a change from current levels which are perceived to be too low, and are represented in qualitative ('eat more/less') or at best semi-quantitative ('five a day', '50% more') form. Derivation of a more precise level akin to micronutrient requirements would require a better knowledge of functional markers related both to health outcomes and to specific plant food (or component) intake, and to improved knowledge about mechanisms of action within the body. Such data are not yet available and any approach must therefore necessarily remain relativistic rather than absolute.

In summary, a consensus has developed amongst national and international expert groups (WHO, COMA, US National Cancer Institute) that for adults a reasonable target for Western societies, based on an increase over baseline, and which would be expected to confer tangible benefits both to individuals and to the population burden of disease, is of the order of at least 400 g/person/day. This is taken to equate to five or more portions of 80 g each (Williams, 1995) (see below). A portion of 80 g ties in well with the average serving size in British households, although serving size is influenced by factors such as age, gender and physical activity level. This approximation is the basis for the 'five a day' campaign in the USA and similar programmes in other developed countries, including the UK. It should be noted that the COMA figure of at least 400 g/person/day is a population goal, whereas the five-a-day message tends to be used as a goal for individuals. In reality, most people's intakes are so low compared with these goals that they can both potentially serve as aspirational goals, with the hope of moving average intakes towards the population goal.

There is insufficient evidence to support recommendations for particular types of fruits or vegetables. No universally accepted convention exists as to which vegetables and fruit should be included in the 400 g or how much of each type. Williams suggested that a way round this was to use 'try to eat five different fruits and vegetables' each day (Williams, 1995). To some extent, there is also inconsistency regarding the inclusion or exclusion of foods such as potatoes, nuts, pulses and dried fruit. For example, in the USA, the five-a-day message includes non-fried potatoes, which are excluded from the fruit and vegetables section

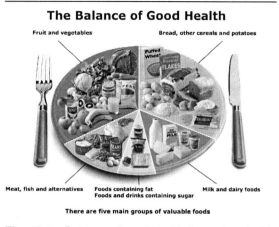

The Balance of Good Health

Fruit and vegetables   Bread, other cereals and potatoes

Meat, fish and alternatives   Foods containing fat   Milk and dairy foods
        Foods and drinks containing sugar

There are five main groups of valuable foods

Fig. 13.1 Balance of good health (reproduced with kind permission of the Food Standards Agency; specific versions for Scotland and Wales are also available).

in the UK guide, appearing instead with other starchy foods. Lack of clarity can cause confusion and uncertainty, and the Food Standards Agency (2001) has recently clarified some of these issues. For example, beans and pulses count as only one portion towards fruit/vegetable intake, however much is eaten in a day. The same applies to fruit juice. In the UK guides, pulses are also included in the meat, fish and alternatives group, along with nuts (see Fig. 13.1).

Painter *et al.* recently compared pictorial national food guides used in 12 countries around the world (Painter *et al.*, 2002). Table 13.2 shows the plant food recommendations for seven of these (and also for Ireland), as interpreted by Painter and colleagues. In some, fruits and vegetables are combined as one food group, whereas in others they are depicted as separate.

A hurdle for many is the decision as to what constitutes a portion. Useful advice has been published (Williams, 1995), which utilises the large body of information available from national surveys about typical portion sizes in Britain (Table 13.3). This work, together with new work on portion sizes conducted for the Department of Health (England) by Leatherhead Food Research Association (Cullum, 2003), has been used as the basis of discussions that the Department of

Health (England) has been having with interested parties, with a view to establishing agreement on what constitutes a portion. Currently, there are no specific recommendations for children, but the concept of 'handfuls' is being considered as a means of helping to identify suitable servings for different age groups. In spring 2003, a logo and associated support materials were launched by the UK government to help promote fruit and vegetables consumption as part of its five-a-day programme (see Section 13.11). These resources will be used in England to support the school fruit scheme (see Table 13.1) and 66 Primary Care Trusts in England will be starting five-a-day community initiatives.

A summary of the five-a-day message of the Department of Health's campaign is as follows (Cullum, 2003):

- eat at least five portions of a *variety* of fruit and vegetables each day
- fresh, frozen, chilled, canned and dried fruit and vegetables all count
- 100% fruit juice and purées count once per day only, even if more than one portion is consumed
- 100% vegetable juice counts once per day only, even if more than one portion is eaten
- vegetable purées (*e.g.* tomato purée) count once per day only, even if more than one portion is eaten (*e.g.* as a component of a pizza or pasta sauce)
- potatoes and other starchy 'staple' foods do not count, although they are important foods which constitute another food group in their own right
- nuts, seeds, coconut, marmalade and jam do not count (nuts and seeds are part of the meat and alternatives food group)
- processed foods containing fruit and vegetables can contribute to five-a-day but nutrition labelling information should be checked as they may also have high levels of fat, salt or sugar
- a portion of fresh, canned or frozen fruit or vegetables is 80 g (as eaten); a portion of 100% juice is 150 mL and a portion of tomato purée is 1 tablespoon. A portion of dried fruit is roughly the amount that would be eaten as a

Table 13.2 Plant food recommendations in seven countries around the world.

	USDA/HHS Food Guide Pyramid	Canada's Food Guide to Healthy Eating	Australian Food Guide to Healthy Eating	The Balance of Good Health of UK	Chinese Food Guide Pagoda	Korean Food Guide Pagoda	German Nutrition Circle	Irish Food Pyramid
Grains	**6–11 servings** A serving: 1 slice of bread; 1 ounce of cereal; ½ cup of cooked rice or pasta	**5–12 servings** A serving: 1 slice of bread; 30 g cereal; ½ cup of cooked rice or pasta	**3–11 samples** A sample: 2 slices of bread; 1⅓ cup of cereal; 1 cup of cooked rice or pasta	**More than 5 portions** A portion: 30 g bread; 30 g cereal; 60 g rice (not specified if cooked or dry)	**300–500 g** (based on raw weight)	**4–5 servings** A serving: 3 slices (100 g) of bread; 90 g cereal; 210 g cooked rice	250–350 g of bread/day or 200–250 g of cooked rice/day or 250–300 g of potatoes/day	**6 or more portions** A portion: 1 bowl of cereal; 1 slice of bread; 3 dessert spoons pasta or rice; 1 medium boiled or baked potato
Vegetables	**3–5 servings** A serving: 1 cup of raw leafy vegetables, ½ cup of other vegetables (cooked or raw), ¾ cup of vegetable juice		**2–9 samples** A sample: 1 cup of salad vegetables; ½ cup (75 g) of cooked vegetables		**400–500 g** (based on raw weight)		200 g/day cooked vegetables & 100 g/day raw vegetables & 75 g/day of salad; 100 g (raw) legumes/month	
Fruit	**2–4 servings** A serving: a medium apple, banana or orange; ½ cup of cooked or canned fruit; ¾ cup of fruit juice		**1–5 samples** A sample: 1 medium apple, banana or orange; ½ cup of fruit juice		**100–200 g**		**250–300 g/day** Minimum two portions fresh fruits	

(cont'd overleaf)

Table 13.2 (Cont'd)

	USDA/HHS Food Guide Pyramid	Canada's Food Guide to Healthy Eating	Australian Food Guide to Healthy Eating	The Balance of Good Health of UK	Chinese Food Guide Pagoda	Korean Food Guide Pagoda	German Nutrition Circle	Irish Food Pyramid
Vegetables & fruit		**5–10 servings** A serving: 1 medium vegetable or fruit; ½ cup of fresh or canned vegetable or fruit; ½ cup of juice		**More than 5 portions** See Section 13.2		**6–7 servings** A serving: 70 g raw vegetable; 100 g fruit; ½ cup of juice		**4 or more servings** 3 dessert spoons cooked or tinned fruit ½ glass of fruit juice 1 medium-sized piece of fresh fruit 3 dessert spoons cooked vegetables Small bowl of home-made vegetable soup

Source: adapted from Painter *et al.* (2002).

Table 13.3 Practical information on portion sizes of fruit and vegetables.

Food type	Description of portion (equivalent to 80 g)*	Examples
Fruit:		
Very large fruit	One large slice	Melon, pineapple
Large fruit	One whole	Apple, banana
Medium fruit	Two whole	Plum, kiwi
Berries	Cupful	Raspberries, grapes
Stewed and canned fruit	Three serving spoonfuls	Stewed apple, canned peaches
Dried fruit	Half a serving spoonful	Apricots, raisins
Fruit juice	Full wine glass (standard size)	Orange juice, fresh or from concentrate
Vegetables:		
Green vegetables	Two serving spoonfuls[†]	Broccoli, spinach
Root vegetables	Two serving spoonfuls[†]	Carrots, parsnips
Very small vegetables	Three serving spoonfuls	Peas, sweetcorn
Pulses and beans	Two serving spoonfuls	Baked beans, kidney beans
Salad	Bowlful	Lettuce, tomato

*The term 'serving spoonful' is used to emphasise that the amounts apply to the quantities served on to a plate as part of a meal or snack, rather than in the raw state.
[†]Recent work conducted for the Department of Health by Leatherhead Food Research Association (Cullum, 2003) indicates that three (15 mL) tablespoons is a more appropriate serving size for vegetables.
Source: Williams (1995).

portion if the fruit or vegetable was fresh, *e.g.* three apricots. For most vegetables, 80 g equates to three heaped tablespoons when cooked.

A staged approach is expected. In stage 1 the Department of Health will focus on publicising the new logo and associated materials (*e.g.* information leaflets, posters and resource packs). In association with this, as stage 2, producers, retailers, processors and the food service industry will be invited to use the logo on fresh (*i.e.* raw), chilled and frozen fruits and vegetables, *i.e.* those to which no other ingredients have been added (*e.g.* fat, salt or sugar). The next stage will be to invite manufacturers and retailers to brand canned and dried products, recognising that criteria will need to be established to ensure that consumers' desire for a 'logo they can trust' is adhered to. Identification of such criteria may help pave the way for stage 4, branding of composite meals, *e.g.* ready meals, for retail and food service, and stage

5, devising an indicator for use by manufacturers to signal the number of portions of fruit and vegetables provided by a product.

Dietary advice to eat more fruits and vegetables should emphasise the advantages of variety rather than focusing on particular types. Although the lack of demonstrable effect of supplements of vitamins C and E and β-carotene may be due to methodological problems with the intervention trials used to assess their effects, the evidence that these particular constituents are specifically responsible for a beneficial health effect of fruits and vegetables is at best equivocal. Nevertheless, an increase in fruit and vegetable consumption would in any case lead to an increase in the intake of these nutrients.

Some studies have observed adverse outcomes associated with large supplements of specific constituents, *e.g.* β-carotene. However, it is highly unlikely that such high intakes would be achievable via diet. Furthermore, blood levels of β-carotene achieved through supplementation are many times higher than those achieved through ordinary diets even for equivalent intakes. Therefore, an increase in intakes of β-carotene consequent on raising consumption of a variety of vegetables would not be expected to carry adverse effects; indeed, observational studies suggest the opposite (Wald, 1987; Wald *et al.*, 1988).

The conclusions in this respect of the COMA Working Group on cancer (Department of Health, 1998b) in relation to the benefits of individual nutrients are more cautious than those of some other commentators. They concluded that the results of the intervention trials reported so far do not support the notion that either vitamin supplements or fortified foods provide an equivalent alternative to increasing the consumption of fruit and vegetables. In addition, efforts to increase the concentration of particular constituents of fruit and vegetables, for instance by selective breeding or genetic manipulation, should be done cautiously with careful evaluation of the possible risks and benefits, including unacceptable changes in taste and other organoleptic properties (see Section 13.5).

13.3 To what extent are the plant food goals being achieved in the UK?

13.3.1 Methodological issues

Before considering achievement of dietary goals, it is worth noting some of the limitations that exist in relation to the available estimates of food intake and the attempts to find associations between components of diet and health.

Surveys reasonably tend to measure and record factors of known or suspected functionality. In themselves, they are not particularly good vehicles for testing hypotheses of causality relating to diet, especially as there is considerable collinearity between various foods, and between foods and food components. Most information has been on recognised macro- and micro-nutrients, but increasingly data are becoming available on many components of plant foods which have not conventionally been regarded as nutrients such as flavonoids and non-provitamin A carotenoids (information about current con-

sumption levels can be found in Section 6.5). Although these data provide an essential background to studies relating to function or outcome, without a clear understanding of their role *in vivo*, interpretation remains difficult.

Interpretation of measures of diet is further compounded by problems relating to methodology. There are several methods commonly used to derive estimates of dietary intake, ranging from 24 h recall through food frequency questionnaires and diary methods, weighed or estimated, to analysis of duplicate portions. All have advantages and disadvantages, and it is important to match the method to the question needing to be answered (Fehily & Johns, 2002). Different methods will be appropriate to characterising an individual's or a group's diet; to habitual compared with recent behaviour; and to free living or experimental settings. Often, although a survey may seek to address many different aspects of diet (group average, individual ranking, absolute intakes for regression), for practical reasons only one method is usually chosen, *e.g.* a food frequency questionnaire if the objective is to rank intakes.

In addition, there is now compelling evidence that all methods to a greater or lesser extent involve systematic bias, specifically under-reporting of energy-rich foods (or those perceived to be) (Poppitt *et al.*, 1998; Heitmann *et al.*, 2000; Lissner *et al.*, 2000). With regard to fruits and vegetables, so-called 'optimistic bias' may result in over-reporting of intakes (Shepherd, 1999). For example, Basiotis *et al.* reported data for a cohort of almost 6000 adults that serve to emphasise the extent to which people overestimate their consumption of particular foods (Basiotis *et al.*, 2000). For different age and gender groups and for different food groups, they compared perceived and actual intakes with recommended intakes (derived from the American *Food Guide Pyramid*). They found that people's perceptions of their food group consumption were very different from their actual consumption, based on information collected via diet diaries. Adults underestimated their consumption of grains, fats, oils and sweets and overestimated their consumption of fruit, milk products and meat and alternatives. For vegetables, women overestimated, thinking they ate 2.5–2.6 servings when in fact their actual intake was 1.7–2.2, depending on age group, whereas men slightly underestimated. The authors suggest that lack of understanding about what constitutes a serving may explain some of the mismatch. The diaries revealed that the actual intakes of fruit ranged from 0.8 to 1.5 servings/day in the women and from 0.6 to 1.3 servings/day in the men, the higher values pertaining to the groups over 51 years of age.

For these and other reasons, although dietary survey data are very important, they should be interpreted with caution.

Because of this, attention has focused on the use of objective biological markers (see Chapter 6), both of diet (exposure) and of outcome (*e.g.* function or risk of disease). There are currently few validated markers of plant food consumption of sufficient precision to act as reliable proxies in epidemiological studies. Attempts have been made to use glucosinolates as a measure of Brassica consumption and lutein for green/yellow vegetables, and recent work has considered β-carotene levels in plasma as a surrogate for fruit and vegetable intake. The data do not yet suggest a valid proxy has been developed.

Equally, there is lack of clarity regarding the precise mechanisms by which plant foods and their components may impact on disease risk (Chapter 4). Consequently, it is difficult to identify intermediate markers of disease risk which can confidently be used to predict outcome.

While there are many exciting developments, it is regrettably still probably too early to be able to use these methodological tools to help draw firm conclusions.

13.3.2 Fruit and vegetables

In 2000, the NFS recorded consumption of fruit (excluding fruit juices) at 110 g/person/day, and of vegetables (excluding potatoes) at 165 g/person/day (DEFRA, 2001). This total of 275 g/day compares unfavourably with recommended levels of intake of at least 400 g/day (World Health Organisation, 1990; Department of Health, 1998b).

The consumption of fruits and vegetables is not equally distributed within society. Geographically in Britain, there is a tendency for households in the south and the west to consume more vegetables and fruit than households in more northern parts (see Chapter 1, Table 1.4). Similarly, within Europe, there is a north–south gradient (Naska *et al.*, 2000). Household budget data retrieved from the Data Food Networking (DAFNE) database, comparing intakes in 10 European countries, have been used to estimate mean and median fruit and vegetable consumption. The data have also been used to identify low consumers of fruit and vegetables, based on the premise that the recommended 400 g/day should comprise 250 g of vegetables and 150 g of fruit (three and two servings, respectively). It is apparent that the majority (over 50%) of people did not comply with the five-a-day recommendations now advocated widely (Table 13.4). The highest proportions achieving the guideline intake of at least 400 g/day were found in both Mediterranean countries surveyed, Spain and Greece, although a large portion of each population failed to reach this level (37% in Greece and 49% in Spain). However, in four of the 10 countries studied (Belgium, Luxembourg, Germany and the UK), more than 80% of the population were identified as low consumers. With the exception of Poland, the proportion of low fruit consumers was significantly lower than the proportion of low vegetable consumers, suggesting that different health promotion strategies may be required if intakes are to be boosted. In Ireland and Norway, low vegetable consumption appeared the norm, however, and did not reflect lower social status, for example, as was typical in the other countries.

Consumers in low-income households, in whatever region, tend to consume less vegetables, and especially less fruit and fruit juices (see Chapter 1, Table 1.4 and Henderson *et al.*, 2002). Young children in their early school years have particularly low intakes of fruits and vegetables compared with the recommendations tailored for their requirements. A recent national survey of children aged 4–18 years (Gregory *et al.*, 2000) revealed that on average children were eating less than half the recommended five portions of fruit

Table 13.4 Percentage of low consumers in 10 countries participating in the Data Food Networking (DAFNE) project.

Country	Fruit and vegetables, <400 g/person/day	Fruit <150 g/person/day	Vegetables <250 g/person/day
Belgium	68	42	85
Germany	69	45	88
Greece	37	32	56
Hungary	72	66	76
Republic of Ireland	88	78	90
Luxembourg	62	41	83
Norway	81	55	93
Poland	78	81	75
Spain	49	30	76
UK	76	68	81

Source: Naska *et al.* (2000) with permission from the British Nutrition Foundation.

and vegetables per day, with one in five having no fruit at all during the study week. Furthermore, 4% of the sample had no vegetables during the survey period. Regional comparisons indicated that boys and girls in Scotland were less likely than children elsewhere in the UK to have eaten various types of vegetables.

Among older children there was some evidence of micronutrient inadequacies (vitamin A, calcium, magnesium, potassium and zinc in boys; vitamin A, riboflavin, folate, iron, calcium and magnesium in girls) (Gregory *et al.*, 2000). A discussion of this can be found in a Briefing Paper, *Nutrition and Schoolchildren* (British Nutrition Foundation, 2002b). In younger children at least, the dietary balance identified in the survey of Gregory *et al.* does not appear to be limiting in specific micronutrients, as linear growth in young children is maintained, and children are now taller than previously recorded, but they are also fatter. Indeed, the degree of increasing adiposity in young children is increasingly cited as a cause of concern with regard to future adult obesity and type 2 diabetes (National Audit Office, 2001).

The dietary consumption patterns are associated with similar variation in plasma levels of those micronutrients whose principal sources are fruits and vegetables, *e.g.* vitamin C and β-carotene. This association with the poorer health experiences of those living in northern parts of England

or Great Britain and of those in lower socio-economic groups has led to the suggestion that these substances may be responsible for the observed health differences. It is, however, at least as likely that they are simply acting as a marker for fruit and vegetable consumption in general, with all the various potentially biologically active substances they contain, as well as the social and lifestyle factors which correlate.

Joffe and Robertson have looked at the potential contribution of increased fruit and vegetable consumption to health gain in the EU (Joffe & Robertson, 2001). The World Health Organisation (World Health Organisation, 1990) has recommended a daily intake of at least 400 g of fruit and vegetables. Using FAO food availability data (the shortcomings of which are discussed in Section 1.3.4); Joffe and Robertson calculated that seven out of 15 EU Member States have a mean recorded intake level that is less than about 70% of the 400 g target, *i.e.* less than 275 g/day). Even in countries such as Greece, which has a relatively high mean consumption (511 g/day), a substantial proportion of the population (37%) fell below the recommended level (see also Table 13.3), and a social gradient in intake was apparent in many countries, including the UK (see Chapter 1, Table 1.4). Joffe and Robertson calculated that over 26 000 deaths before the age of 65 years could be prevented annually in the EU if intakes of these foods increased to the highest current average consumption levels (*e.g.* those found in Spain and Greece).

Data are also available from a range of sources for other countries around the world, *e.g.* the USA, and again demonstrate large variations within populations. Examples are given below. The median intake of fruit and vegetables in the study of Liu *et al.*, a cohort of highly selected women (health professionals), was 6.1 servings per day (Liu *et al.*, 2000). This is similar to the level of intake reported in the Nurses Health Study (Joshipura *et al.*, 1999), but is considerably higher than recent estimates in the general US adult population of 1.7–2.2 and 0.8–1.5 servings per day for fruit and vegetables, respectively, in women. The comparable figures for men were 0.6–1.3 servings per day (Basiotis *et al.*, 2000).

13.3.3 Other plant-derived foods

Although there is a considerable national focus on fruit and vegetables, consumption patterns of other plant-derived foods and associated constituents, such as fibre, are also of interest. Fibre data have been reported in the NFS since 1987, but very little change in intake has occurred since that time (13 g/day in 1987, 12.6 g/day in 2000) (DEFRA, 2001).

Using National Food Survey data, it is possible to compare current and past diets within Britain with the targets represented in the *Balance of Good Health*. Over the past 12 years, the proportion of the average household diet that is derived from fruit and vegetables has shown some progress towards the recommendations. However, the opposite is true for bread and cereals (DEFRA, 2001). The other food groups have shown little change overall, although within specific groups of foods, such as milk and milk products, there have been substantial changes; there has been a considerable rise in low-fat milk consumption with semi-skimmed now exceeding whole milk intake. In interpreting this information, it should be noted that this comparison is judging the proportional contribution each food group makes to total food intake, rather than the absolute amount of each food group consumed.

During the past 50 years, the amount of food consumed, as symbolised by daily energy consumption, has fallen considerably. For example, in 2000, daily energy intake from household food was 1880 kcal/day (including confectionery and soft and alcoholic drinks brought home) in contrast to 2474 kcal/day 50 years ago (DEFRA, 2001).

In 1975, 21% of food intake came from fruit and vegetables and 31% from bread, cereals and potatoes. By 2000 these proportions were almost equal at 28% and 27%, respectively (DEFRA, 2001). The target for the *Balance of Good Health* is that each of these two groups provides about a third of total food intake.

The decline in tea consumption is also worthy of note, as is the considerable increase in home wine intake in Britain (see Figs 1.4 and 1.5).

As is evident from the data presented in Chapter 1, the National Food Survey and other government surveys, such as the NDNS series, indicate that regional and income variations in intake exist (see Table 1.4). Similar variations also exist elsewhere in Europe (Naska *et al.*, 2000), based on data collected around 1990 (see Section 13.3.1). Table 13.5 shows changes by country and hence allows comparison of different regions of Europe.

Table 13.5 Median intake of fruit and vegetables in 10 countries participating in the Data Food Networking (DAFNE) project (g/person/day).

Country	Fruits	Vegetables	Total
Belgium	168	143	316
Germany	168	123	299
Greece	261	219	512
Hungary	98	124	232
Republic of Ireland	80	105	198
Luxembourg	184	124	329
Norway	134	78	228
Poland	68	160	233
Spain	249	140	406
UK	91	128	239

The individual values for fruits and vegetables do not add up to the total value as medians have been used (mean values are also provided in the original paper).
Source: Naska *et al.* (2000).

13.4 Evidence for the effect of interventions

To date, most of the work to identify successful interventions in relation to fruit and vegetables consumption has been conducted in the USA, although studies are now under way in the UK. A review conducted by Sahay and colleagues (Sahay *et al.*, 2000) has identified the following characteristics of successful interventions:

- used participatory models for planning and implementing interventions
- were grounded in theory, most notably social learning theory
- incorporated multiple strategies
- provided essential training and support
- were designed to target a person's stage of change
- involved the family as an important source of support
- were of adequate intensity and duration rather than being one-time events
- gave clear, strongly worded, simple messages
- considered the political climate in which the intervention was being implemented
- kept the lines of communication open between the implementing body and other organisations.

A systematic review of community-based interventions to increase fruit and vegetable consumption (Ciliska *et al.*, 2000) concluded that it appears easier to effect changes in fruit intake than vegetable intake. Multi-component interventions were most successful as were longer term interventions. All of the published studies that met the inclusion criteria had been conducted in the USA.

13.4.1 Campaigns in the USA

Probably the best-known intervention in this area of research is the 'five-a-day' campaign in the USA (Potter *et al.*, 2000). In 1991, the US National Cancer Institute (NCI) objective was that members of the public should increase their consumption of fruit and vegetables to five or more servings per day (Havas *et al.*, 1995). At the outset of the study, median fruit and vegetable intake among US adults was found to be 3.4 servings per day, according to a telephone food frequency questionnaire (Subar *et al.*, 1995). This is similar to current levels in the UK. It is worth noting that data published since that time have demonstrated the difficulties many people have in identifying what constitutes a portion (Eldridge *et al.*, 1999; Basiotis *et al.*, 2000).

As part of the campaign, the NCI funded nine research studies concerned with implementing and evaluating community-based programmes designed to increase fruit and vegetable intake among different segments of the population in Alabama, Arizona, Georgia, Louisiana, Maryland, Massachusetts, Minnesota, North Carolina and Washington. The settings for these projects included the Special Supplement Food Program for Women Infants and Children (WIC Programs), churches, workplaces and schools. The projects were led by multi-disciplinary teams and entailed extensive collaboration among academic, governmental, private sector and voluntary agencies within each State. A feature of the adult-focused projects was the inclusion of peer educators or intervention channels that also targeted the social environment. The impacts of these nine randomised interventions are summarised in Table 13.6. These projects have stimulated a number of similarly structured projects around the country. Such a programme that was conducted in California achieved similar results (Forester *et al.*, 1998).

Published data on evaluations of this programme and other associated work are generally positive (see Table 13.6 and below). For example, improvements in fruit consumption, in particular, among younger children were seen in randomised school-based trials in Minnesota (Perry *et al.*, 1998) and Alabama (Reynolds *et al.*, 2000a), although attempts to improve vegetable consumption among boys were disappointing. Such studies have provided useful information on successful interventions, such as involvement of parents (such that availability of the foods at home can be achieved) and adopting a whole school approach. Not all the work focusing on children has been conducted in schools. For example, a project involving urban boy scouts (Cullen *et al.*, 2000) was used to identify an intervention that

Table 13.6 Summary of the findings of fruit and vegetable interventions in the US five-a-day campaign.

Project title and target group	Intervention	Study design and main outcomes measured	Net change between treatment and control groups, daily servings of fruit, vegetables and juice
Gimme 5, Georgia; 4th–5th graders	2 years of intervention, involvement of classroom, parents and industry	8 school pairs, randomised. 7-day recall 1253 participants	Fruit & veg. 0.20*, fruit 0.12, veg. 0.08
5-a-day Power Plus, Minnesota, 4th–5th graders, 60% in receipt of free/subsidised lunches	2 years of intervention, classroom, parent, school food service and industry involvement	10 school pairs, randomised. 24 h recall, direct observation at lunchtime 441 participants	*24 h recall*: total servings of fruit & veg. 0.58, fruit 0.62*, veg. −0.02; per 1000 kcal: fruit & veg. 0.41*, fruit 0.36*, veg. 0.05. *Direct observation at lunchtime*: total servings fruit & veg. 0.47*, fruit 0.30*, veg. 0.16; per 1000 kcal: fruit & veg. 0.83*, fruit 0.72*, veg. 0.23
Alabama High 5, Alabama; 4th–5th graders	2 years of intervention, classroom activities taught by programme staff, involvement of parents and school food service	14 school pairs, randomised. 7 days of 24 h recall, 5-a-day fruit and vegetable score (also direct observation at lunchtime). Post-test and follow-up measurements 1426 participants	*Post-test (7 days recall)*: fruit & veg. 1.68*, fruit 0.88*, veg. 0.69*. *Follow-up (7 days recall)*: fruit & veg. 0.99*, fruit 0.56*, veg. 0.35*. *Post-test (fruit & veg. score)*: fruit & veg. 1.46*, fruit 0.77*, veg. 0.50*. *Follow-up (fruit & veg. score)*: fruit & veg. 0.85*, fruit 0.50*, veg. 0.23*
Gimme 5: a fresh nutrition concept, Louisiana; 9th–12th graders	3 years of intervention, food service marketing, student workshops, parent involvement	6 school pairs, randomised. Daily consumption of fruit, juice and vegetables; single item self report 1911 participants	Fruit & veg. 0.30
Healthier Eating for the Overlooked Worker, Arizona; lower income males	1.8 years of intervention. Peer education plus general 5-a-day programme versus 5-a-day alone	93 randomised work cliques. As well as pre- and post-test, there was follow up at 6 months. 24 h recall and 7-item 30 day food frequency 695 participants	*24 h recall (post-test)*: fruit & veg. 0.77*, fruit 0.41*, veg. 0.26. *Follow-up*: fruit & veg. 0.41*, fruit 0.06, veg. 0.24. *Food frequency (post-test)*: fruit & veg. 0.41*, fruit 0.24*, veg. 0.19. *Follow-up*: fruit & veg. −0.04, fruit 0.03, veg. −0.08

(cont'd overleaf)

Table 13.6 *(Cont'd)*

Project title and target group	Intervention	Study design and main outcomes measured	Net change between treatment and control groups, daily servings of fruit, vegetables and juice
Black Churches for Better Health, North Carolina; low-income women, 98% African American	20 months of multicomponent intervention: tailored print material, direct education, lay health advisors, community coalitions, church activities, grocery	5 matched randomised county pairs, 49 churches; 7-item 30 day food frequency 2519 participants	Fruit & veg. 0.85*, fruit 0.66*, veg. 0.19*
Maryland WIC 5-a day promotion programme, Maryland; lower income women, 53% African American, 43% white	6 months of intervention: nutrition sessions by peer leaders, print materials and visual reminders, direct mail	WIC sites (16), randomised, 7-item 30 day food frequency. Post-test plus follow up at 1 year 695 participants	*Post-test:* fruit & veg. 0.43*; *Follow-up:* 0.74
Treatwell 5-a-day, Massachusetts; 84% female, attended high school or college	9.5 month multicomponent intervention: worker participation, individual and environmental changes, family component	22 worksites randomised into minimal intervention (8), worksite plus family (78), worksite only (7). 7-item 30 day food frequency 1306 participants	*Worksite and family:* fruit & veg. 0.50* *Worksite only:* 0.20*

*Statistically significant (*p* < 0.05).
Source: information extracted from Potter *et al.* (2000).

could be incorporated into the scouts' programme of activities. A media campaign approach, *Gimme 5*, has also demonstrated that the dietary habits of high school students can be influenced by positive media messages presented in a way that is relevant to the age group (Nicklas *et al.*, 1998). In other studies among older students, assessing knowledge, attitudes and practices in relation to fruit and vegetables, significant ethnic differences in the outcomes were reported (Beech *et al.*, 1999), with white adolescents scoring higher than African Americans. These trends were consistent with those identified in older black populations (McClelland *et al.*, 1998) and in the five-a-day programme in general, in which associations were found between fruit and vegetable consumption and income, education, smoking status, age, gender, marital status and presence of children within the household.

A workplace intervention (Sorensen *et al.*, 1998) demonstrated the importance of incorporation of family-focused interventions, and consumption of fruit and vegetables was directly associated with the level of household support for healthy eating. Work with women participating in WIC Programs has also demonstrated that consumption of fruit and vegetables can be increased with appropriate intervention, even in this hard to reach group (Havas *et al.*, 1998b). Two months after the intervention, mean daily intake had increased by 0.56 ± 0.11 servings (0.13 ± 0.07 in the controls), with the extent of the change being associated with the number of nutrition sessions attended, education, race, and how ready they were to consider changing their diet at baseline (stage of change). One year later, intake had risen by a further 0.27 servings in both the intervention and the control group. Self-efficacy and positive attitudes were found to be the most powerful predictors of achieving an increased intake (Havas *et al.*, 1998a). On balance, however, the programme was less successful in reaching minority and low-income populations than other populations. Overall, the strongest predictors of dietary change were knowledge of the recommendations to eat five or more servings per day, taste preferences and self-efficacy (in particular confidence in one's ability to eat vegetables and fruit in a variety of situations) (Potter *et al.*, 2000).

The campaign benefited from collaboration with private industry, such as producers and retailers of fruit and vegetables, in particular with regard to the expanded communication base and the promotion of national nutritional objectives. In addition, there were successful collaborations with a range of Federal, State and voluntary agencies. The campaign also used advertising and developed relationships with media outlets to generate and inform news stories related to the programme.

It is instructive to consider the outcome measures in such studies. There is no doubt that as a tool to increase general awareness of a simple 'message' such campaigns can be very successful. Often this is an important outcome, especially if awareness is initially low. However, in relation to fruits and vegetables, the awareness in the UK that it is important to eat more of these foods is already high. What is less obvious is why such knowledge is not always converted into action. Psychological theories relating to the reasons for behaviours go some way to furthering understanding of this topic, but only a relatively small proportion of behaviour can be explained in this way (Horwath, 1999).

In summary, evaluation of the US 'five-a-day' campaign has found significant increases in fruit consumption, for example in the school-based interventions (Nicklas *et al.*, 1998; Perry *et al.*, 1998; Baranowski *et al.*, 2000; Potter *et al.*, 2000; Reynolds *et al.*, 2000b), but with the exception of Baranowski *et al.* (2000) little impact on vegetable consumption. In the studies among younger school children (elementary school), the average increase in intake (fruit and vegetables combined) was 0.62 servings per day and the largest was 1.68 servings per day (Potter *et al.*, 2000). Among adults, changes in the workplace, church or family social environment resulted in an average increase of 0.48 servings per day, and the largest effect was 0.85 servings per day (Potter *et al.*, 2000). Baranowski *et al.* suggested that the results perhaps reflect an ability in these targeted school-age populations to mitigate an age-related decline in consumption (Baranowski *et al.*, 2000). In addition, there is now considerable evidence that health information campaigns tend to be more successful amongst those who are already health conscious, principally the better off in higher socio-economic groups. This has the paradoxical effect of improving behaviours on average, but at the expense of widening social inequalities.

During the campaign period, surveys conducted among adults indicated that total consumption of fruit and vegetables (including non-fried potatoes, which are excluded in the UK) increased by 0.12 servings per day, which was not statistically significant. In some groups, *e.g.* 18–35 year olds, the increase was significant (Potter *et al.*, 2000). In their evaluation of the programme, Potter *et al.* concluded that, at national level, there had been a slow though steady increase in vegetable and fruit consumption in the USA during the campaign period but that the ability to infer that this had resulted from the programme was extremely limited, as no non-exposed comparison group existed. Nevertheless, the NCI-funded randomised trials offer persuasive evidence that behavioural interventions can have a modest positive impact on fruit and vegetable intake. The findings of these interventions are summarised in Table 13.6.

13.4.2 National UK campaigns

In England, two national government schemes were announced in 2000 and have undergone a piloting phase (see Table 13.1). These are the school fruit scheme and the five-a-day programme, both of which fall under the auspices of the Department of Health. In addition, there are other more general programmes that target fruit and vegetable consumption in the context of a healthy and varied diet, such as the National Standards for school meals that became mandatory in 2001, and the Healthy Schools programme, responsibility for which is shared by the Department of Health and the Department for Education and Skills. Table 13.1 also outlines activities in other parts of the UK.

In the school fruit scheme, 4–6 year olds in England will be offered a free piece of fruit at morning break, each school day. Pilots began in 2000 to assess the feasibility of the scheme and the expectation is that the scheme will be fully operational by 2004. The first phase of the piloting, 'farm to school gate', was focused on the logistics of supply and delivery of fruit to schools. The second phase concentrated on movements of the fruit supply within the school, and the final phase on strategies to ensure the fruit is eaten, looking at issues such as the need to help smaller children with peeling fruit. Details can be found on the Department of Health's website (www.doh.gov.uk). In order to evaluate the impact of the scheme, work is under way to develop and validate an easy-to-use means of measuring overall intake of fruit and vegetables in young children of this age. This process has also been a feature of the US campaign (Potter *et al.*, 2000).

The scheme in England is government funded. Similar schemes are being piloted elsewhere in the UK but are being funded differently. For example, a scheme in Scotland focusing on preschool children is being funded through the Health Improvement Fund (the revenue accruing from higher tobacco taxation).

The five-a-day programme will target the population as a whole. Pilots have been completed in five areas: Airedale and Craven, County Durham, Hastings, Sandwell and Somerset. The key issues being addressed are as follows: (i) accessibility, availability and affordability, which involves working with shops and other commercial and public food outlets, such as schools and hospitals; (ii) awareness, which entails improving people's knowledge, attitudes, motivation and skills in relation to eating, buying and preparing fruits and vegetables; and (iii) acceptability, making fruit and vegetables the easy choice and an integral part of daily eating patterns. A variety of different interventions (community projects) have been tested across these five areas, including mapping food outlets within a locality, working with retailers and farmers' markets, working with workplaces and leisure services, establishing food co-ops, and working with children via sport-related activities. The evaluation of this work can be found on a dedicated website (www.doh.gov.uk/fiveaday).

Again, similar community projects are running or being evaluated in other parts of Britain under the auspices of regional government structure.

Details of these can be found by looking at a number of websites, including those of Sustain (www.sustainweb.org) and the Health Development Agency (www.hda-online.org.uk).

13.4.3 Local initiatives in the UK

Projects conducted in the UK have often been focused on school-age populations. A project in primary school children (Anderson *et al.*, 2001), which took the form of a whole school intervention, resulted in an average increase in fruit intake from 133 ± 11.9 to 183 ± 17.0 g/day. This was significantly greater than the increase estimated in children in control schools (from 100 ± 11.7 to 107 ± 14.2 g/day). No changes in vegetable consumption or the intake of any other foods was detected. The intervention included increased provision of fruits and vegetables via tuck shops and lunches, tasting opportunities, a range of point of purchase marketing (posters and quizzes), newsletters for parents and children and teacher information sessions. The intervention was also found to have a modest but significant effect on cognitive and attitudinal variables.

Researchers at Bangor University are currently developing and evaluating in schools a schools-based intervention package designed to increase fruit and vegetable consumption in 4–11 year olds. Children are introduced to cartoon characters known as food dudes (Horne *et al.*, 1995) via videos, letters and rewards (stickers and pencils), which encourage them to taste fruit and vegetables. The programme has been shown to double or triple children's consumption of fruit and vegetables at school as well as increase intake at home. Details can be found at www.fooddudes.co.uk. A similar type of approach, *5 a day the Bash Street way*, has been tried in primary schools in Dundee. Adoption of a whole school approach resulted in a modest increase in fruit intake (Anderson *et al.*, 2001).

Researchers in Cardiff have tested whether the provision of fruit tuck shops in primary schools in under-privileged areas is associated with a change in fruit consumption. The research has also attempted to identify effective ways of operating the shops, and this has involved 43 schools, 23 of which have tuck shops with 20 acting as controls (Moore *et al.*, 2000). An after-school 'food club' is the focus for a Newcastle project involving 11–13 year olds in 10 schools (five intervention and five control) (Moynihan *et al.*, 2001; Revill *et al.*, 2001). Another school-based intervention, the Grab 5 project, is focusing on the fruit and vegetable consumption of primary school children. The use of an interactive multi-media medium is being explored in Northern Ireland as a means of positively influencing diet, including fruit and vegetable intake, in 11–14 year olds. Some of these are government funded and progress has been summarised recently (Hughes, 2001).

Several other on-going projects involve adults, such as one, among low-income groups, designed to assess the effects of behaviourally oriented dietary counselling on fruit and vegetable intake, in a primary care setting in South London, and another (the Cookwell Initiative) in Scotland has a cooking skills focus [see Hughes (2001) for a brief summary]. A randomised controlled nurse-led primary care intervention, based in Oxford, in 25–64 year olds, is also under way.

A study among adults (Cox *et al.*, 1998b) showed that well-thought-through interventions not only can increase intakes to target levels but also these increases are sustainable for at least 1 year post-intervention. Intervention advice included the specific association of high fruit and vegetable intake with reduced risk of disease, practicalities regarding shopping and preparation and portion definition. The effects were statistically significant with intakes rising from 324g/day to 557g/day and reflected by validated portion measures after 8 weeks of intervention. Successful strategies chosen by the subjects were conventional, such as fruit as a snack and vegetables with main meals, and they mainly focused on fruit. The dietary change was associated with other beneficial changes such as reduced intake of fat (as % energy) in those with a previously high intake.

A point to note is that the types of interventions referred to above can be very costly considering the number of people they involve, and can be very labour intensive. The sustain-

ability of the effect once the intervention ends
is also an important consideration. In the studies
in the USA, summarised in Table 13.6, that
included a follow-up phase a period of months
after the intervention ended, it was evident that
the size of the effect of the intervention had
diminished.

13.4.4 Barriers to change

Many factors impinge on people's food choices
and behaviours, and for many people there are
important barriers such as mobility (with increasing age), cost (for the less well off), access (for the
socially excluded) and resistance to change
(Williams, 1995; Lechner & Brug, 1997; Cox *et
al.*, 1998a; Trudeau *et al.*, 1998). A greater understanding of the joint and several roles of all these
factors will help to develop rational interventions
to effect change.

In order to explain the observed variation in
vegetable and fruit consumption across countries,
gender and age groups, researchers can apply two
theoretical models: the Attitude, Social influence
and Self-efficacy (ASE) model and the Stage of
Change model. The ASE model is derived from
a number of psychosocial theories, including
social learning theories and cognitive expectancy
theories. A version of the model is illustrated in
Fig. 13.2.

The ASE Model applied to fruit and vegetable
consumption is primarily a function of motivation
or intentions, for example see Brug *et al.* (1995).
A person's attitude toward fruit and vegetables is
a result of the consequences that are expected
from this consumption. Social influences are a
result from subjective norms, examples of important others and direct social support and pressure
related to fruit and vegetable intake. Self-efficacy
is a result of a subjective assessment of abilities
and possibilities related to fruit and vegetable
intake. The model proposes that by introducing
or clarifying more positive consequences of fruit
and vegetable intake, by creating or encouraging
a positive social environment and by making
fruits and vegetables as easily available as possible, higher consumption of fruits and vegetables
can be reached. When applying the ASE model
to nutrition behaviours, lack of awareness of
personal intake levels has been identified as an
important barrier toward dietary change.

The Stages of Change model (Prochaska &
DiClemente, 1983) proposes five separate stages
through which people may progress toward long-
term positive health behaviours: pre-contemplation, contemplation, preparation, action and
maintenance. The model further proposes that
subjects in different stages of change benefit most
from interventions tailored specifically to that
stage. Subjects in pre-contemplation need feed-

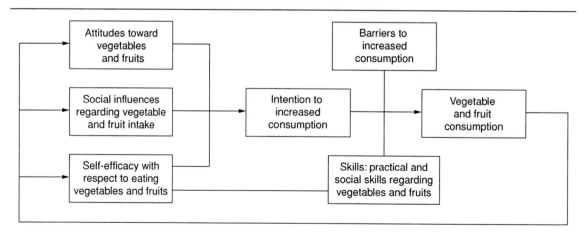

Fig. 13.2   A model for determining factors predictive of fruits and vegetable consumption based on the ASE
model.

back to make them aware of a need to change and attitude information to convince them of the benefits of increased fruit and vegetable consumption. Subjects in the contemplation and preparation stages need skills training, observational learning techniques and environmental change to convince them of the possibilities and their abilities to increase their fruit and vegetable consumption. The model was originally developed for use in smoking cessation, but has subsequently been applied to other forms of behaviour change. A review is available (Horwath, 1999).

Recognised barriers also include consumers' complacency about their present consumption levels, confusion in the interpretation of the messages of health promotion campaigns (*e.g.* what constitutes a portion, see Section 13.2), and the perception that fruit and vegetables provide poor value for money.

Work from the USA has suggested that, where food selection is concerned, nutritional concerns, *per se*, are of less relevance to most people than taste and cost (Glanz *et al.*, 1998). The implication of this is that to increase fruit and vegetable consumption, nutrition programmes should promote such foods as tasty and inexpensive. This in itself poses a problem, as many perceive such foods as poor value for money. The evaluation of the US five-a-day programme also identified taste, along with awareness of the campaign message and self-efficacy, as important determinants (Potter *et al.*, 2000).

Work in Britain (Cox *et al.*, 1998a) has identified a lack of perceived social pressure to increase fruit and vegetable intake and the authors suggest that public health efforts require stronger and broader health messages that incorporate consumer awareness of the current low intakes. Anderson *et al.* assessed the response of low consumers of fruit and vegetables to a nutrition intervention programme (Anderson *et al.*, 1998a). Apparent barriers were lack of support from family and friends, cost and time constraints regarding shopping and preparation practicalities. Also, limited availability of vegetables, salads and fruit in work canteens and take-away outlets were practical obstacles to increasing intake.

Evidence from the USA, Europe and the UK demonstrates that increasing the consumption of vegetables is particularly difficult and may require particular attention and focused strategies because the deficit in relation to current recommendations appears to be more substantial (based on three of the five recommended servings being vegetables). There is clearly more resistance to change vegetable consumption than there is for fruit.

13.5 Looking to the future

In spite of the cautious approach taken by expert committees, a number of investigators are working to enhance the concentrations in certain plants of specific bioactive compounds, on the assumption that such enhancement would carry benefits. However, the absence of reliable evidence for specific benefits from particular substances, together with a lack of evidence of absence of adverse effects (see below), argues for a cautionary approach to these technologies in the same way as for dietary supplements.

Enhancing the content of bioactive compounds in plant foods through selective breeding or genetic improvement is a potent dietary option if such substances are proved to be protective. However, most if not all are bitter, acrid or astringent, and therefore may be unacceptable to consumers at higher concentrations (Drewnowski & Gomez-Carneros, 2000).

In addition to the biological activity of these compounds in humans, which is the cause of the attention they are receiving, they provide a defence for the plant against predators by making them unpalatable, by acting as natural pesticides and toxins or by protecting against oxidative damage from solar radiation (see Chapter 2).

The instinctive rejection of bitter foods, characteristic of those containing alkaloids, may be immutable and developed as crucial to survival. Indeed, selective breeding and a variety of debittering processes (Drewnowski & Gomez-Carneros, 2000) have resulted in the progressive removal of glucosinolates and other substances, *e.g.* from Brussels sprouts. However, attempts to make plant foods more palatable by removing bitter-tasting compounds may at the same time be diminishing their healthful properties as components of such foods, such as glucosinolates (see Chapters 1, 5 and 7), are themselves bitter.

Many structurally unrelated compounds can give rise to a uniform bitter taste, *e.g.* terpenoids, phenols, polyphenols, glucosinolates and also amino acids. For example, bitter phenolic compounds include flavonones and flavones in citrus fruit, neohesperidin found in grapefruit juice, tannins in wine and tea and flavans such as catechins and epicatechins in red wine, tea and cocoa (see Chapter 2). Higher molecular weight polyphenols, such as tannins, are more likely to be astringent and are widespread in foods such as grains, pulses, fruit, tea, wine and a variety of foliage plants. They have long been regarded as 'antinutrients' because they can interfere with protein absorption or reduce iron availability (Drewnowski & Gomez-Carneros, 2000).

13.6 Safety considerations

It is frequently wrongly assumed that just because a substance is naturally present in a plant food, it is harmless or even potentially good for health. Plants have evolved to rely upon elaborate chemical defences to ward off unwanted predators and disease, and as a result have developed an arsenal of substances that are noxious or toxic to bacteria, fungi, moulds, insects and herbivores, and sometimes humans. Most plant species in the world are not edible, many because of the toxins they produce. Plant breeding has resulted in those plants eaten as food having lower concentrations of these toxic components, but this has also led to modern plant foods being more susceptible to disease.

There are many examples of naturally present plant components being harmful to health when consumed in excess (see Table 13.7), but paradoxically many of the information sources on this topic include substances discussed in terms of their potential health effects within this report, for example phytoestrogens and glucosinolates. This paradox raises an important point. It may be the quantity of the substance that is consumed that is of relevance, with different amounts having differing effects on important biochemical pathways, such as induction of Phase II enzymes (see Chapter 4).

Table 13.7 focuses on plants consumed as foods, but the presence of substances that are potentially hazardous to humans is widespread in the plant kingdom. Some of these are likely to be present in small amounts in many herbal remedy preparations and plant-derived medications. For example, comfrey is recognised as a source of the pyrrozilidine alkaloids mentioned in Table 13.7 in relation to honey (www.anzfa.gov.au).

Over the centuries, humans have learned how to avoid or limit exposure. Lectins found in red kidney beans are completely destroyed if the dried beans are soaked for at least 12 h and boiled vigorously for at least 10 min in fresh water. All potatoes contain natural toxicants known as glyco-alkaloids, usually at low levels. The most common glycoalkaloids are solanine and chaconine (which are also found in tomatoes and aubergines, which are members of the same family). This group of substances are anti-cholinesterases and by inhibiting the enzyme cholinesterase, the level of the neurotransmitter acetylcholine accumulates, causing the characteristic symptoms of nausea, vomiting and respiratory difficulties (www.ace.orst.edu/info/extoxnet). Levels are higher in the green parts of potatoes, sprouted potatoes and potatoes stored in the light. The Food Standards Agency advises that severe glyco-alkaloid poisoning is very rare but it is important to store potatoes in a dark, cool and dry place and not to eat green or sprouting potatoes (www.food.gov.uk/safereating).

Genetic engineering has the potential to modify the presence in plants of these naturally occurring toxicants and, as a result, the US Food and Drug Administration encourages developers of genetically modified foods to evaluate the levels and to compare them with the levels in equivalent non-genetically modified plants (Novak & Haslberger, 2000).

In addition to the presence of naturally occurring toxins, some plants used as food can also become contaminated with toxins of fungal origin, resulting in illness. Toxin-producing moulds and fungi grow on most foods if the conditions are

Table 13.7 Toxic substances naturally present in plant foods*.

Food	Active agent	Effects
Potatoes	Solanine is found in high levels in green potatoes, sprouting potatoes and those stored in the light	Nausea, vomiting and respiratory difficulties
Cassava, sorghum	Cyanogens that readily yield cyanide; removed by appropriate processing of the staple (peeling, washing in running water and then cooking or fermenting to inactivate the enzyme and volatilise the cyanide)	Interferes with tissue respiration, causing dysfunction of the central nervous system, respiratory failure and cardiac arrest
Rhubarb leaves	Oxalate	Oxaluria
Many fungi	Various mycotoxins	Mainly toxic effects on the nervous system
Bananas and some other fruits	5-Hydroxytryptamine	Effects on the nervous system
Legumes, uncooked	Haemagglutinins (lectins)	Red cell and intestinal cell damage. The latter reduces nutrient absorption
Cycad nut	Methylazoxymethanol (cycasin)	Liver damage
Ackee fruit	α-Amino-β-methylenecyclopropane propionic acid, which causes accumulation of branched chain amino acids	Hypoglycaemia and a form of food poisoning known as vomiting sickness
Mustard oil	Sanguinarine	Oedema (epidemic dropsy), inhibits the oxidation of pyruvic acid
Nutmeg, mace	Myristicin	Vomiting and colic
Soya beans	Trypsin inhibitors, destroyed by cooking	Impairs protein digestion and availability
Brassica seeds (*e.g.* rapeseed) and seeds of some other cruciferae	Glucosinolates	Goitrogenic effects when consumed in excess
Honey	Alkaloids in circumstances where bees have foraged almost exclusively on alkaloid-containing plants, *e.g. Echium* spp.	Pyrrolizidine alkaloids can cause liver damage
Celery, parsley, parsnips, figs	Coumarins	Light activated substances that can cause skin irritation

*These substances are generally found at very low levels in the food we eat. However, under certain circumstances, as illustrated in the table, levels can be higher and pose a threat to health.
Sources: Passmore and Eastwood (1986); www.fao.org; www.anzfa.gov.au; www.ace.orst.edu/info/extoxnet; www.comm.cornell.edu.

right. They grow fastest in warm, moist conditions and hence growth of the mould species is typically a problem in tropical and subtropical areas. Well-recognised examples are ergotism that results from the consumption of rye (and other cereals) contaminated with the fungus ergot which produces toxins. Contamination of cereal crops (*e.g.* maize) and also peanut crops with moulds and fungi of the genus *Aspergillus* can also result in severe illness as a result of toxins known as aflatoxins, which can cause liver damage. The aflatoxins can be present even when there is no visible sign of mould. Spices are often imported from tropical and subtropical parts of the world and are another potential source of exposure. The law covering contaminants in food has recently been amended to include European Commission maximum levels for total aflatoxins and aflatoxin B in certain spices (for details see www.food.gov.uk/foodindustry/regulations/ria/aflareg).

The toxin ochratoxin, produced by various species of *Aspergillus* and by *Penicillium verrucosum*, is another source of contamination of stored foods and is known to cause kidney damage. It can contaminate cereals but also has been found in grape juice, red wine, coffee, cocoa, nuts, spices and dried fruits (Walker, 2002).

The Food Standards Agency's programme of work for 2000–1 on contaminants in food included several projects on ochratoxin, including surveys of nuts, dried fruit and fig paste, rice, spices, vine fruit and maize and maize products. Also included in the programme is a survey of dioxin levels in fruit and vegetables. Details of these can be found at www.food.gov.uk/science/surveillance.

Regular surveys are also carried out to assess the levels of metal contaminants in foodstuffs. For instance, a recent study assessed levels of arsenic, cadmium, chromium, copper, lead, manganese, mercury, nickel, platinum, tin, titanium and zinc in two types of food that grow wild, fungi and blackberries. The estimated dietary exposures were within relevant guidelines on safe exposures, even for above average adult consumers of wild foods (MAFF, 2000a).

Another potential source of contamination in plant foods is pesticide residues. The use of individual pesticides is subject to government approval in the UK and a surveillance programme monitors their use and the levels present in the food chain. Pesticides are used to kill or control pests and disease carriers, *e.g.* rodents, insects, fungi and plants that might damage the food itself or, indirectly, human health. The role of the surveillance programme is to ensure that pesticide residue levels are not posing a threat to health, *i.e.* they are below the scientifically supported safety limits, which incorporate a large safety factor. For more information about the Advisory Committee on Pesticides, and the Pesticides Residues Committee, see www.pesticides.gov.uk. The Food Standards Agency states on its website that the risk to health from eliminating fruit and vegetables from the diet would far outweigh the risks posed by possible exposure to pesticide residues (www.food.gov.uk/safeeating/pesticides). Concern has been expressed about the theoretical risk posed by consumption of foods exposed to more than one type of pesticide. Although the Agency has been advised that there is no reason to suppose that this would cause a problem, a working party of COT (the independent Committee on the Toxicity of Chemicals in Food, Consumer Products and the Environment) has been established to consider this matter.

One of the mechanisms for assessing risks posed by chemicals in foods is via the Joint FAO/WHO Expert Committee on Food Additives (JECFA), whose brief also includes food contaminants, and the Joint FAO/WHO Meeting on Pesticide Residues (JMPR). To date, JECFA has evaluated more than 1300 food additives and approximately 25 contaminants and naturally occurring toxicants. In 2001, FAO and WHO initiated a joint project to update and consolidate principles and methods for the risk assessment of chemicals in food. Details of the project plan can be found on their websites (www.fao.org and www.who.org/pcs).

A detailed report on hazard characterisation of chemicals in food and diet, which focuses on dose–response, mechanism and extrapolation issues, has recently been published (Dybing *et al.*, 2002). This report is the consequence of a pan-

European initiative and although not directly focusing on plant bioactive substances, it provides a very useful overview of various stages of risk assessment, namely hazard identification and, in particular, hazard characterisation in relation to micronutrients and nutritional supplements on the one hand, and macronutrients and whole foods on the other.

13.7 Policy implications

There are a number of possible ways in which public health policy might approach the improvement of health through increased plant food consumption. Essentially there are two approaches, one that operates at a population level (*e.g.* legislation, fiscal policy or a school-based policy) and another that targets the individual (see Section 13.1). At the simplest level, information can be disseminated, for example through schools, public campaigns and literature available via health care professionals. Information is an essential component of public policy in any area, but alone is often insufficient to effect change as it is often not sufficient simply to increase knowledge. Two specific types of action are discussed below, first the addition of nutrients (or other food constituents) to foods and second food labelling and claims. Consideration is also given to the roles of different players (Section 13.7.3).

13.7.1 Addition of nutrients to foods

Addition of nutrients (or other constituents) to foods, often referred to as fortification, is an approach which is used around the world as a public health measure and as a cost-effective means of ensuring the nutritional quality of the food supply. It has been adopted in the UK for over half a century, yet is not favoured in other parts of Europe where a much less liberal attitude to fortification has been adopted (British Nutrition Foundation, 2002a). Foods with added nutrients are attracting more and more interest and a legislative proposal on the addition of nutrients to foods is under development in Europe.

The addition of nutrients can be classified in several ways. Fortification (or enrichment) refers to the addition of one or more nutrients to a food or drink, whether or not they are normally present, for the purpose of preventing or correcting a demonstrated nutrient deficiency in the population as a whole or in a specific population group. It can be a legal requirement or voluntary. Examples in the UK include the statutory addition of calcium to all types of wheat flour, other than wholemeal, and of vitamins A and D to margarine; the voluntary fortification of breakfast cereals with a range of nutrients, and of bread with folic acid; and the voluntary fortification of salt with iodine. A topical example is the recent decision in the USA to fortify grain products by law with folic acid. A similar approach (to fortify flour) has been considered in the UK (Gibson, 2002) but, for the time being at least, a fortification programme is not expected to take place.

Restoration refers to the addition of nutrients to a food to replace naturally occurring substances lost during the course of good manufacturing practice or during normal handling and storage procedures, to the level present in the edible part of the food before processing. An example of statutory restoration is the addition of thiamin, niacin and iron to all types of wheat flour, other than wholemeal, to restore levels to those present in 80% extraction flour. An example of voluntary restoration is the addition of vitamin C to dehydrated potato products.

Substitution refers to the addition of a nutrient to a substitute product to the levels found in the food that it is designed to resemble in appearance, texture and flavour. Examples are the addition of calcium to soya products marketed as a substitute for milk, or vitamin B_{12} to textured vegetable protein products (positioned as alternatives to meat).

Although the UK has adopted a liberal attitude to the addition of nutrients to foods, claims about such additions may only be made for the so-called scheduled vitamins and minerals, listed in the Food Labelling Regulations 1996, and these claims cannot be medicinal claims, *i.e.* suggesting prevention or treatment of disease. These are the vitamins A, D, E, C, riboflavin, B_6, folic acid, B_{12}, biotin and pantothenic acid, and the minerals calcium, phosphorus, iron, magnesium, zinc and iodine. This situation is likely to stifle product innovation should clear evidence emerge for the benefits of a nutrient not on this list.

13.7.2 Food labelling and claims

Policy can be supported by ensuring that a coherent message is transmitted by all channels, so that labelling and claims, which are a major component of consumers' information relating to food and health, should be governed by common principles to those underpinning the policy objective. This is only possible where there is widespread agreement on those principles, but this appears to be so for increasing fruit and vegetable consumption. While Governmental responsibility for this area lies with the Food Standards Agency, a recently formed coalition of industry, consumer groups and enforcement officers (the Joint Health Claims Initiative, JHCI) has been set up with government approval to develop a process to examine and approve claims (www.jhci.co.uk).

Two classes of claims are envisaged, generic and innovative. Generic claims would apply to widely accepted associations between classes of food or food ingredients and health benefits, such as for unsaturated fatty acids and lowering of blood cholesterol. Innovative claims will apply to specific products developed by manufacturers, which can also be demonstrated to have beneficial effects. Products in the latter category will represent the sort of food currently called 'functional food'. The former will incorporate the more general claims of healthfulness of fruit and vegetables and other plant foods in general. The scheme is expected to be self-financing through manufacturers' fees. The JHCI's Expert Committee is currently reviewing the evidence that underpins a number of potential health claims. It is also compiling a list of nutrient function claims on behalf of the Food Standards Agency. Progress with this work can be found on the JHCI's website.

Although only voluntary and in its early days, this initiative offers the opportunity to ensure that consumers are not unjustly exposed to inappropriate, conflicting or unjustified messages on foods. With regard to plant foods, it will be important to ensure that the reasonable enthusiasm for finding a simple single effective substance is not translated into unreasonably exaggerated claims of efficacy. Unfortunately, the advertising budget for 'generic' products such as fruit and vegetables rarely approaches that for their pseudopharmacological competitors. In such circumstances, it is reasonable to look to the public health agencies to become involved, and this may underpin the appearance of food-related public health policies over the last few years.

A similar initiative, under the auspices of the US Food and Drug Administration, has been in place for some time. The food and health linkages that have been accepted as scientifically supportable by the FDA and can be used in the USA are to be found at www.cfsan.fda.gov. The detailed criteria that apply to each of these linkages are also provided and are summarised in a recent BNF publication (British Nutrition Foundation, 2002a). A number of other countries, including Canada and Australia, are also grappling with the processes that need to be in place in order to assess the validity of health claims (Health Canada, 2001; Food Standards Agency Australia New Zealand, 2002) and the European Union is also giving this matter consideration via the PASSCLAIM project (http://europe.ilsi.org/passclaim/) (International Life Sciences Institute, Europe, 2002). In addition, the European Commission is currently preparing a legislative proposal to cover nutrition claims, functional claims and health claims (see www.europa.eu/int).

Manufacturers naturally respond to consumer demand and consumers also prefer a 'quick fix' which is cheap and easy to incorporate into daily life without a major change in behaviour. In such a climate, it is often difficult to maintain an evidence-based cautionary approach.

A particular case of current interest relates to the growing popularity of organic foods. These are variously perceived as better for the environment, more tasty, safer or more nutritious. However, a recent review by the Food Standards Agency failed to find sufficient evidence to support the claims that organic foods are either safer or more nourishing than their conventional counterparts (see www.food.gov.uk).

13.7.3 Key players

The examples given in Sections 13.7.1 and 13.7.2 are of particular relevance to the food industry. However, other important sectors in achieving dietary change are schools and primary heath care professionals.

Educational and social background are key determinants of people's likelihood of consuming amounts of fruits and vegetables close to recommended levels. With this in mind, it appears that schools have a major role to play in helping to narrow the social variations in consumption, which may contribute to similar variations in health. By adopting a whole school approach to good nutrition that embraces all aspects of school life and not just the formal curriculum, schools could improve children's exposure to different types of food at a young age so that they become familiar [see British Nutrition Foundation (2002b) for more information]. Attention to teaching not only the technology of food at an academic level but also the appreciation of food as a social skill, as in France, might also be valuable. Similarly, it is important for children to learn to cook for themselves as they approach adulthood, in order better to be in control of their daily diet. This is particularly important as many parents now do not have these skills, and they therefore cannot be passed down in the family.

Local and national government have a role in ensuring that an appropriate variety of food of adequate quality is available and accessible to all strata of society. It is likely that aiding the least well off to eat better will reap benefits over time in improved health and reduced healthcare demand. Education-based health promotion strategies tend to favour the better off, and although they can be effective, they may paradoxically widen health inequalities. An important consideration is the training and employment of adequate numbers of public health nutritionists and community dietitians to develop, take forward, evaluate and disseminate local and national initiatives, which are based on robust evidence.

Government has a special role in promoting the need for an evidence-based approach and supporting the research needed to develop new evidence-based interventions, and in particular ensuring that such interventions are properly evaluated in order to help understand the important drivers for improved nutrition.

13.8 Conclusions

There is a large body of generally consistent evidence from ecological, prospective and case control epidemiological studies, and also supportive evidence from laboratory data, that a change in the current diet in the UK and elsewhere to favour plant foods including fruits, vegetables and fibre-rich starchy foods would result in improved personal and public health. However, not all the data point in the same direction, and change is difficult to effect. A major need will be to ensure that public understanding does not run ahead of the evidence base in the inevitable search for easy, quick and cheap remedies. Public policy has a number of levers that can be used to help ensure a coherent approach to developing the science base and public information synchronously. The responsibility for ensuring this happens falls to politicians and health professionals to lead, but also to the media, industry and others to act responsibly.

13.9 Research recommendations

- There is a need to develop better methods of characterising both habitual plant food consumption, and risk of disease through use of biomarkers.
- There is a need to understand better the roles of individual constituents of plant foods, and combinations of them, in promoting health and preventing disease.

- There is also a need to investigate whether effects differ with dose, and to identify mechanisms of action.
- There is a need to develop effective methods of altering the dietary patterns of communities and of groups within them, particularly in relation to social inequalities.
- There is a need to characterise better the adverse effects seen in some groups following consumption of high doses of micronutrients.

13.10 Key points

- Public health nutrition operates at several levels: collection of information on diet and nutrition status in the population; analysis of data; knowledge and understanding of the principles underlying the relationship of nutrition to health; and the development, implementation and evaluation of interventions to improve nutrition in the community.
- There are systems in place for advising Government on the links between nutrition and health, and academic courses for training nutritionists to utilise relevant information. However few authorities recognise a need for appropriately trained nutritionists as part of their approach to improving health in the community.
- There are several sources of information at a national level on diet and nutrition status in the population. Health experience in the community is unequally distributed in society, with those worse off having poorer health, and this inequality is mirrored by lower consumption of plant foods, in particular fruit, and to a lesser extent vegetables. Similar inequalities are found in many other countries within Europe and beyond.
- There are several different approaches that could be taken to influence population eating behaviours. They are not mutually exclusive, and in some situations may be complementary.

- Evaluation of the US 'five-a-day' campaign (which employed a variety of strategies) has found significant increases in fruit consumption but little impact on vegetable consumption, suggesting that different approaches may be required for the two types of food, and that different barriers to change may exist.
- Policies to improve health often focus on public information ('five-a-day') provision, which tends to widen inequality. The determinants of social variation are likely to be more structural, and structural programmes are needed to address them. Educational programmes in schools to address inequalities from an early age by fostering healthy attitudes and providing children with skills to control their own diets and lifestyles are important components. Educating GPs in particular (but also other health professionals) in nutrition and its health implications is an important step forward.
- National and local government have a responsibility to ensure that all strata of society have access to reliable information, are educated to utilise such information and have access to affordable food of adequate quality and variety to construct a healthy diet for themselves and their families. Current policies and policies in the UK and elsewhere address these issues in an incomplete and piecemeal fashion. Research resources

- addressing the biological and social questions should be enhanced.
- Looking to the future, enhancing the content of bioactive compounds in plant foods through selective breeding or genetic improvements is a potent dietary option if such substances are proved to be of health benefit. However, the majority of compounds are bitter, acid or astringent and this may restrict the amounts tolerated.
- There are many examples of naturally present plant components being harmful to health, but paradoxically a number of these (*e.g.* glucosinolates, phytoestrogens) are now in the spotlight from a health improvement perspective. It is likely that the amount consumed is of crucial relevance, with different amounts having different effects on important biochemical pathways.
- Many scientific questions remain unanswered, for instance relating to biological markers of diet and of risk of diet-related disease.

- A key message of this Task Force is the need to eat plenty of plant foods, including a variety of different vegetables and fruit. However, this should be placed in the context of a varied diet, given that the substances of interest are found in every food group (*e.g.* phytoestrogens in pulses and cereals; CLA and sphingolipids in dairy products and meat; and long-chain *n*-3 PUFA, derived from phytoplankton, in fish), and a broad selection of substances in plant foods, ranging from herbs and condiments through fruits and vegetables, to tea and wine. It is not yet possible to tease out particular compounds, or indeed foods, as more important than others. Different compounds have different but equally important effects on cell functions and hence a variety of them needs to be consumed. Hence it is impossible to be precise about which particular foods to target or the amounts required for 'optimum' health.

14
Conclusions of the Task Force

It has been recognised for some time that diets rich in fruits and vegetables are associated with positive health benefits and lower risk of chronic diseases, such as some cancers and cardiovascular disease. In the search for the specific constituents that confer this benefit, attention was initially focused on constituent nutrients with antioxidant properties. However, more recently, attention has turned to the diversity of other constituents of edible plants, such as flavonoids and allied phenolics and polyphenolics; carotenoids and other terpenoids; and alkaloids and sulphur-containing compounds. These various classes of compound comprise the main focus of this report, which attempts to summarise current knowledge about the health benefits of plant-derived bioactive compounds.

The conclusions reached by the Task Force are presented below, in chapter order. The recommendations of the Task Force can be found in Chapter 15.

14.1 Chapter 1

- In this report, the term plant foods is used to describe fruits, vegetables, cereals, pulses, nuts, seeds, herbs and spices, and also plants that have been processed in some way to yield foods and drinks whose origin is primarily plant-based (*e.g.* oils, various hot and cold beverages, chocolate, condiments).
- Information on national food consumption patterns is available from a variety of sources, in particular government surveys, *e.g.* the UK's National Food Survey (now Expenditure and Food Survey) and the National Diet and Nutrition Survey Programme. From these sources, it is evident that UK fruit and vegetable consumption, for example, varies with socio-economic group (being lower in the lowest social classes) and to a lesser extent with region.
- Information is also available on intakes of the various nutrients provided by plant foods (*e.g.* vitamins C and E; folate; minerals, *e.g.* iron, calcium, selenium, potassium, magnesium; and unsaturated fatty acids) and to a lesser extent there is information available on other substances such as carotenoids and flavonoids.
- There is now a considerable body of evidence that shows that diets rich in plant foods are generally associated with lower disease risks. In the search for the specific constituents that confer this benefit, attention has to date been focused on constituents with antioxidant properties, initially vitamins E and C and the carotenoids, but increasingly other plant-derived antioxidants, such as flavonoids have become the focus.
- Whether or not a plant constituent is provided in a bioavailable form in a food is crucial to the food's nutritional value. Interactions can also occur between the constituents present in foods, for example polyphenols present in plant-derived foods can inhibit uptake of iron from the same or other foods.

14.2 Chapter 2

- A diverse variety of organic compounds are to

be found in edible plants. Some compounds (primarily metabolites) have essential roles in the plant, being associated with photosynthesis, respiration and growth and development. Others (secondary metabolites) protect against herbivores and microbial infection, act as attractants for pollinator and seed-dispersing animals, as allelopathic agents, as UV protectants or as signal molecules in the formation of nitrogen-fixing root nodules in legumes.

- In recent years, the potential for some secondary metabolites to carry health benefits for humans has attracted considerable interest.
- Plant secondary metabolites can be divided into three major groups: flavonoids and allied phenolic and polyphenolic compounds (about 8000 compounds); terpenoids (about 25 000 compounds); and alkaloids (about 12 000 compounds) and sulphur-containing compounds.
- Flavonoids are the most numerous of the phenolics and are found throughout the plant kingdom, concentrated mainly in the epidermis of leaves and the skin of fruits. The group includes flavonols (*e.g.* myricetin and quercetin), flavones (*e.g.* luteolin and apigenin), flavan-3-ols (*e.g.* catechin, epicatechin, proanthocyanidins), anthocyanidins (*e.g.* cyanidin), flavanones (*e.g.* hesperidin, narigen) and isoflavones (*e.g.* genistein and daidzein). The principle non-flavonoid phenolic compounds are hydroxycinnamates (*e.g.* caffeic acid and ferulic acid), stilbenes (*e.g.* *trans*-resveratrol) and phenolic acids (*e.g.* tannins).
- Carotenoids (tetraterpenoids) are the best-known members of the terpenoid family. However, there are more than 25 000 terpenoids in all, many of which have recognised medicinal effects or are flavouring agents. Plant sterols are triterpenoids.
- There are 12 000 or so alkaloids, which contain one or more nitrogen atoms. It is now known that alkaloids were the active ingredients in numerous potions and poisons used over the centuries, and many alkaloids (*e.g.* codeine) are still in use today as prescription drugs. Most alkaloids are synthesised from certain amino acids. However, two well-known alkaloids, caffeine and theobromine, are derived from purine nucleotides.

- A variety of sulphur-containing compounds are also present, including the glucosinolates found in plants of the Brassica family and all the derivatives of the sulphur-containing amino acid cysteine, found in members of the onion family.

14.3 Chapter 3

- It is important to recognise the strengths and weaknesses of data derived from epidemiological studies, in general, and from specific types of study.
- Eating patterns characterised by an abundance of fruit, vegetables and other plant foods are associated with a reduced risk of chronic disease, *e.g.* cardiovascular disease (coronary heart disease and stroke) and some cancers. A less extensive amount of information is also available for type 2 diabetes, age-related macular degeneration, cataract, and chronic obstructive pulmonary disease. Although these findings have been supported by many studies, the association is usually of moderate strength.
- The search for the active components in these foods has met with limited success; specific constituents responsible for the association have yet to be identified, and so have not been widely investigated in epidemiological studies.
- Research has been focused on the antioxidants vitamins C and E and β-carotene, although a few studies have also looked at other carotenoids and some of the polyphenols (*e.g.* flavonoids) that are among the main subjects of this report. Promising and generally consistent results have been reported in animal and *in vitro* studies but, to date, convincing evidence from human intervention and epidemiological studies is sparse. The evidence that antioxidants such as vitamins E and C and β-carotene specifically are responsible for the beneficial effects of fruit and vegetables is at best equivocal.
- The need for caution when it comes to advocating supplements of individual substances provided by plant foods has been clearly underlined by the findings of several intervention studies that demonstrated that large doses of β-carotene may actually be detrimental to the health of certain groups, *e.g.* heavy smokers.

- There is a need for soundly constructed prospective studies and related mechanistic studies, designed to identify active components in plant foods, their long-term health effects and their mode of action. Identification of these would enable dietary advice to be more specific.

14.4 Chapter 4

- Our understanding of the pathogenic processes underlying cancers and CVD is developing rapidly and is leading to improved pharmacological means of preventing and treating these disorders.
- In parallel with these developments, it has become apparent that there is a very large range of bioactive compounds present in plant-derived foods and drinks that may have protective effects against these disorders.
- The potential of these compounds to be beneficial to human health appears significant, but many mechanisms of action are likely to be involved.
- In order to provide clear dietary guidelines aimed at maximising these potential protective effects, it will be necessary more clearly to understand the importance and relevance of the different protective pathways and the efficacy of the different compounds in modulating these pathways.
- Epidemiological data are consistent with the possibility that constituents of fruit and vegetables may play specific roles in prevention of the pathogenesis of certain cancers and CVD.
- The pathophysiological processes involved in the formation of tumours and in CVD are becoming increasingly well understood.
- *In vitro* and cell culture studies have indicated multiple potential steps in the pathophysiological processes at which various plant constituents might act to prevent the formation of tumours or occurrence of CVD.
- Little evidence has been presented demonstrating that any such effects occur *in vivo* and many of the studies have used experimental conditions that do not approximate to nutritional intake levels.

14.5 Chapter 5

- The mucosal surfaces of the alimentary tract are unique in their direct exposure to food constituents at levels that are often far in excess of those achieved at systemic sites. In the colon, this exposure is extended to include a complex variety of bacterial metabolites, which include both harmful and potentially protective factors.
- The interior of the human alimentary tract provides an ideal environment for colonisation by micro-organisms. Although the stomach and small intestine are relatively sterile, the large intestine contains a rich commensal microflora, strategically located, downstream from the main sites of digestion and absorption. The microflora is an important source of substances derived from undigested plant components, which may act as protective factors against colorectal and systemic disease.
- The colonic microflora derive their energy from two sources, undigested food and endogenous secretions. Most of the bacteria of the human colon utilise carbohydrate as a source of energy, although not all can degrade polysaccharides directly. Around 30 g of bacteria are produced for every 100 g of carbohydrate fermented, and it has been estimated that somewhere between 20 and 80 g of undigested carbohydrate enter the human colon every day.
- The large intestine is subject to a range of functional, structural and infectious diseases, the most important of which are the inflammatory conditions of unknown cause, Crohn's disease and ulcerative colitis, and colorectal carcinoma, which is the second most common cause of death from cancer in many industrialised societies
- The lactic acid bacteria have long been considered beneficial to health. Evidence for the subtle biological effects of such bacteria is accumulating but, in general, the importance of these for the prevention of disease remains to be established. Some plant foods, *e.g.* artichokes, onions, garlic and chicory, contain prebiotic substances. These cannot be digested by human enzymes, but can be broken down and utilised by some colonic microflora, therefore modify-

ing the profile of gut bacteria. The general principle of manipulating the balance of the colonic microflora by dietary intervention is an area that requires further intensive study.

- The major carbohydrate fermentation pathway for colonic bacteria leads to the formation of the short-chain fatty acids acetate, propionate and butyrate. The colonic epithelial cells are adapted to utilise butyrate preferentially as a source of energy, and butyrate stimulates the growth of normal colon cells and suppresses proliferation of cancer cells *in vitro*. Butyrate also induces apoptosis (programmed cell death) in tumour cells. These and other findings have prompted interest in the development of functional food products containing readily fermentable substrates, such as resistant starch, that could augment the supply of butyrate to the colonic epithelium.

- The Brassica vegetables (cabbage, broccoli, Brussels sprouts) provide some of the best-documented examples of induction of potentially anticarcinogenic defence mechanisms by plant secondary metabolites in food. At least part of their effect appears to be due to colonic bacterial metabolism. Some food-borne glucosinolates remain intact in cooked vegetables, and pass to the colon where they are degraded. Their biologically active breakdown products (isothiocyanates) then become available for interactions with colonic epithelial cells, and for uptake into the circulation via the colonic mucosa.

- The human diet contains a rich variety of phenolic substances that originate from plant-derived foods and drinks, amongst the most important of which are the flavonoids. These are generally present in the form of water-soluble but relatively inactive glycosides, some of which are efficiently absorbed in the upper part of the alimentary tract. A proportion of the unabsorbed flavonoids pass through the small intestine unabsorbed and become available for bacterial metabolism in the colon but the physiological effects of the bacterial metabolites of flavonoids in humans are unknown.

- The isoflavones are diphenolic compounds found principally in soya products, that bear a structural similarity to mammalian oestrogen. The parent species are broken down by the intestinal microflora to yield the aglycones genistein and daidzein, which can be transported across the intestinal mucosa into the circulation. In some individuals, another bacterial product, the isoflavan equol, is produced. A second important group of diphenolic phytoestrogens, the lignan precursors matairesinol and secoisolariciresinol, occur in cereal seeds and vegetables. As with the isoflavones, these compounds are degraded by colonic bacteria to yield the active lignans enterolactone and enterodiol, which can be taken up by mucosal epithelial cells and transferred to the circulation. Much of the importance of phytoestrogens lies in their ability to exert weak hormone-like activity. They may also exert potentially beneficial direct effects on the epithelial cells of the colon through suppression of protein kinases and cyclooxygenases. Further research is needed to assess these effects.

- A great deal remains to be discovered about the biochemistry and ecology of the colon, and about the physiological response of the colon epithelial cells to their environment. Biologically active substances derived from plant foods are an important part of that environment. There may be much to gain through the manipulation of this complex system by dietary intervention.

14.6 Chapter 6

- In order to assess the bioavailability of a food component, it is necessary to have information about the amount that enters the blood circulation intact following consumption of the food, *i.e.* following digestion and absorption. This knowledge is essential in order to understand the potential role of dietary components in the prevention of disease.

- There remains a need for a comprehensive and thorough survey of the occurrence in food and progress through the body of the various types of bioactive compounds (*e.g.* flavonoids and allied compounds, terpenoids, alkaloids, nitrogen-containing alkaloids and sulphur-containing compounds) using selective, sensitive and well-standardised methods, which are applicable to blood, plasma, urine and tissues.

- Although intestinal absorption can be high, there is evidence of extensive metabolism of absorbed flavonoids, as changes in plasma antioxidant capacity generally considerably exceed changes in levels of the parent flavonoid in plasma. Absorption from the colon, following the action of colonic bacteria on ingested flavonoids and related compounds, is thought to be important in contributing to antioxidant capacity in plasma but little is known about the precise role of the microflora in the bioavailability of such substances and, apart from a limited understanding of why flavonol glycosides are better absorbed than their aglycones, little is known about the influence of other structural parameters.

- For the flavonoids and carotenoids in particular, research is beginning to provide information on the amounts of selected compounds in foods, and typical intakes in a number of populations world wide. However, compared with the flavonoids, much more is known about the absorption and transport of carotenoids. Assessment of relative bioavailability is also receiving considerable research attention. Functional markers for carotenoids are required, however, to enable research into potential health benefits to progress.

- Flavonoids (*e.g.* flavonols, flavones, flavan-3-ols, flavanones and isoflavones) account for about two-thirds of the dietary phenols, with phenolic acids accounting for the remainder. The main sources are fruit, beverages (fruit juice, wine, tea, coffee, cocoa and beer) and chocolate. Vegetables, dry legumes and cereals also contribute. The total intake of phenols is estimated to be about 1 g/day.

- The potential beneficial effects of flavonoids justify a thorough understanding of the bioavailability in humans of these abundant dietary constituents. The limited data available suggest that dietary concentrations are potentially high enough to give biological effects.

- The five most commonly occurring carotenoids in blood are β-carotene, lycopene, lutein, β-cryptoxanthin and α-carotene. The main

dietary sources of these are, respectively, carrots, tomatoes/tomato products, peas, citrus fruit and carrots. Average intake of total carotenoids in UK adults is 14.4 mg/day, with the largest contributions coming from β-carotene and lycopene.

- A beneficial role for plant sterol and stanol esters, in relation to reducing plasma cholesterol, has been established. Their action hinges on their very low absorption rates and their structural similarity to cholesterol and hence their competition in the micellar phase with dietary and endogenous cholesterol, reducing uptake of the latter.

- More data are required on the absorption and endogenous metabolism of phytoestrogens in humans, and clarification is also needed of the biological activity of the metabolites. It is necessary to identify the key gut micro-organisms responsible for the conversion of the plant constituents to the biologically active derivatives, and the factors that determine their occurrence in the gastrointestinal tract. The interactions of phytoestrogens with each other and with endogenous steroids should also be investigated further.

- Glucosinolates are sulphur-containing compounds found in Brassica vegetables. Disruption of the plant tissue (*e.g.* by chopping or cooking) releases myrosinase which converts the glucosinolates to a number of substances including isothiocyanates. There is also evidence that conversion to isothiocyanates can occur in the colon; ability to degrade glucosinolates is widespread among bacteria. There is growing interest in these breakdown products and animal evidence that they may have anti-cancer effects.

- Interest is growing in the hydroxycinnamates (*e.g.* caffeic and ferulic acids) and hydroxybenzoates (ellagic acid). Although there is some information about the uptake and metabolism of hydroxybenzoates in humans, further research in this area is required.

14.7 Chapter 7

- In the growing plant, bioactive compounds have roles in metabolism and in the interaction of the plant with the environment. The occurrence of the compounds of potential nutritional interest varies throughout the plant kingdom from the widespread carotenoids to the glucosinolates (found only in the Cruciferae).

- Polyphenols and carotenoids provide colour to stems, leaves, flowers and fruits. The carotenoids provide yellows with some orange and red while the polyphenolics, most notably the anthocyanins, are more numerous and provide a greater range of colours from orange to blue.
- Some bioactive compounds affect insect predation, some act as feeding deterrents to certain species of insect but to others insect larvae are attracted.
- Some bioactive compounds have antifungal and antibacterial activities and their presence in the plant may contribute to resistance to pathogen attack.
- The role of bioactive compounds in protecting crops poses a dilemma. It is the very compounds that make a crop less palatable that have ensured their survival in different environments. However, levels of some of these compounds tend to be lower in modern plant varieties because they have been deliberately bred out (*e.g.* the bitter-tasting glucosinolates in Brussels sprouts). More attention needs to be given to the changes in plant composition that have occurred given the potential health benefits of these constituents.
- It is important to be aware of the sheer numbers of compounds. Attention tends to be focused on a few representatives of each class, but 25 000 members of the terpene family have been identified, around 8000 phenolics and there are even 250 different sterols.
- The bioactive compound content of individual fruits and vegetables is affected by variety, soil, climatic conditions, agricultural methods, physiological stress under which they are grown, degree of ripeness, storage conditions and period of storage before consumption. Not all references have recognised the resultant variability, and results from a single unnamed variety have often been taken as representative of the species.

- The levels of bioactive compounds also vary within the plant; within fruits many are concentrated in the skin, and within vegetables in the outer leaves. The content determined by analysis will therefore depend on the amount discarded and exactly which part of the plant is analysed.
- Bioactive compounds, including those contributing to colour, are known to be present in fruits and vegetables. Together with the vitamins and minerals, they may be the basis for the beneficial effects of these foods. The fact that particular bioactive compounds are highlighted should not be taken as an indication that these are the only ones associated with the foodstuff.
- The epidemiological evidence for the benefit of consuming diets that are high in fruit and vegetables is quite compelling but the evidence for specific vegetables, and indeed specific compounds, is less convincing.

14.8 Chapter 8

- In addition to their macronutrient content, cereals, nuts and pulses contain a number of potentially bioactive substances, in particular selenium, folates and other bioactive compounds from the phytoestrogen class. The presence of bioactive substances in this food group adds further weight to their proposed beneficial effects for human health. However, further research is required, particularly in relation to the phytoestrogens, in order to define specific health benefits and optimal intakes.
- High consumption of cereals, nuts and pulses may be associated with a decreased risk of diseases such as cardiovascular disease and some cancers, but so far many of the specific food constituents that might be responsible for these associations have yet to be identified. To date, research interest has concentrated on folate, selenium, phytoestrogens and fibre (which is not considered in detail in this report).
- Selenium is found in many plant foods, and both cereals and nuts can be important sources. In humans, it is an essential component of a

number of enzymes, *e.g.* glutathione peroxidase, and recent research has been focused on cancer protection and cardiovascular benefits. Cereals and pulses are contributors to folate intake. This micronutrient has recently been recognised as important in protecting against neural tube defects in fetal life and as a potential influence on cardiovascular risk via an effect on reducing blood homocysteine levels.

- Phytoestrogens comprise a range of structurally dissimilar compounds with the common characteristic of being able to bind to oestrogen receptors in humans. The group includes isoflavones, lignans and stilbenes, which function as anti-fungal agents in plants.
- Relatively little is known about the factors that influence the bioavailability and the pharmacokinetic profile of phytoestrogens.
- Through their ability to bind to oestrogen receptors, it has been suggested that phytoestrogens may be beneficial in post-menopausal women in relation to menopausal symptoms, and risk factors for heart disease and osteoporosis. A role in breast cancer has also been suggested.
- The richest source of isoflavones is soya beans (although they are also present in chick peas and kidney beans). They are either present as the aglycone (genistein or daidzein) or as various glycoside conjugates (*e.g.* daidzin and genistin).
- Isoflavone supplements seem to be relatively ineffective in managing menopausal hot flushes, whereas isoflavone-rich foods appear to have a beneficial effect that exceeds that of a placebo, although the impact is much less than that seen with HRT. A key issue is whether consumption needs to be life-long (as in Japan, where soya consumption is high) to be effective.
- Soya has a recognised modest ability to reduce plasma cholesterol levels. The cholesterol-lowering effect appears to be the result of a combination of components acting together; isoflavones together with soya protein appear to have a greater effect than soya protein alone. Other effects of isoflavones have also been proposed including a direct effect on the arterial wall. Clinical data to determine the effects of isoflavones in relation to osteoporosis are still lacking; however, recent short-term human data are not as supportive as the available mechanistic data and animal data for a positive effect of isoflavones on bone health. The data with regard to bone health are still unclear, and the risks versus benefits of phytoestrogens in relation to breast cancer are unresolved.

- The role of phytoestrogens in infant health has been a controversial matter, as isoflavones are present in high concentrations in soya infant formula. Assessment of this matter is currently being addressed by the UK Government's Committee on Toxicity of Chemicals in Foods, Consumer Products and the Environment (COT).
- In Europe, owing to the frequency of consumption, cereals, nuts and pulses makes a significant contribution to intake of many of these bioactive compounds. However, information on their absorption, metabolism and mechanisms of action at physiologically relevant levels is required to design appropriate human intervention studies to define optimal doses for health benefits.

14.9 Chapter 9

- In many biological systems, extracts of tea have a wide range of effects with potential health benefits. In cell culture and animal models they may inhibit oxidation of low-density lipoproteins and prevent mutations and have been shown to be anti-carcinogens. Much of this activity is ascribed to the polyphenolic components of tea, in particular the catechin derivatives. More studies are required to establish the bioavailability of these compounds and their effects *in vivo* before any health benefits can be established with certainty. The impact of these compounds when consumed as part of a normal diet and in amounts normally consumed by humans is not yet clear.
- Most studies on the health effects of coffee have been focused on the diverse actions of caffeine on cellular metabolism. There is little evidence that coffee exacerbates or decreases the risk of heart disease and cancer. However, animal models suggest possible anti-carcinogenic activity of the coffee phenolics chlorogenic and caffeic acid.

- Cocoa as a beverage is less widely consumed than either tea or coffee, and its nutritional impact is likely to be relatively small. Cocoa powder is a rich source of minerals and contains a range of polyphenols, in particular catechin-type polymers. It is not yet clear whether the antioxidant activity of these compounds confer health benefits.
- Any health benefits arising from alcoholic beverages have to be considered within the context of the well-known adverse affects of excessive alcohol consumption. With this caveat, there is substantial evidence that moderate intakes of alcoholic beverages may reduce the risk of heart disease. Although such effects have generally been attributed to ethanol *per se*, additional benefits may be linked to the many polyphenols in red wine, some of which are absorbed through the gut and have potentially promising effects *in vitro*.
- Scotch whisky contains many phenolic compounds extracted from the wood during maturation in casks. The antioxidant potential of whisky is similar to that of wine and its consumption transiently raises the antioxidant activity of plasma. However, there are few data to suggest that this translates into an overt health benefit.
- Beer contains phenolic compounds and its antioxidant potential is similar to that of wine. Consumption of beer transiently increases the antioxidant activity of plasma, and phenolics in beer inhibit the oxidation of low-density lipoproteins and DNA damage *in vitro*. Whether these effects result in protection from heart disease and cancer is not clear. Beer also contributes to the intake of several essential micronutrients.

14.10 Chapter 10

- Plant lipids provide energy, carry vitamins and contain essential fatty acids.
- Plant and plant-derived lipids are important for maintaining the function and integrity of cell membranes. They also participate in the regulation of cholesterol metabolism and they are precursors of eicosanoids which act as local

hormones and are involved in wound healing, inflammation, platelet aggregation and in signal transduction mechanisms within cells.
- Dietary fatty acids are important modulators of a number of physiological processes involved in atherosclerosis and so also influence risk for CVD. They are also implicated in the aetiology and prevention or amelioration of cancer. A number of plant and plant-derived fatty acids and lipids are reported to have beneficial, ameliorating or preventative effects on biomarkers of various disease states in animals and humans.
- A raised blood cholesterol concentration is a risk factor for CVD. Determining the proportion of total cholesterol found in LDL and HDL particles is an important index of overall CVD risk. High levels of HDL cholesterol reduce the risk of atherosclerosis and heart disease, whereas high levels of LDL cholesterol increase the risk. A high fat intake, and in particular a high intake of SFA, has been associated with a raised blood cholesterol level. However, some SFA present greater risks than others.
- Increasing the proportion of unsaturated fatty acids in the diet can reduce blood cholesterol and TAG levels. Substitution of SFA with MUFA or PUFA has been found to lower LDL but not HDL cholesterol, even when total fat and energy intakes are maintained. MUFA are less susceptible than PUFA to oxidation, and high MUFA diets may decrease the susceptibility of the LDL particle to oxidation, reducing its atherogenicity.
- The long-chain *n*-3 PUFA of marine phytoplankton and algae that are concentrated in the body oils of fish have well-documented inhibitory effects on the inflammatory arm of the immune system. They regulate the expression of genes responsible for cytokine production and modulate the type of eicosanoids produced by cells (type 3 prostaglandins and type 5 leukotrienes), which attenuates inflammation and regulates the propensity for blood clotting (thrombus formation). The pattern of eicosanoid production may explain the effect of these fatty acids on cancer development and progression because PGE2 is an angiogenic

factor and new vascularisation is important for tumour growth. Long-chain *n*-3 PUFA also reduce plasma TAG concentrations significantly thereby attenuating another risk factor for CVD.

- Although it has been proposed that the unique antioxidant properties of the phenolic compounds present in olive oil may contribute to the beneficial effects of the Mediterranean diet, the evidence is insufficient to draw any conclusions.
- The effects of CLA and other conjugated fatty acids derived from plant linoleic and linolenic acids appear similar to those observed for *n*-3 PUFA. CLAs have also been shown to induce apoptosis in different types of human cancer cells by regulating pro- and anti-apoptotic oncogene expression. The same could also be the case for other plant-derived PUFA with conjugated double bonds in their structures.
- Data from animal studies demonstrating anti-cancer effects, reductions in body fat mass and improved lipid profiles have led to interest in the potential role that CLA might have for human health. However, with the exception of body fat reduction, the results of studies reported to date have been inconsistent. This is probably due to the different doses, the mix of isomers used and the characteristics of the subjects studied. There may also be synergism or antagonism between different CLA isomers.
- Sphingolipids are a structurally diverse class of complex, polar lipids present in all eukaryotic and some prokaryotic cell membranes. Consequently they are ubiquitous in human foods of both animal and plant origin. Sphingolipids are similar in structure to glycerophospholipids but utilise sphingosine as the 'backbone' of the diacyl ester rather than glycerol. Studies *in vitro* and animal models have shown that plant- and animal-derived sphingolipids such as sphingosine-1-phosphate regulate the function of cancer cells and endothelium, and so may be beneficial in preventing cancer, particularly bowel cancer, and also vascular disease.
- Refining of vegetable oils significantly reduces the content of sterols, and the potential to lower serum cholesterol through a normal diet.

- Plant sterol and stanol esters significantly reduce serum cholesterol levels by inhibiting cholesterol uptake and facilitating its elimination. With respect to cholesterol lowering, results suggest that a daily intake of up to 2 g/day of plant stanol or sterol esters is effective, and that higher doses may not increase their efficacy. Sterol and stanol esters appear to be equally effective.

14.11 Chapter 11

- Chocolate is derived from the cocoa plant, which is a source of theobromine, caffeine and a range of other bioactive substances. In particular, polyphenolics and phenolic acids comprise about 14% of the weight of the dried cocoa bean, with at least 60% of these being procyanidin oligomers of epicatechin (a flavan-3-ol). The hydroxycinnamates caffeic, ferulic and 4-coumaric acids are also present in the unfermented cocoa bean.
- Procyanidin levels have generally been shown to be higher in dark (plain) chocolate and epicatechin levels in blood have been shown to rise after dark chocolate consumption.
- There is an increasing body of largely *in vitro* evidence that the consumption of cocoa derivatives has the potential to increase the antioxidant capacity of the plasma and the potential to modify beneficially a number of processes thought to be associated with cardiovascular disease, *e.g.* LDL oxidation, inhibition of peroxynitrite and inhibition of platelet activity.
- It should be noted that much of this work has been conducted *in vitro* and needs to be corroborated in *ex vivo* or *in vivo* human studies.
- It should also be remembered that any potential benefits have to be considered in context. Chocolate, and products containing it, are often energy-dense and contain relatively high amounts of fat and sugar, and thus should be eaten in moderation (see Balance of Good Health in Chapter 13).
- Herbs and spices have been used for culinary purposes all over the world for thousands of years, for flavouring, preserving and colouring foods.

- The culinary use of plants as herbs and spices utilises all parts of the plan – leaves, stems, roots, seeds, seed pods and flowers. Thus a range of bioactive substances present in plants will be consumed in this way.
- Herbs and spices also have a long history of use as medicines, perfumes cosmetics, insect repellents and antiseptics. Many 'modern' mass-produced drugs have their origins in plant extracts and are based on knowledge gained over centuries of traditional use.
- In Western societies there is a resurgence of interest, or a new interest in the properties of herbs and spices, in the traditional use of herbs and spices as medicines.
- The use of herbs and spices for medicinal purposes, and more recently in *in vitro* and *in vivo* studies for potentially beneficial effects on CVD and cancer, usually requires tincture or essences or very concentrated extracts in the form of powders, granules and gels to be used. Thus intakes or 'doses' are much higher than would be so as a result of culinary use.
- The bioactive compounds contained in plants used as herbs and spices (and condiments such as horseradish sauce and mustards) are more immediately obvious than many other bioactive compounds, because many of them are aromatic, and released by the plant simply by being brushed or crushed.
- The bioactive compounds found in herbs and spices are mostly terpenoids and it is these oils that are responsible for flavours, taste and aromas.
- The bioavailability of bioactive compounds in herbs and spices is readily apparent because of their use as medicines. However their properties, bioactivity and possible effects *in vivo* when used in very small amounts required for culinary purposes, and as part of typical recipes, remain to be established.
- Although herbs and spices are eaten in very small amounts on an absolute basis, in many cultures they are essential to traditional recipes, and so are consumed regularly; the cumulative intake may therefore be important. Furthermore, until recently people would have used only those herbs and spices that were

locally grown and available. Today they are much more widely consumed by many more people.

14.12 Chapter 12

- Research on bioactive substances in foods is constantly expanding and developing. The emphasis has been on discovering and classifying their function in plants and their importance for human nutrition. In many cases, knowledge of the effects of storage, processing and cooking is very limited.
- The processing of plant crops has resulted in a wider choice of nutritious, good-quality produce being available all year round in a convenient form for the consumer.
- Retention of bioactive substances depends on their chemical and physical properties, the type of food in which they are found and the storage conditions and the processes used. As a rule, the higher the processing/cooking temperature, the longer is the holding time, and the greater the exposure to oxygen, the more detrimental is the effect on the content of fruit and vegetables.
- Bioactive substances can be classified as water-soluble (flavonoids, vitamin C and folate) or fat-soluble (carotenoids, other terpenoids and sterols). The main method of losing water-soluble substances is by leaching into the cooking medium, whereas fat-soluble substances are lost through oxidative degradation.
- Careful harvesting and keeping fresh plant foods at chilled temperatures and protected from exposure to air during storage minimise the losses of bioactive substances. Blanching the plant products before freezing greatly improves the retention during frozen storage.
- During processing and cooking, the retention of water-soluble substances can be maximised by using the minimum amount of water, starting cooking with boiling water and cooking for a minimum amount of time. Losses are lower with steaming, frying or microwaving than with traditional boiling. In canning, a high proportion of water-soluble components is usually lost.

- Fat-soluble bioactive substances are basically stable during heat treatments, but rearrangements in their structure may occur. Addition of oil during cooking increases the retention and bioavailability of some of these compounds.
- Plant breeding may have an important role in developing plants with modified levels of bioactive compounds, and information about the optimal levels required for plant protection and human health will require further research.

14.13 Chapter 13

- Public health nutrition operates at several levels: collection of information on diet and nutrition status in the population; analysis of data; knowledge and understanding of the principles underlying the relationship of nutrition to health; and the development, implementation and evaluation of interventions to improve nutrition in the community.
- There are systems in place for advising government on the links between nutrition and health, and academic courses for training nutritionists to utilise relevant information. However few authorities recognise a need for appropriately trained nutritionists as part of their approach to improving health in the community.
- There are several sources of information at a national level on diet and nutrition status in the population. Health experience in the community is unequally distributed in society, with those worse off having poorer health, and this inequality is mirrored by lower consumption of plant foods, in particular fruit, and to a lesser extent vegetables. Similar inequalities are found in many other countries within Europe and beyond.
- There are several different approaches that could be taken to influence population eating behaviours. They are not mutually exclusive, and in some situations may be complementary.
- Evaluation of the US 'five-a-day' campaign (which employed a variety of strategies) has found significant increases in fruit consumption but little impact on vegetable consumption, suggesting that different approaches may

be required for the two types of food, and that different barriers to change may exist.
- Policies to improve health often focus on public information ('five-a-day') provision, which tends to widen inequality. The determinants of social variation are likely to be more structural, and structural programmes are needed to address them. Educational programmes in schools to address inequalities from an early age by fostering healthy attitudes and providing children with skills to control their own diets and lifestyles are important components. Educating GPs in particular (but also other health professionals) in nutrition and its health implications is an important step forward.
- National and local government have a responsibility to ensure that all strata of society have access to reliable information, are educated to utilise such information and have access to affordable food of adequate quality and variety to construct a healthy diet for themselves and their families. Current policies and policies in the UK and elsewhere address these issues in an incomplete and piecemeal fashion. Research resources addressing the biological and social questions should be enhanced.
- Looking to the future, enhancing the content of bioactive compounds in plant foods through selective breeding or genetic improvements is a potent dietary option if such substances are proved to be of health benefit. However, the majority of compounds are bitter, acid or astringent and this may restrict the amounts tolerated.
- There are many examples of naturally present plant components being harmful to health, but paradoxically a number of these (*e.g.* glucosinolates, phytoestrogens) are now in the spotlight from a health improvement perspective. It is likely that the amount consumed is of crucial relevance, with different amounts having different effects on important biochemical pathways.
- Many scientific questions remain unanswered, for instance relating to biological markers of diet and of risk of diet-related disease.
- A key message of this Task Force is the need to eat plenty of plant foods, including a variety of

different vegetables and fruit. However, this should be placed in the context of a varied diet, given that the substances of interest are found in every food group (*e.g.* phytoestrogens in pulses and cereals; CLA and sphingolipids in dairy products and meat; and long-chain *n*-3 PUFA, derived from phytoplankton, in fish), and a broad selection of substances in plant foods, ranging from herbs and condiments through fruits and vegetables, to tea and wine. It is not yet possible to tease out particular compounds, or indeed foods, as more important than others. Different compounds have different but equally important effects on cell functions and hence a variety of them needs to be consumed. Hence it is impossible to be precise about which particular foods to target or the amounts required for 'optimum' health.

15
Recommendations of the Task Force

The majority of the individual chapters finish with a set of recommendations for future research. There is, perhaps inevitably, considerable overlap between chapters. To avoid unnecessary repetition, this chapter has been structured to provide an overview of the research recommendations made throughout the report, rather than listing the recommendations from individual chapters. In Section 15.2, some more general recommendations are made, directed at health professionals, industry, the media, funding bodies, and policy makers.

15.1 Priorities for future research

15.1.1 Bioavailability

More information is needed about the bioavailability in humans of bioactive substances in plant foods in order to help establish whether the effects reported *in vitro* are relevant *in vivo*. There is a need to ascertain the levels of bioactive substances in a wide range of fruits, vegetables, other plant foods such as cereals, nuts, pulses and plant oils, and beverages (alcoholic and non-alcoholic), and their intake as well as the extent to which these are absorbed and able to reach target tissues. The available evidence indicates that large differences exist but that certain foods may be especially rich in potentially bioavailable and bioactive substances.

Specific requirements are:

• Studies of the bioavailability of these plant constituents and the factors that influence absorp-

tion, distribution and tissue uptake, and the likely impact of these substances on metabolic processes. For example:

(i) Are they metabolised to any extent in the gastrointestinal tract, and to what extent does this involve the colonic flora? (see Section 15.1.3).

(ii) Do the dietary components and their metabolites provide any benefit during passage through the gastrointestinal tract? Some compounds may have important local effects in the gastrointestinal tract and may not need to be systemically absorbed to be active (see Section 15.1.3).

(iii) To what extent are they absorbed, in what form and where – small intestine or large intestine? (see Section 15.1.3)

(iv) What is the fate of compounds that are absorbed? How long do they survive in the bloodstream? Do they or their metabolites reach specific tissues and are they further metabolised there? Are they deactivated and removed from the bloodstream, *e.g.* by excretion in urine? What is the mechanism of action on specific degenerative processes? Does consumption of any particular product have a demonstrable benefit in the long term?

• Better understanding of the interaction of these substances, both with each other, and with physiological processes (in health and disease): it is important to understand the synergies and interactions of plant bioactive substances from various sources, including spices and herbs.

- Better understanding of the potential for adverse effects.
- Studies to identify which constituents in plant foods contribute to the potential health benefits now being recognised for these foods.
- More information about the range of levels that are found in commercial varieties, the compositional changes in plants as a consequence of modern plant breeding methods and the implications of these for potential health effects, better information about the effects of storage, processing and cooking (both industrial and domestic scale) on the bioactive plant compounds found in commonly eaten foods. Such data should be collected using a large and representative sample of plant-based foods.
- Continued search for other plant-derived compounds of value to human health.

15.1.2 Methodology including biomarkers, mechanistic studies and intervention studies

There is a need to determine which bioactive compounds and which commonly consumed foods contribute to the health effects, so that health messages can be sharpened and alternative strategies developed to meet healthy eating objectives, especially for those consumers who are unable to (or do not choose to) increase their intakes of fruit and vegetables. Assessment of the biological effects of specific plant components is currently confounded by numerous technical barriers. To establish whether the effects reported *in vitro* are relevant *in vivo*, the following priorities exist:

- The basic mechanisms of action of these bioactive substances need to be worked out, along with an understanding of how the activity of these compounds in isolation differs from their activity when delivered in their natural (plant) milieu, and how this activity can be modified by the effects of other plant substances, by food processing and preparation methods, by gut bacteria and by the amount consumed.
- More information is required on the effects of plant constituents, *in vivo* and *in vitro*, at concentrations relevant to their feasible levels of intake from foodstuffs.

- Development and validation of biomarkers of intermediate endpoints, both biological response markers and early disease markers, and emphasis on the relevance of the biomarker to the disease endpoint. In some instances, however, it will be necessary to use morbidity and mortality data where there are uncertainties about the relevance of surrogate biomarkers to the pathogenetic process (*e.g.* oxidation markers).
- Application of these validated biomarkers to soundly constructed prospective studies, trials and parallel mechanistic studies, designed to identify active components in plant foods, their mode of action in maintaining health and well-being and any interactions that occur between them. Identification of these would enable dietary advice to be given with even greater assurance.
- Better methods for characterising both habitual plant food consumption and risk of disease through the use of biomarkers. This will require comprehensive food composition databases for bioactive plant substances in order to assess the range of likely intakes of individual compounds in a diversity of populations.
- Development of practical and feasible tests for the measurement of biological effects, which take account of the need for high-sensitivity measurements of small changes in endpoint.
- Use of novel approaches to develop appropriate and relevant models of cancer pathogenesis and CVD, in which food constituents can be studied over a realistic timespan.
- Development of non-invasive methods for determining the metabolism of compounds *in vivo*.
- Understanding of nutrient–gene interactions and other factors that influence inter-individual variation in response to intake of specific foods and constituents of foods. New genomic and metabolomic technologies need to be embraced.
- Understanding of the risk versus benefit profile of bioactive compounds present in plant foods, in order to identify safe and efficacious levels, and to ensure a balanced scientific view is available for consumers.

- There is a need to establish more clearly the balance between risks and benefits of consuming alcohol-containing beverages.
- Long-chain *n*-3 fatty acids have been shown to carry benefits with regard to cardiovascular disease. There is a need to identify the mechanisms and conditions that give optimum conversion of ALNA to EPA and DHA.
- Controlled dose–response studies of pure isomers of CLA, so that their potential effects (beneficial and adverse) on health-related outcomes can be clearly defined. Studies investigating any synergism or antagonism between active isomers can then be conducted. Other PUFA with various conjugated double bonds also occur in plants and the study of their likely benefit in nutrition and their potential use in functional foods needs to be actively pursued.
- Investigation of the potential role of complex phospholipids, such as sphingolipids (sphingosine-1-phosphate and ceramides) in human health, and investigation of the potential to provide an effective dose of plant sterol esters in the normal diet, by enhancing understanding of the effects of the range of sterols and stanols present in plants.
- Development of effective methods (social, economic and political) for altering the dietary patterns of communities and of groups within them, particularly in relation to social inequalities.
- Better characterisation of the adverse effects seen in some groups following consumption of high doses of micronutrients (*e.g.* β-carotene).

15.1.3 Gastrointestinal influences

There is already evidence that the gut bacteria have the ability to metabolise food residues that escape digestion in the stomach and small intestine. Understanding of the relevance of this for plant bioactive substances is in its infancy.

- Much remains to be discovered about the biochemistry and ecology of the colon, and about the physiological responses of the colon epithelial cells to their environment.

- In view of the current interest in the development of functional food products containing poorly absorbed but readily fermentable substrates, further research is needed to assess the true biological role of butyrate, both as a stimulant to mucosal cell proliferation and as an inducer of potentially beneficial programmed cell death in colorectal epithelial cells.
- The glucosinolates (found in Brassica vegetables such as cabbage, broccoli and Brussels sprouts), and the polyphenols (derived from many other fruits, vegetables and beverages) provide promising evidence of potentially anti-carcinogenic defence mechanisms. At least part of their effect appears to be due to colonic bacterial metabolism, but the significance of inter-individual variation in bacterial flora remains unknown. Studies on the effects of the human gut flora need to be integrated into future research on protective factors derived from plant foods.

15.2 General recommendations

15.2.1. Recommendations to health professionals

Health professionals have a key role in helping their patients and clients make sense of the wealth of new research regarding plant foods and health that is reaching them on a daily basis through newspapers, magazines, television and radio. This report is intended to help update professionals on this complex area of research and in particular to highlight the limitations of current knowledge, the implications of this for the types of health messages that can be derived and the research questions that still need to be addressed.

15.2.2 Recommendations to industry

It is crucial that claims about the health-promoting properties of foods and drinks are evidence-based, consistent with peer-reviewed scientific thinking and communicated in a responsible way to the public. Industry's support of the Joint Health Claims Initiative is an important step forward in this respect. Noting that progress has already been made, industry needs to take a responsible attitude to promoting foods with implied health claims where the evidence is equivocal. Industry sectors should undertake research more actively and demonstrate the potential of their manufactured foods to contribute to healthy eating by studying the effects of processing on constituent levels and bioavailability. The plant breeding sectors should consider the composition of the plants more carefully in the development of new varieties. Research on how to increase the appeal of fruits and especially vegetables is urgently required, as is the need to provide snacks that are appealing to all and are rich in nutritional benefits.

15.2.3 Recommendations to the media

There is a desperate need for more responsible reporting in some sectors. The constant search for a new angle on diet and health results in the public being bombarded by one out-of-context story after another. Too often reports have been given of experimental data that have been derived from studies undertaken in *in vitro* or *in vivo* in animals that have not been shown to be effective human models, or of effects that are only observable at doses that do not reflect those levels of intake that could be considered physiological. Little wonder the public perceives that the scientists keep changing their minds if the experimental limitations of the results are not included in media reports. On the other hand, the results of these studies do need to be translated into simple, although accurate and practical advice for the consumer, and the increasingly responsible attitude of some sectors of the media is welcomed by the Task Force.

15.2.4 Recommendations to research funding bodies

In order to sharpen public health messages about plant foods and health, there is a need for more precise and detailed information about the functions of different plant constituents *in vivo* in humans. Such information may prove to be of considerable health importance given the already well-established association between plant food consumption, in general, and health. It will be very important that such research effort encompasses a broad range of potential mechanisms, *e.g.* effects on the immune system and inflammatory response, effects on markers of endothelial damage, modulation of Phase I and Phase II enzymes and effects on gene expression and cell signalling. Furthermore, more emphasis should be directed to understanding the bioavailability and functions of plant constituents at a tissue and cellular level, and the impact on these of factors such as genotype, age and ill health. More research on the economic effects of agricultural and food policies on price, availability, supply and demand is required. The effects of horticultural grading standards on price and availability should be evaluated as well as the impact of the loss of local markets.

15.2.5 Recommendations to policy makers

Policies across a wide range of government departments and agencies need to be evaluated in terms of their effectiveness in encouraging the greater consumption of plant-derived foods, focusing on dietary variety, and healthy eating messages based on *foods* rather than *components* of foods. These departments include agricultural departments, Food Standards Agencies, health departments and departments of education. Research into effective means of changing behaviour at policy, community and individual levels should be encouraged. Agricultural support policies should encourage production and effective distribution of fruits and vegetables. Education departments need to enhance their activities in promoting healthy eating messages in schools, both in terms of educating children, and in providing them with practical skills in relation to choosing, purchasing and preparing foods. This should be achieved through appropriate Initial Teacher Education, opportunities in the formal school curriculum, and adoption by schools of a whole school approach and food policy.

16
Plant Foods: Answers to Commonly Asked Questions

The purpose of this chapter is to provide a flavour of the report by briefly summarising the findings in simple terms and to cross reference this information to the more detailed text. In addition, a summary of the conclusions of each chapter can be found in Chapter 14. In this report, the term 'plant foods' is used to describe fruits, vegetables, cereals, pulses, nuts, seeds, herbs and spices, and also plants that have been processed in some way to yield foods and drinks whose origin is primarily plant based (*e.g.* oils, hot and cold beverages, and chocolate) (see Table 1.1 in Chapter 1).

1. What is behind the recent interest in substances present in edible plants?

There is now a considerable body of evidence that shows that diets rich in plant foods are generally associated with lower disease risks, in particular cardiovascular disease (coronary heart disease and stroke) and some cancers, but also age-related eye conditions such as cataract and macular degeneration, and chronic lung disorders (Chapter 3). In the search for the specific constituents that confer this benefit, attention has to date largely focused on constituents with antioxidant properties, *e.g.* vitamins E and C and β-carotene. Whilst promising and consistent results have been reported in animal and *in vitro* studies (*e.g.* tissue culture), convincing evidence for a role for substances with antioxidant properties from human intervention and epidemiological studies is sparse and at best equivocal. Attention has therefore turned to the diversity of other constituents of edible plants such as flavonoids,

carotenoids and sulphur-containing compounds. These are described in Chapter 2 and summarised in Question 4.

2. Which nutrients are provided by plant foods?

A wide range of nutrients and other substances can be provided by plant foods, including vitamins with antioxidant properties (*e.g.* vitamins C and E and carotenoids such as β-carotene), folate and other B vitamins, a wide range of minerals including potassium and iron, essential fatty acids and dietary fibre. In addition, there are known to be tens of thousands of other substances, referred to in the report as bioactive compounds, which have been suggested to have beneficial properties with respect to human health. These and their dietary sources are summarised in Table 1.6 of Chapter 1. Chapter 1 also includes information on typical daily intakes of the major nutrients. Intake information for other bioactive compounds can be found in Chapter 6.

3. What are plant bioactive compounds and why are they present in plants?

Foods of plant origin contain many bioactive compounds which are not normally considered 'nutrients', *i.e.* compounds that have not yet been shown to be essential for life, but which may have possible benefits to human health. These plant constituents have been variously called bioactive substances, phytochemicals or phytoprotectants. In this report, the terms bioactive substances and bioactive compounds have been used throughout.

Within the plant, these bioactive substances have various roles in metabolism and in the interaction of the plant with the environment (Chapter 2). Some provide colour to stems, leaves, flowers and fruits, some protect against attack by insects and other predators as feeding deterrents, while others attract insect larvae for reproduction purposes. Some bioactive substances have antifungal and antibacterial activities, providing resistance to infection by mildew and other fungi (see Chapter 2). Furthermore, it is now recognised that a group of compounds known as alkaloids, which are widely dispersed in the plant kingdom, were the active ingredients in numerous potions and poisons used over the centuries and many are still in use today as prescription drugs.

4. How many of these bioactive compounds exist in plants?

Many tens of thousands of these bioactive compounds have been identified in foods that are commonly eaten. Classification is usually based on chemistry and in this report we use three groups: (i) flavonoids and allied phenolic and polyphenolic compounds (about 8000 compounds are known to exist); (ii) terpenoids (*e.g.* carotenoids) (about 25 000 terpenoids have been identified); and (iii) alkaloids (there are about 12 000 alkaloids) and sulphur-containing compounds. These groups are described in detail in Chapter 2.

5. Why might bioactive substances be good for health?

The concept that intakes of vitamins and minerals at levels above those that prevent clinically observable deficiency may protect against chronic disease began to emerge in the 1980s. More recent is the concept that other micro-constituents may also be protective against diseases that remain the major causes of premature death in our society, even in the absence of a known deficiency state. Diets rich in fruit, vegetables and other plant foods are associated with a decreased risk of diseases such as heart disease and cancer. Many plant foods are good sources of a whole range of vitamins and minerals but the presence of these

alone does not seem to explain the health properties of these foods (Chapters 1 and 3). The search is on for the plant constituents that convey these health benefits and also identification of their mechanisms of action. It has been suggested that it is the presence of these bioactive substances that provides the basis for the beneficial effects of plant foods on health. Hopes were initially pinned on substances with antioxidant properties, but it is now recognised that a wide variety of mechanisms is likely to be important (Chapter 4).

6. Which fruits and vegetables are best and how many should we eat?

If the popular press were to be used as a guide, it may well seem that specific fruits and vegetables have been identified as being of particular importance, *e.g.* cherry tomatoes, broccoli, garlic or bananas. However, this type of reporting is misleading. While there is good evidence to support the consumption of diets rich in fruit and vegetables, as yet no particular plant or plant component has emerged as being especially important in terms of health. Nevertheless, considerable progress has been made in identifying the groups of plant foods that provide different classes of bioactive substance. For example, some plant families such as the Brassica species (*e.g.* cabbage, cauliflower, broccoli and Brussels sprouts) and the Allium species (*e.g.* onion, garlic, leeks and chives) contain relatively high levels of specific groups of bioactive substances, namely glucosinolates and other sulphur-containing compounds, respectively (see Chapters 2, 6 and 7). On the other hand, many other substances (*e.g.* flavonoids, see Chapters 2, 6 and 7) are widely dispersed in the plant kingdom.

Considerable research effort has gone into identifying the health effects of these types of substance in animal experiments and *in vitro* studies using human tissues such as blood and human cell lines in tissue culture. But extrapolation of these findings to human health is highly unreliable and studies in people are required to corroborate the findings. So, despite a wealth of fascinating research, it is still not possible to specify particular fruits and vegetables as being especially important. The advice with regard to consumption of fruit and vegetables should therefore focus on variety, to ensure that a wide array of bioactive substances is consumed; the equivalent of at least five 80 g portions or 400 g per day is recommended (see Chapter 13 for information).

7. Apart from fruit and vegetables, which other foods contain bioactive substances?

Cereals, nuts and pulses all contain bioactive substances. It is recommended that the majority of the diet should consist of plant foods, *i.e.* fruit and vegetables and starchy carbohydrate foods, such as bread, rice, pasta, breakfast cereals and potatoes. The *Balance of Good Health*, depicted in Chapter 13, shows the proportions of these foods and of other food groups, which comprise a healthy balanced diet. Around the world, similar food guides have been published. Other plant-derived foods and drinks considered in this report include soya and soya products (Chapter 8), chocolate (derived from cocoa beans) (Chapter 11), alcoholic drinks (Chapter 9), tea (Chapter 9), coffee (Chapter 9), oils and cholesterol-lowering spreads (both in Chapter 10).

8. What action do these bioactive substances have in the body and how might they protect against disease?

It is now recognised that these substances may function via a number of mechanisms (Chapter 4). However, a popular theory concerns bioactive compounds with antioxidant properties. It has been shown by experiments conducted in animals and *in vitro* experiments (conducted using human samples such as blood or cells) that many of these bioactive substances have antioxidant properties. This applies in particular to the flavonoids and carotenoids, for example (described in Chapter 2). Substances with antioxidant properties are important for health as cells in the body contain many potentially oxidisable substrates such as polyunsaturated fatty acids, proteins and DNA. Antioxidant defence systems protect cells from

the potentially injurious effects of free radicals, which are naturally produced within the body as part of the body's defence against bacteria, for example, but are also derived from exposure to cigarette smoke and pollutants. If exposure to free radicals exceeds the protective capacity of the body's antioxidant defence system, then damage to cells may occur, leading to the development of disease (Chapter 4). Free radical damage has been implicated as a factor in a number of diseases including heart disease, cancer, cataracts and stroke (Chapter 3). A number of vitamins and minerals are important for the functioning of the defence systems and there may be additional protection from other bioactive substances. Attention has been focused on the flavonoids (present in *e.g.* tea, red wine, chocolate, onions and apples). It would seem logical that if these substances are to be effective, they have to reach vulnerable tissue sites, which necessitates absorption through the gut wall and transport via the bloodstream. Currently, little is known about the absorption and subsequent transport and metabolism of most bioactive substances once they have been consumed. This information is urgently required in order to establish their significance as promoters of health (Chapters 4, 6, 7 and 9). It is also likely that substances with antioxidant properties are active via other mechanisms, *e.g.* reducing the stickiness of blood platelets, which are involved in blood clotting (Chapter 4).

9. How many of these bioactive substances do we need to eat to prevent disease?

To date there is no easy answer to this question. Evidence for specific protective effects of either individual or groups of bioactive substances within the body is still being gathered, so 'watch this space'. Chapters 7–11 summarise current knowledge regarding the presence of bioactive compounds in dietary components such as fruit, vegetables, pulses, tea, wine and chocolate. In particular, it is not known to what extent specific bioactive substances are absorbed, transported to body tissues, metabolised and active in the body once they are consumed. To date, it has been shown that a number of substances can pass from the gut into the bloodstream and that the anti-oxidant capacity of the blood (or some other measure of their presence) is increased as a result, but the biological implications of this are generally unclear. Therefore, until more information becomes available, the importance of dietary variety should be stressed in relation to plant food consumption. The most compelling evidence is for the consumption of fruit and vegetables to help protect against disease (Chapter 3). The World Health Organisation recommends that people should try to consume at least 400 g of fruit and vegetables per day, which has been translated to at least five 80 g portions (see Chapter 13).

10. How bioavailable are these substances?

The term 'bioavailability' refers to the extent to which any dietary component is absorbed into the blood stream and then subsequently becomes available for use by body tissues (see Chapter 6). Studies to date have provided evidence that a range of bioactive substances can be absorbed, as they have been shown to be present in the blood after inclusion in the diet, but, with few exceptions, little is known about the extent to which they are subsequently utilised by various tissues in the body. This aspect is currently being investigated by researchers around the world and their findings will have important implications for dietary recommendations and health promotion messages.

It is of interest that plant sterols are very poorly absorbed and it is this property that has caused them to gain prominence as ingredients within products designed to help reduce blood cholesterol levels. The mechanism of action is suppression of cholesterol absorption. Cholesterol is present in the gut via the diet and also as a result of secretion of cholesterol via the bile; the absorption of dietary cholesterol and the reabsorption of the bile-secreted cholesterol are both suppressed by the presence of plant sterols (and stanols) in the diet (see Chapter 10).

11. Why are the bacteria in our gut important for health?

The large intestine provides an ideal environment for a diversity of bacteria which feed on undigested plant components to produce substances, which may for example subsequently promote the health of the colon and protect against infection (see Chapter 5). The lactic acid bacteria in particular are thought to be beneficial for health and more evidence for the positive effects of these bacteria is accumulating, although their importance in terms of disease prevention remains to be established.

Most absorption of dietary components takes place in the small intestine, but it is now recognised that further absorption of dietary components can take place in the large intestine (colon), courtesy of the resident bacteria. The colon contains 10^{12} bacteria/cm^3 which produce enzymes capable of stripping some dietary components of their attached sugars, enabling further absorption of these smaller molecules to take place The bacteria are also able to break down the complex molecules that make up dietary fibre, that would not otherwise be digested, to simple compounds such as the short-chain fatty acid butyrate, recognised as important in maintaining the health of the cells lining the colon, and another known as propionate that has been shown to be involved in reducing blood cholesterol levels (see Chapter 5). The fate of the diversity of derivatives formed by these processes, and their health potential is a topic attracting considerable research interest.

12. How does the evidence for the protective effects of these substances compare to the negative effects of excessive intakes of other components of the diet, such as saturates and salt?

There is strong evidence that decreasing the contribution of saturates to dietary energy is followed by a fall in the concentration of blood cholesterol (LDL cholesterol in particular) and in the risk of heart disease. Therefore, it is recommended that the average contribution of saturates to dietary energy is reduced to 11% of dietary energy intake. This evidence comes from numerous animal, *in vitro*, *in vivo* and human epidemiological and intervention studies. There is also increasing evidence for causal relationships between the consumption of sodium, a principal component of salt, and both the level of blood pressure and the rise in blood pressure with age. A number of other factors, *e.g.* body weight and alcohol intake, also influence blood pressure. Therefore, it is recommended that the average intake of salt in the adult population is reduced from the current level of 9 g per day to 6 g per day.

The evidence that eating diets containing plenty of fruit and vegetables is associated with a reduced risk of disease has also been supported by many epidemiological studies, and this has led to the recommendation of eating at least 400 g (five 80 g portions) of fruit and vegetables every day. However, the association remains of moderate strength. Evidence for possible mechanisms for the effect comes from animal and *in vitro* studies, but there is little direct evidence available from human studies. Therefore, despite considerable research effort, specific constituents responsible for this association have yet to be identified.

A study known as the DASH study, which set out to identify dietary patterns that had a beneficial effect on blood pressure, demonstrated the most effective approach was a diet rich in fruit and vegetables, modest in its salt content and including low fat dairy products (Appel *et al.*, 1997; Sacks *et al.*, 2001).

13. What is the average intake of bioactive substances in the UK?

Until recently, reliable information has been scarce, but databases are now being developed world-wide which allow estimation of UK intakes. In the USA, a database on the polyphenol composition of foods consumed in North America has been established and a database for carotenoids is now available, together with information about current intakes of the major carotenoids across Europe (Chapter 6). Also available are databases listing sources of isoflavones, in both the USA and Europe.

Average UK intakes of flavonoids have been estimated for the six food groups most likely to contain significant levels, *i.e.* various categories of vegetables, fruit and fruit products and beverages (including samples of red and white wine). Estimated total intake of flavonoids was 30 mg/day, with the flavonol quercetin contributing 64% of the total. Beverages contributed 82% of the total intake of these flavonoids; this was mainly attributed to tea, as wine provided very little of the particular flavonoids studied.

The five most commonly occurring carotenoids in blood are β-carotene, lycopene, lutein, β-cryptoxanthin and α-carotene. A new EU-funded survey indicates that the main sources of these, in the UK, are carrots, tomatoes/tomato products, peas, citrus fruit, and carrots, respectively. Median intake of total carotenoids in the UK is 14.38 mg/day in adults, with the largest contributions coming from β-carotene (5.55 mg/day) and lycopene (5.01 mg/day).

Typical intakes of dietary sterols (Chapter 10) are 140–400 mg/day and might be as high as 1000 mg/day in those with a high intake of vegetable oils.

14. How does this compare to intakes in other countries?

It is to be expected that the relationships between the predominant flavonoids and their sources will vary between populations, and that there will be wide inter- and intra-individual variations in intakes of individual compounds, because of the substantial differences that occur in dietary patterns around the world. For example, in the Netherlands, the average daily intake of three flavonols (quercetin, kaempferol and isorhamnetin) and two flavones (luteolin and apiginin) has been estimated at 25.9 mg, the major sources being tea (61%), onions (13%) and apples (10%). The average intake of a particular flavonoid, quercetin, was 16 mg/day, provided mostly in tea (48%), onions (29%) and apples (7%). In a US study, the contribution from tea was proportionately less, but the overall intake similar to that of the Dutch at about 20 mg/day. A small study in Welsh middle-aged men found an average intake of 26 mg/day (Chapter 6). Analysis of data from a study looking at the diets consumed in Japan, the Netherlands, the former Yugoslavia, the USA, Finland, Italy and Greece in the early 1960s found that red wine was the main source of quercetin for the Italians, tea the dominant source in Japan and the Netherlands, and onions in Greece, the former Yugoslavia and the USA. Flavonol intake was highest in Japan (64 mg/day) and lowest in Finland (6 mg/day) (Chapter 6). It should be noted that for the Dutch data, because a limited range of dietary flavonoids was measured, and because the calculation was based on aglycones rather than conjugates, the figure of 25.9 mg/day is likely to be an *underestimate* of total flavonoid intake. At the other end of the scale, a flavonoid intake of over 1000 mg/day in the USA has been suggested. This figure is based on all phenols being glycosides (*i.e.* conjugates) and is likely to be an *overestimate* of flavonoid consumption.

Intakes of phytoestrogens are highest in China and Japan, especially in those consuming their traditional diet, which is rich in soya. However, the rapidly changing eating habits in Japan and China now make it difficult to generalise accurately about the intake of isoflavones in these countries. Recent estimates indicate intakes of 20–50 mg/day, but this may vary between urban and rural areas and with other lifestyle factors. In Western populations, the average daily dietary intake of phytoestrogens is typically negligible (<1 mg/day) (see Chapters 6 and 8 and Question 22).

15. How do transport, storage conditions, preparation and cooking methods affect the content of these substances in foods?

Knowledge of the effects of storage, processing and cooking on the levels of bioactive substances in a food is limited but depends on their chemical and physical properties, the type of food in which they are found and how the food is processed. As a general rule, the higher the processing or cooking temperature, the longer the food is stored and the greater the exposure of the food to oxygen, the more the level of the substances will decrease.

Therefore, it is best to keep plant foods at chilled temperatures, in air-tight containers during storage. When freezing plant foods, they should first be blanched to reduce the loss of bioactive substances. During processing and cooking, the loss of bioactive substances can be reduced by using the minimum amount of water, *e.g.* steaming instead of boiling. Adding oil when cooking at high temperatures can also reduce their loss. A high proportion of some of the bioactive substances will be lost in canning. However, it is a mistake to think that canned, frozen or cooked vegetables are less healthy than fresh or raw vegetables. In many cases processing can have a positive effect; freezing can preserve the amount of a bioactive substance and some bioactive substances can be released and made more bioavailable by cooking. For example, boiling carrots helps break down the tough plant cell wall and releases the carotenoids, making them more easily absorbed by the body (see Chapter 12).

16. Does the content of these substances vary between varieties of the same food?

Considerable variations have been reported because the amount of bioactive substances present in individual fruits and vegetables is affected by variety, soil, climatic conditions, agricultural methods and degree of ripeness (Chapter 7). These substances are often concentrated under the skin in fruits or in the outer leaves in vegetables and so measurements will also be influenced by the part of the plant tested. Furthermore, some substances are found in higher concentrations in plants that have been attacked by insects or disease, as their role is to defend the plant in such circumstances (Chapter 2). Therefore, no single measurement can be taken as representative of a particular food.

17. Are plants being bred to contain higher levels of these substances?

There is currently considerable interest in the potential to enhance the bioavailability of various bioactive substances in plants, via conventional breeding techniques as well as by genetic modification technology. Studies are needed to evaluate whether modification of the amount of a bio-active substance present in a plant will affect other attributes such as yield, post-harvest stability and storage, taste or processing qualities. It will also be important to know whether enhancement of one bioactive substance reduces the bioavail-ability of another, perhaps more critical, substance. It should also be recognised that many such substances, because of their function in plants (see Question 3), are bitter or astringent, and increasing the level may make the food unpalatable, and consequently some plant breeding has aimed to reduce the levels (see Chapter 13).

18. Which drinks contain high levels of bioactive substances?

Tea is a rich source of polyphenolic compounds and in many biological systems (*e.g.* animal models and cell culture) extracts of tea have been demon-strated to have a wide range of effects with poten-tial health benefits (Chapter 9). For example in such systems they have been shown to inhibit oxi-dation of low-density lipoproteins (Chapter 4), prevent mutations and to be anti-carcinogens. Much of this activity has been ascribed to the polyphenolic compounds of tea, in particular the catechin derivatives (Chapter 2). More studies are required to establish the bioavailability of these compounds and their effects *in vivo* before any health benefits can be established with certainty. The impact of these compounds when consumed as part of a normal diet and in amounts normally consumed by humans is not yet clear.

Coffee also contains a number of phenolic compounds, including chlorogenic acid and caf-feic acid, which have been shown to have anti-cancer properties in animal studies. However, until recently, most studies on the health effects of coffee have been focused on the diverse actions of caffeine on cellular metabolism. There is little evidence that coffee exacerbates or decreases risk of heart disease or cancer. Cocoa is also a rich source of phenolic compounds (similar to those found in tea) in addition to being a rich source of minerals. However, it is much less widely consumed as a drink than either tea or

coffee and therefore its nutritional benefit is likely to be small. See Chapter 9 for more details.

Red wine (and other forms of alcoholic drink) is often quoted as being good for the heart and there is in fact substantial evidence that low to moderate intakes of alcohol may reduce the risk of heart disease, particularly in middle-aged and older people (Chapters 1 and 9). Although such effects have generally been attributed to the alco-hol *per se*, additional benefits may be linked to the presence of bioactive substances. Red wine con-tains many polyphenols (found in the skin of grapes, giving them their red colour), which are known to be absorbed through the gut. These polyphenols display both antioxidant and anti-cancer properties *in vitro*. Like red wine, both beer and Scotch whisky also contain many pheno-lic compounds (the phenolic compounds in the whisky are extracted from the wooden casks in which they are matured). As with red wine, when either beer or whisky is consumed, antioxidant activity in the blood rises for a short time. In cell culture tests, the phenolics in beer have been shown to inhibit the oxidation of low-density lipoproteins and to prevent DNA damage. Also, modest consumption of beer has been shown to be associated with a reduced risk of heart disease. It is important to note that any benefits arising from the consumption of alcoholic beverages must be considered within the context of the well-known adverse health effects of excessive alcohol consumption.

19. Should people who avoid alcoholic drinks be encouraged to consume small amounts?

Given the well established adverse effects of alco-hol on health (particularly with regard to certain forms of cancer), it is not appropriate to encour-age people who choose to avoid alcohol to start to take alcoholic beverages for their health. On the other hand, 1–2 units of alcohol per day are associated with modest heart health benefits compared with abstaining, particularly in people beyond middle age. The evidence suggests that much of the benefit seems to be due to the alcohol itself (Chapter 3). However, bioactive substances present in these beverages may have an additional effect, and people who choose not to drink alcohol can obtain good intakes of a variety of bioactive substances from many other sources, including beverages such as tea, coffee and fruit juices, and by consuming plant-derived foods in their daily diets.

20. Is there any difference to health between drinking tea or coffee?

The simple answer is that we don't yet know. Both tea and coffee have been found to contain bioactive substances, which have been suggested to confer health benefits (see Question 18). However, the substances present are very different and might be expected to operate through different mechanisms and so perhaps affect different systems of the body. In tea, the major class of substances present is flavan-3-ols (*e.g.* catechins) and in coffee the main substances are phenolics such as chlorogenic acid and caffeic acid. These compounds contribute to the antioxidant capacity of these beverages and in some *in vitro* systems the antioxidant capacity is similar. Both beverages provide substantial amounts of caffeine (Chapter 9) and tea also contains a related compound, theobromine, the amounts present being dependent in part on the strength of the beverage.

There is some, but inconclusive, evidence for a benefit to heart health from tea drinking, and while there have been some studies associating adverse effects to coffee drinking, these are likely to be due to confounding by associated smoking. There is good evidence that boiled coffee contains a fraction that increases blood cholesterol, although no sound link with heart disease has been established.

21. Why is the Mediterranean diet considered a healthy diet?

Features of traditional Mediterranean diets include an abundance of fruit and vegetables, regular intakes of fish, modest meat consumption, moderate wine drinking, a physically active lifestyle and reliance on olive oil as a fat source. Each of these food categories has been shown to contribute a range of nutrients and other bioactive substances. Furthermore, heart disease rates are lower in southern European (Mediterranean) countries than in northern Europe. However, the pattern of nutrients and bioactive substances provided by such diets can be simulated by other diets rich in plant foods – a Mediterranean diet is just one option for eating healthily.

22. Are vegetarians healthier than people who consume meat?

Vegetarian diets are often thought of by the media and the general public as being more healthy. However, often it is not the diet that is more healthy, it is the people; those who follow vegetarian diets are often more healthy than those who do not, simply because they pay more attention to other heath issues; they tend to be non-smokers, drink alcohol only in moderation (or not at all) and have active lifestyles. The diet itself may be no more or no less healthy than a diet that includes meat, and with so many different interpretations of a vegetarian diet (ranging from just avoiding red meat through to a strict vegan diet where all foods of animal origin are excluded), it is difficult to make comparisons (see Chapter 3).

In an omnivorous diet, animal foods normally provide substantial amounts of food energy, protein, calcium, iron, zinc and vitamins A, D and B_{12}. A well-planned and varied vegetarian diet can provide sufficient energy and adequate amounts of these nutrients, but problems arise if those foods excluded are not replaced by suitable alternatives to supply these nutrients. Meat is a good source of protein, iron, zinc and B vitamins, and the iron and zinc in meat are in a form that is very easily absorbed by the body. Lack of iron in the diet or poor absorption of iron can eventually lead to iron deficiency anaemia, which is one of the commonest causes of chronic ill health in young women in the UK. However, if red meat is avoided it can be replaced with other sources of protein (*e.g.* milk, nuts, eggs, cereals, pulses *e.g.* soya) and iron (*e.g.* pulses, nuts, dark green vegetables and fortified cereal foods). Including a source of vitamin C (*e.g.* citrus fruit or orange juice) can help to absorb the iron from these non-meat sources.

On the other hand, vegetarian diets, and in particular vegan diets, tend to be higher in fibre and lower in fat, in addition to being higher in fruit and vegetables, and so are more likely to include the recommended minimum of five portions per day. Therefore, meat eaters should be encouraged to eat more fruit and vegetables and less fat (*e.g.* by choosing lean cuts of meat).

Nutrition advice should promote a well-balanced diet that provides a variety of foods, including plenty of fruit and vegetables. For those who eat meat and processed meat, the advice is to choose lean cuts of meat and remove visible fat. Average total intakes of no more than 90 g per day of red meat and processed meat have been recommended by the government's advisory committee, COMA, and those regularly consuming a higher intake should consider a reduction.

23. What are the effects on health of eating soya?

Soya is a rich source of particular substances, which are structurally similar to mammalian oestradiol and known as phytoestrogens. These include the isoflavones daidzein and genistein, which have been shown to act as weak oestrogens (Chapters 2 and 8). Phytoestrogens have both oestrogenic and anti-oestrogenic effects in that they compete with oestradiol to bind with the oestrogen receptors. However, on binding they fail to stimulate a full oestrogenic response. Through their ability to bind to oestrogen receptors, it has been suggested that phytoestrogens may be beneficial in post-menopausal women in relation to menopausal symptoms and risk factors for heart disease and osteoporosis. A role in breast cancer has also been suggested. Isoflavone supplements seem to be relatively ineffective in managing hot flushes, whereas isoflavone-rich foods appear to have a beneficial effect that exceeds that of a placebo, although the impact is much less than seen with HRT. Soya foods in which the natural isoflavones have been retained have been shown to reduce plasma cholesterol levels modestly when soya protein is consumed at levels of at least 25 g/day. The data with regard to bone health are still unclear, and the risks versus benefits of phytoestrogens in relation to breast cancer is unresolved.

Isoflavones also have other properties not related to their ability to mimic oestrogen, which are common to other plant polyphenols, *e.g.* flavonoids.

A key issue is whether consumption needs to be lifelong (as in Japan, where soya consumption is high in those following a traditional diet) to carry real benefit. Epidemiological evidence shows that people living in China and Japan, who have higher phytoestrogen intakes as the traditional diet contains substantial amounts of soya products, also have a low incidence of a number of cancers, heart disease and menopausal symptoms. There is no evidence that these are directly linked to diet, but should diet prove to be influential, it will be important to establish whether it is lifelong intake or intake at particular life stages that matters.

The risks and benefits of long-term phytoestrogen consumption by infants and young children from soya infant formula is a controversial issue. Currently, breast milk or cows' milk formula are recommended for infant feeding, unless there is a clear indication that soya-based formula is required on medical grounds. This matter has recently been considered by the UK Government's Committee on Toxicity of Chemicals in Foods, Consumer Products and the Environment (COT).

There are a number of different soya products available including textured vegetable protein, tofu, tempeh and soya drinks, all of which can make a useful contribution to nutrient intake. If soya products are used to replace animal sources of protein, such as meat or milk, it is important to ensure that adequate amounts of the nutrients that these animal-derived foods contain (particularly iron, calcium, zinc and vitamin B_{12}) are provided by other foods and drinks. A recent Briefing Paper from the British Nutrition Foundation provides an update on soya and health (British Nutrition Foundation, 2002c).

24. Which fats and oils should be included in the diet?

Although fat is a major source of dietary energy and a carrier of fat-soluble vitamins, the only specific requirement for fat in the diet is that for the essential fatty acids linoleic acid (an *n*-6 polyunsaturate) and α-linolenic acid (an *n*-3 polyunsaturate). Furthermore, many people eat too much fat and on balance the British diet is too rich in saturates and an adjustment needs to be made in favour of unsaturated fatty acids, namely monounsaturates and polyunsaturates.

The essential fatty acids cannot be made in the body and so have to be provided by diet. Linoleic acid is found in greatest natural abundance in vegetable and seed oils (*e.g.* sunflower, soya and corn oils, and the spreads commercially derived from them). These are also the richest sources of α-linolenic acid, which is also found in nuts (*e.g.* walnuts, brazil nuts, almonds and peanuts) and seeds (*e.g.* sunflower, sesame and poppy) and meat. A number of other polyunsaturates that occur in plant and fish oils are also thought to be particularly beneficial to health, although these can be made, at least to a limited extent, by the body. They include arachidonic acid, docosahexaenoic acid (DHA) and eicosapentanoic acid (EPA). DHA and EPA belong to the *n*-3 family and are principally obtained ready-made from oily fish. Arachidonic acid belongs to the *n*-6 family and is obtained mainly from vegetable oils and products made from them. Both EPA and arachidonic acid are the substances from which important molecules known as eicosanoids are formed, these being local mediators, *e.g.* in inflammation and immune responses. As a rule of thumb, eicosanoids formed from EPA tend to have less potent effects than those derived from arachidonic acid. In this context, concern has been expressed in recent years about the balance between *n*-3 (or ω-3) and *n*-6 (or ω-6) fatty acids in the diet. It has been suggested that a shift towards *n*-3 fatty acids might favour health, particularly cardiovascular health. For more details, see Chapter 10.

In food terms, this means selecting oils such as rapeseed oil or olive oil, which are rich in monounsaturates, whilst continuing to also include moderate amounts of the *n*-6 fatty acids. It is worth noting that these days most oils labelled as 'vegetable oil' are often based on rapeseed oil. Rapeseed oil has the additional advantage of also being rich in the essential *n*-3 fatty acid α-linolenic acid. Spreads and other products made from fats derived from these oils can be useful additions to a healthy balanced diet and help reduce saturates intake, provided overall fat intake is moderated. Eating oil-rich fish such as mackerel, sardines or salmon once a week can boost long chain *n*-3 fatty acid intake. Specific advice on oily fish consumption exists for pregnant women and for children (www.food.gov.uk).

25. What is the difference between ordinary olive oil and extra virgin olive oil?

The oil obtained from olives by pressing, without further treatment, is called extra virgin olive oil. Compared with other forms of olive oil, produced from the residual pulp after the first pressing, it contains a wide range of bioactive substances including terpenic and phenolic acids that have antioxidant properties. The main fatty acid is oleic acid, a monounsaturated fatty acid, which is mostly present attached to glycerol molecules in the form of triglycerides (triacylglycerols). Extra virgin olive oil contains no more than 1 g of free oleic acid per 100 g. Virgin olive oil (made from a subsequent pressing) is said to retain a perfect flavour if the free oleic acid content does not exceed 1.5 g per 100 g. Ordinary (refined) olive oil may contain up to 3.0 g per 100 g and has a slight off-flavour. Refined olive oil is obtained from the residual pulp. It tends to have a more intense colour and a weaker aroma. Phenolic acids present in virgin olive oil are almost completely destroyed during the refining process because they are polar compounds and removed by water.

Although it has been suggested that the antioxidant properties of the phenolic compounds present in virgin olive oil may contribute to the health effects associated with the Mediterranean diet, supportive evidence is not yet available (Chapter 10).

26. What is CLA and what does it do?

Conjugated linolenic acid, CLA, is a collective term for a mixture of substances related to the essential fatty acid linoleic acid. They are found only in the meat of ruminant animals, *e.g.* beef and lamb, and in cows' milk and its products, *e.g.* cheese. The effects of CLA and other conjugated fatty acids derived from linoleic and α-linolenic acids appear similar to those observed for *n*-3 fatty acids. Data from animal studies suggesting anti-cancer effects, ability to reduce body fat and to improve lipid profiles have led to a flurry of interest in CLA. With the exception of body fat reduction, the results of human studies to date have been inconsistent, although this may in part be explained by the use of different isomers of CLA in the various studies (Chapter 10).

27. How do plant sterol and stanol esters work?

Plant sterols are found naturally in a variety of plant foods, and plant stanols are the saturated (hydrogenated) derivatives (Chapter 10). Sterol and stanol esters are now added to several spreads and to a range of other products. In this form, they have been shown to reduce serum cholesterol levels significantly by inhibiting cholesterol uptake in the gut and by facilitating its elimination. Typical reductions of 10–15% in total cholesterol and 20% for LDL cholesterol have been achieved with intakes of plant sterols/stanols around 2 g per day, with the best effect being seen in those with the highest cholesterol levels.

28. Chocolate contains bioactive substances, but what about its fat content?

It is correct that there is a growing body of evidence that the cocoa bean, and chocolate made from it, contain a number of bioactive substances, similar to those in tea, which have been shown in *in vitro* studies to have potential health effects (Chapter 11). This work now needs to be corroborated in human studies. Chocolate is derived from cocoa butter, which contains the fatty acids stearic and oleic acids, with a smaller contribution from palmitic acid and traces of several other fatty acids. Stearic acid is regarded as a neutral fatty acid in respect to its effect on blood cholesterol levels, which neither increase nor decrease. Stearic acid has also been shown to be less throm-

bogenic (reduces the risk of blood clot formation) than other saturates. Oleic acid is also beneficial in terms of blood cholesterol levels, although the saturated fatty acid palmitic acid tends to raise cholesterol levels (Chapter 10).

29. Can eating too many of these bioactive substances be harmful to health?

The best known example of adverse effects of high levels of dietary supplements concerns the carotenoid (a terpenoid) β-carotene, where a detrimental effect on lung cancer incidence was evident in high-risk subjects, namely heavy smokers and former asbestos workers (see Chapter 1). It is worth noting that the dose given was substantially higher than would be achieved by diet. Apart from this, few studies have been done. However, it has long been known that just because a substance is 'natural' does not signify that it is safe (Chapter 13). Indeed, many of the active ingredients in poisons are plant-derived substances such as alkaloids (Chapters 2 and 13).

30. Can taking nutritional supplements or herbal remedies be as beneficial as eating fruit and vegetables?

The results of the intervention trials reported so far do not support the notion that either vitamin supplements or fortified foods provide an equivalent alternative to increasing the consumption of fruit and vegetables. This is likely to be because it is the cocktail effect of the many substances present in whole foods that confer the health properties that have been evident for decades for diets rich in fruits and vegetables, or that the substances tested are not those responsible.

31. What action is being taken to increase fruit and vegetable intake?

Whilst research continues to identify the active ingredients in plant foods, it remains important for health professionals to emphasise the need to eat more of these foods, in particular to achieve the target of at least five 80 g servings of a variety of fruits and vegetables daily. Current intakes are on average between two and three servings, depending on the population group considered. Government-funded campaigns are under way such as the School Fruit Scheme for 5–7 year olds in England and the five-a-day campaign launched in 2003 (Chapter 13). Similar activities are taking place in other parts of the UK. Evidence from the UK and the USA indicates that persuading people to eat more fruit is often easier than persuading them to increase vegetable intake (Chapter 13), and this is supported by data for trends in consumption over recent decades (Chapter 1). It may be necessary to employ different types of strategy to improve levels of vegetable intake, given that these foods provide a different selection of nutrients and bioactive substances than fruit. Also, particular attention needs to be paid to identifying strategies that are relevant and practical for low income groups, among whom intakes of these foods are typically lower (Chapter 1). Educational programmes in schools to address inequalities from an early age by fostering healthy attitudes and providing children with skills to control their own diets and lifestyles are important components.

32. In a nutshell, what is the take-home message from this report?

Eat plenty of plant foods, including a variety of different vegetables and fruits. Having recognised the benefit of diets rich in fruit, vegetables and other plant foods, the hunt has been on for the active ingredient(s) that convey these properties. Despite a vast amount of research, the answer still eludes scientists, although knowledge has already expanded in terms of the sources and function *in vitro* of the many compounds found naturally in plants. A substantial body of evidence now exists to support the claim that various bioactive substances can pass through the gut wall into the bloodstream. The challenge for the future is to establish that this process is associated with biological effects within humans and is able to convey health benefits. To date, most of the evidence collated in this respect has been derived from animal studies or *in vitro* experiments, and needs to be corroborated in humans in an experimental design that takes account of typical dietary patterns and realistic consumption levels of the bioactive substances of interest.

33. What are the research priorities for these bioactive substances and the foods that contain them?

Research into the possible health benefits of bioactive substances continues to have considerable potential but there remain many challenges, not least of which is the need to substantiate in humans the findings from other biological systems. Future research (Chapter 15) should be focused on establishing the bioavailability of these substances including the factors that affect absorption, distribution and their metabolism within the body. Research should also be focused on how these different substances affect disease processes: the roles of individual substances and also combinations of them need to be established with respect to beneficial effects on health. There is also a need to identify and understand possible adverse effects following high consumption of some of these substances. Finally, effective methods should be developed for altering the dietary patterns of people who would benefit from eating more fruit, vegetables and other plant foods, particularly among those groups where social inequalities exist and intakes are low (see Chapter 1).

Appendix
Projects on Plant-derived Substances Funded by the European Commission's Fourth and Fifth Framework Programmes

The following is a list of research projects on plant bioactive compounds in plant foods and drinks which have been funded by the European Commission's 4th and 5th Framework research programmes.

Information about these projects may be obtained from the project website, or by searching the FLAIR-FLOW Europe IV website www.flair-flow.com or the Cordis website www.cordis.lu.

Framework Programme 4 Projects

Understanding the biological effects of dietary complex phenols and tannins and their implications for the consumer's health and well being
Project number: FAIR-CT95-0653
Website: www.surrey.ac.uk/SBS/nutrition/nutritionhome.htm

Phenolic phytoprotectants – role in preventing initiation, promotion and progression of cancer
Project number: FAIR-CT95-0894
No website

Tomatoes and lycopene (TOMATE)
Project number: FAIR-CT97-3233
Website: www.tomate.org

Vegetal oestrogens in nutrition and skeleton (VENUS)
Projects number: FAIR-PL98-4456
Website: www.venus-ca.org

Model systems, *in vitro* and *in vivo*, for predicting the bioavailability of lipid soluble components of food (MODEM)

Project number: FAIR-CT97-3100
No website

Effects of food-borne glucosinolates on human heath (EFGLU)
Project number: FAIR-CT97-3029
www.ifrn.bbsrc.ac.uk/Diet/GItract_EFGLU.html

Natural antioxidants from olive oil processing waste water (WWANTOX)
Project number: FAIR-CT97-3039
Website: www.unimi.it/

Wine and cardiovascular disease (WCVD)
Project number: FAIR-97-3261
No website

Framework Programme 5 Projects

Garlic and health (G&H)
Project number: QLK1-1999-000498
Website: www.plant.wageningen-ur.nl/projects/GarlicandHealth/

Functional properties, bioactivities and bioavailability of phytochemicals, especially anthocyanins, from processed foods (ANTHCYANIN BIOACTIV)
Project number: QLK1-1999-00124
www.honeybee.helsinki.fi/mmkem/ek/tutkimus/antho.html

The role of dietary phytoestrogens in the prevention of breast and prostate cancer (PHYTOPREVENT)

Project number: QLK1-2000-00266
Website: www.phytoprevent.org

European research in functional effects of dietary antioxidants (EUROFEDA)
Project number: QLK1-1999-00179
Website: www.ifr.bbsrc.ac.uk/eurofeda

Health implications of natural non-nutrient antioxidants (polyphenols): bioavailability and colon carcinogenesis (POLYBIND)

Project number: QLK1-1999-00505
Website: www.ifrn.bbsrc.ac.uk/Polybind/polybind.html

Food Safety in Europe: risk assessment of chemicals in food (FOSIE)
Project number: QLK1-1999-00156
www.ilsi.org/misc/fosie/Project/project.htm

Glossary

Accuracy   Refers to whether or not a measurement is correct. A correct measure should be both accurate and precise.

Acute   Refers to a condition of short duration that starts quickly and has severe symptoms (*cf.* Chronic). Acute conditions can either resolve, or progress to become chronic.

Atherosclerosis   The process by which fatty and fibrous deposits cause narrowing and hardening of the arteries.

Blinding   In the context of clinical trials, whenever participants (single blind trial) or both participants and researchers (double blind trial) are kept unaware of 'treatments' given or received.

Cancer   A wide variety of diseases characterised by uncontrolled growth of tissue.

Carcinogen   A compound that is capable of inducing cancer, commonly by interaction with DNA.

Cardiovascular disease (CVD)   A disease of the heart or circulation. This broad term encompasses coronary heart disease, peripheral vascular disease and stroke.

Chronic   Refers to a persistent or recurring condition. The disease may or may not be severe, often starts gradually, and changes are slow (*cf.* Acute).

Clinical significance   This refers to the magnitude of an effect, expressed in terms such as relative risk (see Chapter 3). Unlike statistical significance it is not dependent on sample size, but requires a clinical or public health judgement on what is a large effect. A statistically significant result may nonetheless be too small

to warrant any changes in treatment or other policies, *i.e.* it is not clinically significant.

Confidence intervals   (See Precision).

Conjugated   Joined to.

Coronary heart disease (CHD)   Disease that results from the build-up of fatty deposits on the lining of the coronary arteries. It may cause angina, a heart attack or sudden death.

Disease   Any abnormality of bodily structure or function, other than those arising directly from physical injury. A disease can be acute or chronic, communicable or non-communicable.

Enzymes   Proteins that speed up (catalyse) a metabolic reaction in vivo or *in vitro*.

Epidemiology   The study of the distribution of health and illness within human populations.

Esters   Compounds formed by the reaction between an acid and an alcohol. For example, fats and oils are esters of glycerol (an alcohol) and long-chain fatty acids.

Glycoproteins   Proteins conjugated with carbohydrate groups.

Glycosides   Compounds made up of a molecule to which is attached a sugar molecule. Glycoside linkages can be hydrolysed, and the compound split to yield the separate components. The non-sugar component is the aglycone (see Chapters 2 and 6).

Hydrolyse   To split a complex compound into its constituent parts by the action of water, either chemically, or catalysed by the addition of acid or alkali.

In vitro   *In vitro* means 'in glass', and is used to indicate observations made experimentally in a 'test-tube' as distinct from living conditions (*in* *vivo*). *In vitro* studies may also use tissues derived from plants or animals, including humans (sometimes referred to as *ex vivo* studies) and micro-organisms.

In vivo *In vivo* experimental studies are carried out in whole living animals, including humans.

Incidence This is a measure of the number of new cases of a disease occurring during a specified period of time (*cf.* Prevalence).

Isomers Molecules that contain the same atoms, but differently arranged, so that their chemical and biological properties differ. Different isomers are often depicted by prefixes such as α, β, $(+)$, $(-)$, P, O.

Meta-analysis A statistical analysis that combines the results of individual studies used in a systematic review, producing a quantitative summary across the different studies. This technique is commonly used for randomised controlled trials, or therapies or interventions.

Morbidity The condition of being diseased.

Mutagen A compound that can modify DNA. Many mutagens are also carcinogens.

Non-communicable disease Unlike a communicable disease, an NCD is not infectious, *i.e.* it cannot be transmitted from one person to another. NCDs of particular relevance to this report include cardiovascular disease and cancer.

Phase I metabolism The first phase of metabolism of 'foreign' compounds. Generally regarded as detoxification reactions, but they may also convert inactive precursors into metabolically active compounds, and be involved in the activation of precursors to carcinogens (see Chapters 4 and 6).

Phase II metabolism The second phase of the metabolism of foreign compounds in which the activated derivatives from in Phase I metabolism are conjugated with amino acids to yield water-soluble derivatives that can be excreted in bile or urine (see Chapters 4 and 6).

Precision In the context of estimation, this term refers to the magnitude of standard errors. This is reflected in the width of the confidence intervals (CIs) constructed around the same estimates. Wide CIs reflect a lot of uncertainty about the value and arise from small sample sizes and/or large variability. A measurement can be precise, but not accurate.

Prevalence This is a measure the total number of existing cases of a disease or condition at a particular point in time or during some specified time period. Prevalence is usually expressed as a percentage of the total population, or per 1000, 10 000 or 100 000 people (*cf.* Incidence).

Primary prevention Primary prevention strategies aim to prevent the occurrence of a disease, *i.e.* reducing the incidence of a disease in the population. Examples relevant to this report include encouraging the consumption of fruits and vegetables to reduce the risk of heart disease and cancer (see Chapter 13).

Secondary prevention The aim of secondary prevention is to reduce the risk of progression of an established disease, *e.g.* the use of n-3 fatty acids in individuals with heart disease to reduce the risk of a subsequent heart attack (see Chapters 1, 3, 10 and 13).

Stroke (cerebrovascular disease) Damage to part of the brain resulting from a breakdown in the blood supply (ischaemia) or haemorrhage.

Systematic review A review of the methods and results from all individual studies which focus on a particular research question and conform to set criteria. These include the identification and selection of studies, assessment of their validity and description of results, and use of special statistical methods to obtain overall single estimates known as meta-analysis.

References

Abdelali H, Cassand P, Soussotte V *et al.* (1995) Effect of dairy products on initiation of precursor lesions of colon cancer in rats. *Nutrition and Cancer*, **24**, 121–32.

Abu-Amsha R, Croft KD, Puddey IB, Proudfoot JM, Beilin LJ (1996) Phenolic content of various beverages determines the extent of inhibition of human serum and low density lipoprotein oxidation *in vitro*. *Clinical Science*, **91**, 449–58.

Acheson D (1998) *Independent Inquiry into Inequalities in Health Report*. London: HMSO.

Ackermann RT, Mulrow CD, Ramirez G *et al.* (2001) Garlic shows promise for improving some cardiovascular risk factors. *Archives of Internal Medicine*, **161**, 813–24.

Adams H, Vaughan JG, Fenwick GR (1989) The use of glucosinolates for cultivar identification in swede, *Brassica napus* L. var. *napobrassica* L. *petem*. *Journal of the Science of Food and Agriculture*, **46**, 319–24.

Adamson GE, Lazarus SA, Mitchell AE *et al.* (1999) HPLC method for the quantification of procyanidins in cocoa and chocolate samples and correlation to total antioxidant capacity. *Journal of Agricultural and Food Chemistry*, **47**, 4184–8.

Aggarwal BB, Ahmed N, Mukhtar H (2002) Spices as potent antioxidants with therapeutic potential. In: *Handbook of Antioxidants*, 2nd edn (eds. E Cadenas, L Packer), pp. 437–72. New York: Marcel Dekker.

Ainsworth P (1994) Chemistry in the kitchen – fruit and vegetables 2. *Nutrition and Food Science*, **6**, 19–21.

Akabi K, Hirose M, Hoshiya T *et al.* (1995) Modulating effects of ellagic acid, vanillin and quercetin in a rat medium term multi-organ carcinogenesis model. *Cancer Letters*, **94**, 113–21.

Akihisa T, Kokke WCMC, Tamura T (1991) Naturally occurring sterols and related compounds from plants. In: *Physiology and Biochemistry of Sterols* (eds. G Patterson, W Nes), pp. 172–228. Champaign, IL: American Oil Chemists Society.

Akiyama T, Ishida J, Nakagawa S *et al.* (1987) Genistein, a specific inhibitor of tyrosine-specific protein kinases. *Journal of Biological Chemistry*, **262**, 5592–5.

Al MDM, van Houwelingen AC, Hasart THM, Hornstra G (1994) The relationship between essential fatty acid status of mother and child and occurrence of pregnancy-induced hypertension. *World Review of Nutrition and Dietetics*, **75**, 110–13.

Albanes D, Heinonen OP, Huttunen JK *et al.* (1995) Effects of alpha-tocopherol and beta-carotene supplements on cancer incidence in the Alpha-Tocopherol, Beta-Carotene Cancer Prevention Study. *American Journal of Clinical Nutrition*, **62** (Suppl 6), 1427–30S.

Alberts DS, Martinez ME, Roe DJ *et al.* (2000) Lack of effect of a high-fiber cereal supplement on the recurrence of colorectal adenomas. Phoenix Colon Cancer Prevention Physicians' Network. *New England Journal of Medicine*, **342**, 1156–62.

Albi T, Lanzon A, Guinda A, Perez-Camino MC, Leon M (1997) Microwave and conventional heating effects of some chemical and physical parameters of edible fats. *Journal of Agricultural and Food Chemistry*, **45**, 3000–3.

Albrecht JA, Schafer HW, Zottola EA (1990) Relationship of total sulphur to initial and retained ascorbic acid in selected cruciferous and non-cruciferous vegetables. *Journal of Food Science*, **55**, 181–3.

Allman-Farinelli M (1999) Food groups. In: *Essentials of Human Nutrition* (eds. J Mann, A Truswell), pp. 351–7. Oxford: Oxford University Press.

Almeida MHG, Fragoso RA, Leitao MCA, Nascimento AC (1998) *Polyphenol Communications*, **98**, 403–4.

Ames BN (1989) Mutagenesis and carcinogenesis: endogenous and exogenous factors. *Environmental and Molecular Mutagenesis*, **14** (Suppl 16), 66–77.

Andersen ML, Outtrup H, Skibsted LH (2000) Potential antioxidants in beer assessed by ESR spin trapping. *Journal of Agricultural and Food Chemistry*, **48**, 3106–11.

Anderson AS, Cox DN, McKellar S *et al.* (1998a) Take Five, a nutrition education intervention to increase fruit and vegetable intakes: impact on attitudes towards dietary change. *British Journal of Nutrition*, **80**, 133–40.

Anderson AS, Adamson A, Hetherington MM *et al.* (2001) Results from a school-based nutrition education intervention aimed at increasing fruit and vegetable intake in primary-school aged children. *Proceedings of the Nutrition Society*, **60 OCB**, 143A.

Anderson JJ, Ambrose WW, Garner SC (1998b) Biphasic effect of genistein on bone tissue in the loss in ovariectomized, lactating rat model. *Proceedings of the Society for Experimental Biology and Medicine*, **217**, 345–50.

Anderson JW, Garrity TF, Wood CL *et al.* (1992) Prospective randomised controlled comparison of the effects of low-fat and low-fat plus high-fiber diets on serum lipid levels. *American Journal of Clinical Nutrition*, **56**, 887–94.

Anderson JW, Johnstone BM, Cook-Newell ME (1995) Meta-analysis of the effects of soy protein intake on serum lipids. *New England Journal of Medicine*, **333**, 276–82.

Anderson JW, Allgood LD, Lawrence A *et al.* (2000) Cholesterol lowering of psyllium intake adjunctive to diet therapy in men and women with hypercholesterolemia: meta analysis of 8 controlled trials. *American Journal of Clinical Nutrition*, **71**, 472–9.

Andersson A, Karlstrom B, Mokson R, Versby B (1999) Cholesterol-lowering effects of a stanol ester-containing low-fat margarine used in conjunction with a strict lipid-lowering diet. *European Heart Journal*, Suppl, S80–S90.

Ang CYW, Livingstone GE (1974) Nutritive losses in the home storage and preparation of raw fruits and vegetables. In: *Nutritional Qualities of Fresh Fruits and Vegetables* (eds. PL White, N Selvey), pp. 121–32. New York: Futura.

Anon (1897) *The Gardeners Chronicle*, ii, 19.

Anthony MS, Clarkson TB, Hughes CL, Morgan TM, Burke GL (1996) Soyabean isoflavones improve cardiovascular risk factors without affecting the reproductive system of peripubertal rhesus monkeys. *Journal of Nutrition*, **126**, 43–50.

Apgar JL, Tarka SM (1999) Methylxanthines. In: *Chocolate and Cocoa: Health and Nutrition* (ed. I Knight), pp. 153–73. Oxford: Blackwell Science.

Appel LJ, Moore TJ, Obarzanek E *et al.* (1997) A clinical trial of the effects of dietary patterns on blood pressure. DASH Collaborative Research Group. *New England Journal of Medicine*, **336**, 1117–24.

Arab L (ed.) (2000) *The Efficacy and Safety of Medicinal herbs*. Public Health Nutrition, Vol. 3. Oxford: CABI on behalf of the Nutrition Society.

Arimoto-Kobayashi S, Sugiyama C, Harada N *et al.* (1999) Inhibitory effects of beer and other alcoholic beverages on mutagenesis and DNA adduct formation induced by several carcinogens. *Journal of Agricultural and Food Chemistry*, **47**, 221–30.

Armstrong B, Doll R (1975) Environmental factors and cancer incidence and mortality in different countries, with special reference to dietary practices. *International Journal of Cancer*, **15**, 617–31.

Arteel GE, Sies H (1999) Protection against peroxynitrite by cocoa polyphenol oligmers. *FEBS Letters*, **462**, 167–70.

Arts ICW, Hollman PCH, Kromhout D (1999) Chocolate as a source of tea flavonoids. *Lancet*, **354**, 488.

Arts IC, Hollman PC, Feskens EJ, Bueno de Mesquita HB, Kromhout D (2001a) Catechin intake might explain the inverse relation between tea consumption and ischaemic heart disease: the Zutphen Elderly Study. *American Journal of Clinical Nutrition*, **74**, 227–32.

Arts ICW, Hollman PCH, Feskens EJM, Bueno de Mesquita HB, Kromhout D (2001b) Catechin intake and associated dietary and lifestyle factors in a representative sample of Dutch men and women. *European Journal of Clinical Nutrition*, **55**, 76–81.

Ascherio A, Hennekens C, Willett WC *et al.* (1996) Prospective study of nutritional factors, blood pressure, and hypertension among US women. *Hypertension*, **27**, 1065–72.

Ashihara H, Crozier A (1999) Biosynthesis and degradation of caffeine and related purine alkaloids. In: *Advances in Botanical Research*, Vol. 30 (ed. J Callow), pp. 177–205. London: Academic Press.

Ashihara H, Crozier A (2001) Caffeine: a well known but little mentioned compound in plant science. *Trends in Plant Science*, **6**, 407–13.

Astley SB, Lindsay DG (2002) European Research on the Functional Effects of Dietary Antioxidants – EUROFEDA. *Molecular Aspects of Medicine*, **23**, 1–291.

ATBC (1994) The effect of vitamin E and beta carotene on the incidence of lung cancer and other cancers in male smokers. The Alpha-Tocopherol, Beta Carotene Cancer Prevention Study Group. *New England Journal of Medicine*, **330**, 1029–35.

Atkinson RL (1999) Conjugated linoleic acid for altering body composition and treating obesity. In: *Advances in Conjugated Linoleic Acid Research*, Vol. 1 (eds. M Yurawecz, M Mossoba, J Kramer, M Pariza, G Nelson), pp. 348–53. Champaign, IL: American Oil Chemists Society.

Aviram M, Eias K (1993) Dietary olive oil reduces low-density lipoprotein uptake by macrophages and decreases the susceptibility of the lipoprotein to undergo lipid peroxidation. *Annals of Nutrition and Metabolism*, **37**, 75–84.

Axelson M, Kirk DN, Farrant RD *et al.* (1982) The identification of the weak oestrogen equol [7-hydroxy-3-(4'-hydroxyphenyl)chroman] in human urine. *Biochemical Journal*, **201**, 353–7.

Azen SP, Qian D, Mack WJ *et al.* (1996) Effect of supplementary antioxidant vitamin intake on carotid arterial wall intima-media thickness in a controlled clinical trial of cholesterol lowering. *Circulation*, **94**, 2369–72.

Aziz AA, Edwards CA, Lean MEJ, Crozier A (1998) Absorption and excretion of conjugated flavonols, including quercetin-4'-O-β-glucoside and isorhamnetin-4'-O-β-glucoside, by human volunteers after the consumption of onions. *Free Radical Research*, **29**, 257–69.

Bakalinsky AT, Nadathur SR, Carney JR, Gould SJ (1996) Antimutagenicity of yogurt. *Mutation Research*, **350**, 199–200.

Balentine DA, Wiseman SA, Bouwnes LC (1997) The chemistry of tea flavonoids. *Critical Reviews in Food Science and Nutrition*, **37**, 693–704.

Bandoniene D, Murkovic M (2000) On-line HPLC–DPPH screening method for evaluation of radical screening phenols extracted from apples (*Malus domestica* L.). *Journal of Agricultural and Food Chemistry*, **50**, 2482–7.

Banni S, Martin JC (1998) Conjugated linoleic acid and metabolites. In: *Trans Fatty Acids in Human Nutrition* (eds. JL Sebedio, WW Christie), pp. 261–302. Dundee: The Oily Press.

Banni S, Heys SD, Wahle KWJ (2003) Conjugated linoleic acids (CLAs) as anti-cancer nutrients: studies *in vivo* and cellular mechanisms. In: *Advances in CLA Research*, Vol. 2 (ed. J-L Sebedio, WW Christie, R Adlof). Champaign, IL: American Oil Chemists Society.

Baranowski T, Davis M, Resnicow K *et al.* (2000) Gimme 5 fruit, juice, and vegetables for fun and health. *Health Education Behaviour*, **27**, 96–111.

Barnes S, Kirk M, Coward I (1994) Isoflavones and their conjugation soy foods: extraction conditions and analysis by HPLC–mass spectrometry. *Journal of Agricultural and Food Chemistry*, **42**, 2466–74.

Barra S, Franceschi S, Negri E, Talamini R, La Vecchia C (1990) Type of alcoholic beverage and cancer of the oral cavity, pharynx and oesophagus in an Italian area with high wine consumption. *International Journal of Cancer*, **46**, 1017–20.

Barth MM, Hong Z (1996) Packaging design affects antioxidant vitamin retention and quality of broccoli florets during postharvest storage. *Postharvest Biology and Technology*, **9**, 141–50.

Basiotis PP, Lino M, Dinkins JM (2000) *Consumption of Food Group Servings: People's Perceptions Versus Reality. Insight 20.* Washington, DC: USDA Center for Nutrition Policy and Promotion; www.usda.gov/cnpp.

Basu S, Smedman A, Vessby B (2000) Conjugated linoleic acid induces lipid peroxidation in humans. *FEBS Letters*, **468**, 33–6.

Bauernfeind J (1980) Tocopherols in foods. In: *Vitamin E: a Comprehensive Treatise* (ed. L Machlin), pp. 99–167. New York: Marcel Dekker.

Bazzano LA, He J, Ogden LG *et al.* (2001) Legume consumption and risk of coronary heart disease in US men and women: NHANES I Epidemiologic Follow-up Study. *Archives of Internal Medicine*, **161**, 2573–8.

Bearden MM, Pearson DA, Rein D *et al.* (2000) Potential cardiovascular health benefits of procyanidins present in chocolate and cocoa. In: *Caffeinated Beverages: Health Benefits, Physiological Effects and Chemistry. ACS Symposium Series 754* (eds. T Parliament, C Ho, P Schieberle) pp. 177–87. Washington, DC: American Chemical Society.

Beech BM, Rice R, Myers L, Johnson C, Nicklas TA (1999) Knowledge, attitudes, and practices related to fruit and vegetable consumption of high school students. *Journal of Adolescent Health*, **24**, 244–50.

Bender DA, Bender AE (1999) *Benders' Dictionary of Nutrition and Food Technology*. Cambridge: Woodhead Publishing.

Bernalier A, Dore J, Durand M (1999) Biochemistry of fermentation. In: *Colonic Microbiota, Nutrition and Health* (eds. G Gibson, M Roberfroid), pp. 37–53. Dordrecht: Kluwer.

Berry RE, Tatum JH (1986) Bitterness and immature flavour in grapefruit juices and their changes with processing and storage. *Journal of Food Science*, **51**, 1368.

Bertelli AAE, Giovannini L, Stradi R *et al.* (1996) Kinetics of *trans*- and *cis*-resveratrol (3,4',5-trihydroxystilbene) after red wine oral administration in rats. *International Journal of Clinical Pharmacological Research*, **16**, 77–81.

Bhattacharyya AK, Connor WE (1974) β-Sitosterol and xanthomatosis. A newly described lipid storage disease in two sisters. *Journal of Clinical Investigation*, **53**, 1033–43.

Bhushan B, Thomas P (1990) Effect of gamma irradiation and storage temperature on lipoxygenase activity and carotenoid disappearance in potato tubers. *Journal of Agricultural and Food Chemistry*, **38**, 1586–90.

Bingham SA, Pignatelli B, Pollock JRA *et al.* (1996) Does increased endogenous formation of *N*-nitroso compounds in the human colon explain the association between red meat and colon cancer? *Carcinogenesis*, **17**, 515–23.

Bixler RG, Morgan JN (1999) Cacao bean and chocolate processing. In: *Chocolate and Cocoa: Health and Nutrition* (ed. I Knight), pp. 43–60. Oxford: Blackwell Science.

Björkhem I, Boberg KM (1995) Inborn errors in bile acid synthesis and storage of sterols other than cholesterol. In: *The Metabolic Bases of Inherited Disease*, 16th edn (eds. C Scriver, A Beaudet, W Sly, *et al.*), pp. 2973–3099. New York: McGraw-Hill.

Blacklock CJ, Lawrence JR, Wiles D *et al.* (2001) Salicylic acid in the serum of subjects not taking aspirin. Comparison of salicylic acid concentrations in the serum of vegetarians, non-vegetarians, and patients taking low dose aspirin. *Journal of Clinical Pathology*, **54**, 553–5.

Blankson H, Stakkestad JA, Fagertun H *et al.* (2000) Conjugated linoleic acid reduces body fat mass in overweight and obese humans. *Journal of Nutrition*, 130, 2943–8.

Block G (1992) The data support a role for antioxidants in reducing cancer risk. *Nutrition Reviews*, **50**, 207–13.

Bloom C (1998) *All About Chocolate: the Ultimate Resource for the World's Favorite Food*. New York: Macmillan.

Blostein-Fujii A, DiSilvestro RA, Frid D, Katz C (1999) Short term citrus flavonoid supplementation of type II diabetic women: no effect on lipoprotein oxidation tendencies. *Free Radical Research*, **30**, 315–20.

Blot WJ, McLaughlin JK, Chow WH (1997) Cancer rates among drinkers of black tea. *Critical Reviews in Food Science and Nutrition*, **37**, 739–60.

Bobak M, Hense HW, Kark J *et al.* (1999) An ecological study of determinants of coronary heart disease rates: a comparison of Czech, Bavarian and Israeli men. *International Journal of Epidemiology*, **28**, 437–44.

Bobak M, Skodova Z, Marmot M (2000) Effect of beer drinking on risk of myocardial infarction: population based case-control study. *British Medical Journal*, **320**, 1378–9.

Bodmer WF (1999) 1998 Runme Shaw Memorial Lecture: Somatic evolution of cancer. *Annals of the Academy of Medicine, Singapore*, **28**, 323–9.

Bohm BA (1998) *Introduction to Flavonoids*. Amsterdam: Harwood Academic Publishers.

Bonithon-Kopp C, Kronborg O, Giacosa A, Rath U, Faivre J (2000) Calcium and fibre supplementation in prevention of colorectal adenoma recurrence: a randomised intervention trial. European Cancer prevention Organisation Study Group. *Lancet*, **356**, 1300–6.

Booth C, Hargreaves DF, Hadfield JA, McGown AT, Potten CS (1999a) Isoflavones inhibit intestinal epithelial cell proliferation and induce apoptosis *in vitro*. *British Journal of Cancer*, **80**, 1550–7.

Booth C, Hargreaves DF, O'Shea JA, Potten CS (1999b) *In vivo* administration of genistein has no effect on small intestinal epithelial proliferation and apoptosis, but a modest effect on clonogen survival. *Cancer Letters*, **144**, 169–75.

Borchers AT, Keen CL, Hannum SM, Gershwin ME (2000) Cocoa and chocolate: composition, bioavailability and health implications. *Journal of Medicinal Food*, **3**, 77–105.

Bornside GH (1978) Stability of human fecal flora. *American Journal of Clinical Nutrition*, **31**, 5141–4.

Bots ML, Elwood PC, Salonen JT *et al.* (2002) Level of fibrinogen and risk of fatal and non-fatal stroke. EUROSTROKE: a collaborative study among research centres in Europe. *Journal of Epidemiology and Community Health*, **56** (Suppl I), LI14–I18.

Bourne LC, Rice-Evans CA (1997) The effect of the phenolic antioxidant ferulic acid on the oxidation of low density lipoprotein depends on the pro-oxidant used. *Free Radical Research*, **27**, 337–44.

Bourne LC, Rice-Evans CA (1998) Urinary detection of hydroxycinnamates and flavonoids in humans after high dietary intake of fruit. *Free Radical Research*, **28**, 429–38.

Bourne L, Paganga G, Baxter D, Hughes P, Rice-Evans C (2000) Absorption of ferulic acid from low-alcohol beer. *Free Radical Research*, **32**, 273–80.

Boushey CJ, Beresford SA, Omenn GS, Motulsky AG (1995) A quantitative assessment of plasma homocysteine as a risk factor for vascular disease. Probable benefits of increasing folic acid intakes. *Journal of the American Medical Association*, **274**, 1049–57.

Bravo L (1998) Polyphenols: chemistry, dietary sources, metabolism and nutritional significance. *Nutrition Reviews*, **56**, 317–33.

British Nutrition Foundation (1992) *Task Force Report: Unsaturated Fatty Acids: Nutritional and Physiological Significance*. London: Chapman and Hall.

British Nutrition Foundation (1995a) *Task Force Report: Iron, Nutritional and Physiological Significance*. London: Chapman and Hall.

British Nutrition Foundation (1995b) *Task Force Report: Trans Fatty Acids*. London: British Nutrition Foundation.

British Nutrition Foundation (1999) *Briefing Paper: n-3 Fatty Acids and Health*. London: British Nutrition Foundation.

British Nutrition Foundation (2001a) *Briefing Paper: Selenium and Health*. London: British Nutrition Foundation.

British Nutrition Foundation (2001b) *Task Force Report: Adverse Reactions to Foods*. Oxford: Blackwell Science.

British Nutrition Foundation (2002a) *Briefing Paper: Food Labelling and Health*, London: British Nutrition Foundation.

British Nutrition Foundation (2002b) *Briefing Paper: Nutrition and Schoolchildren*, London: British Nutrition Foundation.

British Nutrition Foundation (2002c) *Briefing Paper: Soya and Health*. London: British Nutrition Foundation.

British Nutrition Foundation (2004) *Task Force Report: Cardiovascular Disease: Diet, Nutrition and Emerging Risk Factors* (ed. S Stanner). Oxford: Blackwell Publishing.

Brocklyn JR Van, Lee MJ, Menzeleev R *et al.* (1998) Dual actions of sphingosine-1-phosphate: extracellular through the Gi-coupled receptor Edg-1 and intracellular to regulate proliferation and survival. *Journal of Cell Biology*, **142**, 229–40.

Brown JE, Wahle KWJ (1990) Effect of fish oil supplementation on lipid peroxidation and whole-blood aggregation in man. *Clinica Chimica Acta*, **193**, 147–56.

Brown L, Rimm EB, Seddon JM *et al.* (1999) A prospective study of carotenoid intake and risk of cataract extraction in US men. *American Journal of Clinical Nutrition*, **70**, 517–24.

Brug J, Lechner L, De Vries H (1995) Psychosocial determinents of fruit and vegetable consumption. *Appetite*, **25**, 285–96.

Bruswick D (1993) Genotoxicity of phenolic antioxidants. *Toxicology and Industrial Health*, **9**, 223–30.

Budi-Santosa FX, Wei LS (1996) Effect of variety, dehulling, and storage on the activity of soy beta-glucosidases during soaking. *IFT Annual Meeting, Book of Abstracts*, ISSN 22, 1082–236.

Bullen CL, Tearle PV, Willis AT (1976) Bifidobacteria in the intestinal tract of infants: an *in vivo* study. *Journal of Medical Microbiology*, **9**, 325–7.

Burns J, Gardner PT, McPhail DB *et al.* (2000) Antioxidant activity, vasodilation capacity and phenolic content of red wines. *Journal of Agricultural and Food Chemistry*, **48**, 220–30.

Burr GO, Burr MM (1930) On the nature and the role of fatty acids essential in nutrition. *Journal of Biological Chemistry*, **86**, 587–621.

Bushman JL (1998) Green tea and cancer in humans: a review of the literature. *Nutrition and Cancer*, **31**, 151–9.

Butler LG (1989) Effects of condensed tannins on animal nutrition. In: *Chemistry and Significance of Condensed Tannins* (eds. R Hemmingway, J Karchesy), pp. 391–402. New York: Plenum Press.

Buttriss J (1997) Food and Nutrition: attitudes, beliefs and knowledge in the United Kingdom. *American Journal of Clinical Nutrition*, **65** (6 Suppl), 1985S–1995S.

Buttriss J (2001) Herbals; what does the future hold? *Nutrition Bulletin*, **26**, 251–3.

Buttriss JL, Hughes J, Kelly CNM, Stanner S (2002) Antioxidants in food: a summary of the review conducted for the Food Standards Agency. *Nutrition Bulletin*, **27**, 227–36.

Calder PC (1995) Fatty acids, dietary lipids and lymphocyte functions. *Biochemical Society Transactions*, **23**, 302–9.

Calder PC (2002) Conjugated linoleic acid in humans – reasons to be cheerful? *Current Opinion in Clinical Nutrition and Metabolic Care*, **5**, 123–6.

Cao GH, Prior RL (1999) Anthocyanins are detected in human plasma after oral administration of an elderberry extract. *Clinical Chemistry*, **45**, 574–6.

Carlson SE, Werkman SH, Peeples JM, Wilson WM (1994) Growth and development of premature infants in relation to ω-3 and ω-6 fatty acid status. *World Review of Nutrition and Dietetics*, **75**, 63–9.

Carroll YL, Corridan BM, Morrissey PA (1999) Carotenoids in young and elderly healthy humans: dietary intakes, biochemical status and diet-plasma relationships. *European Journal of Clinical Nutrition*, **53**, 644–53.

Cassidy A (1996) Physiological effects of phyto-oestrogens in relation to cancer and other human health risks. *Proceedings of the Nutrition Society*, **55** (1B), 399–417.

Cassidy A, Bingham S, Setchell KDR (1994) Biological effects of isoflavones present in soy in premenopausal women: implications for the prevention of breast cancer. *American Journal of Clinical Nutrition*, **60**, 333–40.

Cassidy A, Faughnan M (2000) Phytoestrogens through the lifecycle. *Proceedings of the Nutrition Society*, **59**, 489–96.

Cassidy A, Hanley B, Lamuela-Raventos RM (2000) Isoflavones, lignans and stilbenes – origins, metabolism and potential importance to human health. *Journal of the Science of Food and Agriculture*, **80**, 1044–62.

Cesano A, Visonneau S, Scimeca JA, Kritchevsky D, Santoli D (1998) Opposite effects of linoleic acid and conjugated linoleic acid on human prostatic cancer in SCID mice. *Anticancer Research*, **18**, 1429–34.

Chan W (1998) Stimulating thoughts: caffeine and food. *Nutrition Bulletin*, **23**, 226–33.

Chan W, Brown J, Buss DH (1994) *Miscellaneous Foods. 4th Supplement to the Fifth Edition of McCance, Widdowson's The Composition of Foods*. Cambridge: Royal Society of Chemistry and London: Ministry of Agriculture, Fisheries and Food.

Chasan-Taber L, Willett WC, Seddon JM *et al.* (1999a) A prospective study of vitamin supplement intake and cataract extraction among U.S. women. *Epidemiology*, **10**, 679–84.

Chasan-Taber L, Willett WC, Seddon JM *et al.* (1999b) A prospective study of carotenoid and vitamin A intakes and risk of cataract extraction in US women. *American Journal of Clinical Nutrition*, **70**, 509–16.

Chen TS, Song YO, Kirshen AJ (1983) Effects of blanching, freezing and storage on folacin content of spinach. *Nutrition Reports International*, **28**, 317–24.

Cheney SL (1999) Analysis and nutrient databases. In: *Chocolate and Cocoa: Health and Nutrition* (ed. I Knight), pp. 63–75. Oxford: Blackwell Science.

Cheynier V, Doco T, Fulcrand H *et al.* (1997) ESI-MS analysis of polyphenolic oligomers and polymers. *Analysis*, **25**, M32–7.

Chin S, Liu W, Storkson JM, Ha YL, Pariza MW (1992) Dietary sources of conjugated dienoic isomers of linoleic acid, a newly recognized class of anticarcinogens. *Journal of Food Composition and Analysis*, **5**, 185–97.

Chiu BC, Cerhan JR, Gapstur SM *et al.* (1999) Alcohol consumption and non-Hodgkin lymphoma in a cohort of older women. *British Journal of Cancer*, **80**, 1476–82.

Cho E, Hung S, Willett WC *et al.* (2001) Prospective study of dietary fat and the risk of age-related macular degeneration. *American Journal of Clinical Nutrition*, **73**, 209–18.

Chou TM, Benowitz (1994) Caffeine and coffee: effects on health and cardiovascular disease. *Comparative Biochemistry and Physiology*, **109C**, 173–89.

Christen WG, Glynn RJ, Hennekens CH (1996) Antioxidants and age-related eye disease. Current and future perspectives. *Annals of Epidemiology*, **6**, 60–6.

Christian MS, Brent RL (2001) Teratogen update: evaluation of the reproductive and developmental risks of caffeine. *Teratology*, **64**, 51–78.

Chu Y-H, Chang C-L, Hsu H-F (2000) Flavonoid content of several vegetables and their antioxidant activity. *Journal of the Science of Food and Agriculture*, **80**, 561–6.

Churella HR, Yao BC, Thomson WAB (1976) Soybean trypsin inhibitor activity of soy infant formulas and its nutritional significance for the rat. *Journal of Agricultural and Food Chemistry*, **24**, 393–7.

Ciliska D, Mies E, O'Brien MA *et al.* (2000) Effectiveness of community-based interventions to increase fruit and vegetable consumption. *Journal of Nutrition Education*, **32**, 341–52.

Clark RJ, Macrae R (eds.) (1993) *Coffee. Volume 1. Chemistry*. Barking: Elsevier Applied Science.

Clarke R, Daly L, Robinson K *et al.* (1991) Hyperhomocysteinemia: an independent risk factor for vascular disease. *New England Journal of Medicine*, **324**, 1149–55.

Clausen MR, Mortensen PB (1994) Kinetic studies on the metabolism of short-chain fatty acids and glucose by isolated rat colonocytes. *Gastroenterology*, **106**, 423–32.

Clausen MR, Mortensen PB (1995) Kinetic studies on colonocyte metabolism of short chain fatty acids and glucose in ulcerative colitis. *Gut*, **37**, 684–9.

Clifford AJ, Ebeler SE, Ebeler JD *et al.* (1991) Delayed tumor onset in transgenic mice fed an amino acid-based diet supplemented with red wine solids. *American Journal of Clinical Nutrition*, **64**, 748–56.

Clifford MN (2000a) Anthocyanins – nature, occurrence and dietary burden. *Journal of the Science of Food and Agriculture*, **80**, 1063–72.

Clifford MN (2000b) Chlorogenic acids and other cinnamates – nature, occurrence, dietary burden, absorption and metabolism. *Journal of the Science of Food and Agriculture*, **80**, 1033–43.

Clifford MN (2000c) Miscellaneous phenols in foods and beverages – nature, occurrence and dietary burden. *Journal of the Science of Food and Agriculture*, **80**, 1126–37.

Clifford MN, Scalbert A (2000) Ellagitannins – nature, occurrence and dietary burden. *Journal of the Science of Food and Agriculture*, **80**, 1118–25.

Cnattingius S, Signorello LB, Anneren G *et al.* (2000) Caffeine intake and the risk of first-trimester spontaneous abortion. *New England Journal of Medicine*, **343**, 1839–45.

Cobbett W (1985) *Rural Rides*. London: Penguin Classics.

Cohen LA (2002) Nutrition and prostate cancer: a review. *Annals of the New York Academy of Sciences*, **963**, 148–55.

Collie-Deguid ESR, Wahle KWJ (1996) Inhibitory effect of fish oil n-3 long chain polyunsaturated fatty acids on the expression of endothelial cell adhesion molecules. *Biochemical and Biophysical Research Communications*, **220**, 969–74.

Collin BH, Horska A, Hotten PM, Riddoch C, Collins AR (2001) Kiwifruit protects against oxidative DNA damage in human cells and in vitro. *Nutrition and Cancer*, **39**, 148–53.

Committee on Toxicology of Chemicals in Food, Consumer Products and the Environment (2002) Statement on the reproductive effects of caffeine. www.food.gov.uk, 13 March 2002.

Conaway CC, Getahun SM, Liebes LL *et al.* (2000) Disposition of glucosinolates and sulforaphane in humans after ingestion of steamed and fresh broccoli. *Nutrition and Cancer*, **38**, 168–78.

Corvazier E, Maclouf J (1985) Interference of some flavonoids and non-steroidal anti-inflammatory drugs with oxidative metabolism of arachidonic acid by human platelets and neutrophils. *Biochimica et Biophysica Acta*, **835**, 315–21.

Coward I, Barnes NC, Setchell KDR, Barnes S (1993) Genistein and daidzein and their b-glucoside conjugates: antitumor isoflavones in soybean foods from American and Asian diets. *Journal of Agricultural and Food Chemistry*, **41**, 1961–7.

Cox DN, Anderson AS, Lean ME, Mela DJ (1998a) UK consumer attitudes, beliefs and barriers to increasing fruit and vegetable consumption. *Public Health Nutrition*, **1**, 61–8.

Cox DN, Anderson AS, Reynolds J *et al.* (1998b) Take Five, a nutrition education intervention to increase fruit and vegetable intakes: impact on consumer choice and nutrient intakes. *British Journal of Nutrition*, **80**, 121–31.

Craig WJ (1999) Health promoting properties of common herbs. *American Journal of Clinical Nutrition*, **70** (Suppl), 491S–9S.

Craig WJ (2001) Herbal remedies that promote health and prevent disease. In: *Vegetables, Fruits, and Herbs in Health Promotion* (ed. R Watson) pp. 179–204. Boca Raton, FL: CRC Press.

Crosby AJ, Wahle KWJ, Duthie GG (1996) Modulation of glutathione peroxidase (GSHPx) activity in human vascular endothelial cells by fatty acids and the cytokine interleukin-1b. *Biochimica et Biophysica Acta*, **1303**, 187–92.

Croteau R, Kutchan TM, Lewis NG (2000) Natural products (secondary metabolites). In: *Biochemistry and Molecular Biology of Plants* (eds. B Buchanan, W Gruesome, R Jones), pp. 1250–1318. Rockville, MD: American Society of Plant Physiologists.

Crouse JR, Morgan T, Terry JG, *et al.* (1999) A randomized trial comparing the effect of casein with that of soy protein containing varying amounts of isoflavones on plasma concentrations of lipids and lipoproteins. *Archives of Internal Medicine*, **159**, 2070–6.

Crozier A (1997) Decaff. *Biological Sciences Review*, **10**, 40–1.

Crozier A, Lean MEJ, McDonald MS, Black C (1997) Quantitative analysis of the flavonoid content of commercial tomatoes, onions, lettuces and celery. *Journal of Agricultural and Food Chemistry*, **45**, 590–5.

Crozier A, Burns J, Aziz AA *et al.* (2000) Antioxidant flavonols from fruits, vegetables and beverages: measurements and bio-availability. *Biological Research*, **33**, 78–8.

Cullen KW, Eagan J, Baranowski T, Owens E, de Moor C (2000) Effect of à la carte and snack bar foods at school on children lunchtime intake of fruit and vegetables. *Journal of the American Dietetic Association*, **100**, 1482–6.

Cullum A (2003) Increasing fruit and vegetable consumption: the 5-a-day programme. *Nutrition Bulletin*, **28**, 159–63.

Cumming RG, Mitchell P, Smith W (2000) Diet and cataract: the Blue Mountains Eye Study. *Ophthalmology*, **107**, 450–6.

Cummings JH (1987) Dietary fibre. *American Journal of Clinical Nutrition*, **45**, 1040–3.

Cummings JH, Banwell JG, Englyst HN *et al.* (1990) The amount and composition of large bowel contents. *Gastroenterology*, **98**, A408.

Cuskelly GJ, McNulty H, Scott JM (1996) Effect of increasing dietary folate on red-cell folate: implications for prevention of neural tube defects. *Lancet*, **347**, 657–9.

Czubayko F, Beumers B, Lammsfuss S, Lutjohann I, von Bergmann KA (1991) A simplified micromethod for quantification of fecal excretion of neutral and acidic sterols for outpatient studies in humans. *Journal of Lipid Research*, **32**, 1861–7.

Damianaki A, Bakogeorgou E, Kampa M *et al.* (2000) Potent inhibitory action of red wine polyphenols on human breast cancer cells. *Journal of Cellular Biochemistry*, **78**, 429–41.

Das NP (1969) Studies on flavonoid metabolism. Degradation of (+)-catechin by rat intestinal contents. *Biochimica et Biophysica Acta*, **177**, 668–70.

Davidek J (ed.) (1995) *Natural Compounds of Foods. Formation and Change During Food Processing and Storage*. London: CRC Press.

Davies AP, Goodsall C, Cai Y *et al*. (1998) Black tea dimeric and oligomeric pigments. In: *Plant Polyphenols 2. Chemistry, Biology, Pharmacology, Ecology* (eds. G Gross, R Hemmingway, T Yoshida), pp. 697–724. Indian Bend, OR: Kluwer Academic.

Daxenbichler ME, Etten CH Van, Williams PH (1980) Glucosinolate products in commercial sauerkraut. *Journal of Agricultural and Food Chemistry*, **28**, 809–11.

Day AJ, Mellon F, Barron D *et al*. (2001) Human metabolism of dietary flavonoids: identification of plasma metabolites of quercetin. *Free Radical Research*, **35**, 941–52.

De Deckere EA , Korvor O, Verschuren PM, Katan MB (1998) Health aspects of fish and *n*-3 polyunsaturated fatty acids from plant and marine origin. *European Journal of Clinical Nutrition*, **52**, 749–53.

De Deckere EA, van Amelsvoort JM , McNeill GP, Jones P (1999) Effects of conjugated linoleic acid (CLA) isomers on lipid levels and peroxisome proliferation in the hamster. *British Journal of Nutrition*, **82**, 309–17.

De la Cruz-Carcia C, Gonzalez-Castro MJ, Oruna-Conccha MJ *et al*. (2000) The effects of various culinary treatments on the content of organic acids of green beans. *Deutsche Lebensmittel-Rundschau*, **95**, 323–6.

de Lorgeril M, Renaud S, Mamelle N *et al*. (1994) Mediterranean alpha-linolenic acid-rich diet in secondary prevention of coronary heart disease. *Lancet*, **343**, 1454–9.

de Lorgeril M, Salen P, Martin JL *et al*. (1999) Mediterranean diet, traditional risk factors, and the rate of cardiovascular complications after myocardial infarction: final report of the Lyon Diet Heart Study. *Circulation*, **99**, 779–85.

de Rijke YB, Demacker PN, Assen NA *et al*. (1996) Red wine consumption does not affect oxidizability of low-density lipoproteins in volunteers. *American Journal of Clinical Nutrition*, **63**, 329–34.

de Vries JH, Janssen PL, Hollman PC, van-Staveren WA, Katan MB (1997a) Consumption of quercetin and kaempferol in free-living subjects eating a variety of diets. *Cancer Letters*, **114**, 141–4.

de Vries JHM, Jansen A, Kromhout I *et al*. (1997b) The fatty acid and sterol content of food composities of middle-aged men in seven countries. *Journal of Food Composition and Analysis*, **10**, 115–41.

Debry G (1994) *Coffee and Health*. London: John Libbey.

DEFRA (2001) *National Food Survey 2000*. London: The Stationery Office.

Dekker M, Verkerk RR, Jongen WMF (2000) Predictive modelling of health aspects in the food production chain: A case study on the glucosinolates in cabbage. *Trends in Food Science and Technology*, **11**, 174–81.

Delcourt C, Cristol JP, Leger CL, Descomps B, Papoz L (1999) Associations of antioxidant enzymes with cataract and age-related macular degeneration. The POLA Study. Pathologies Oculaires Liées à l'Age. *Ophthalmology*, **106**, 215–22.

Denke MA (1995) Lack of efficacy of low-dose sito-stanol therapy as an adjunt to a cholesterol-lowering diet in men with moderate hypercholesterolemia. *American Journal of Clinical Nutrition*, **61**, 392–6.

Department for Education and Employment (2000). The Education (Nutritional Standards for School Lunches) (England) Regulations 2000, Statutory Instrument 2000, No. 1777.

Department of Health (1988) *Acheson Committee of Inquiry into the Future Development of the Public Health Function and Community Medicine*. London: HMSO.

Department of Health (1991) *Dietary Reference Values for Food Energy and Nutrients for the UK. Report on Health and Social Subjects No. 41*. London: HMSO.

Department of Health (1994) *Nutritional Aspects of Cardiovascular Disease. Report on Health and Social Subjects No. 46*. London: HMSO.

Department of Health (1995) *Sensible Drinking: Report of an Inter-departmental Working Group, December 1995*. Wetherby: Department of Health.

Department of Health (1998a) *Health Survey for England: the Health of Young People '95–'97*. London: The Stationery Office.

Department of Health (1998b) *Nutritional Aspects of the Development of Cancer. Report on Health and Social Subjects No. 48*. London: HMSO.

Department of Health (1999a) *Health Survey for England: Cardiovascular Disease '98*. London: The Stationery Office.

Department of Health (1999b) *Saving Lives: Our Healthier Nation*. London: HMSO.

Department of Health (2000a) *Folic Acid and the Prevention of Disease. Report on Health and Social Subjects No. 50*. London: The Stationery Office.

Department of Health (2000b) *The NHS Cancer Plan*. London: Department of Health.

Department of Health (2000c) *The NHS Plan*. London, The Stationery Office.

Department of Health (2000d) *National Service Framework for Coronary Heart Disease*. London: Department of Health.

Department of Health (2000e) *The National School Fruit Scheme*. London: Department of Health.

Department of Health (2001a) *Health Survey for England: The Health of Minority Ethnic Groups '99*, London: The Stationery Office.

Department of Health (2001b) *National Service Framework for Diabetes*. London: Department of Health.

Department of Health and Children (1998) *Healthy Food Magazine*. Autumn, Health Promotion Unit, Republic of Ireland.

Depeint F, Gee JM, Williamson G, Johnson IT (2002) Evidence for consistent patterns between flavonoid structures and cellular activities. *Proceedings of the Nutrition Society*, **61**, 97–103.

DeSouza SC, Eitenmiller RR (1986) Effects of processing and storage on the folate content of spinach and broccoli. *Journal of Food Science*, **51**, 626–8.

Dewick PM (2002) *Medicinal Natural Products. A Biosynthetic Approach*, 2nd edn. Chichester: Wiley.

Dick AJ, Redden PR, DeMarco AC, Lidster PD, Grindley TB (1985) Flavonoid glycosides of Spartan apple peel. *Journal of Agricultural and Food Chemistry*, **35**, 529–31.

Diplock AT, Charleux J-L, Crozier-Willi G *et al.* (1998) Functional food science and defence against reactive oxygen species. *British Journal of Nutrition*, **80** (Suppl 1), S77–S112.

Disler PB, Lynch SR, Charlton RW *et al.* (1975) The effect of tea on iron absorption. *Gut*, **16**, 193–200.

Divi RL, Doerge DR (1996) Inhibition of thyroid peroxidase by dietary flavonoids. *Chemical Research in Toxicology*, **9**, 16–23.

Divi RL, Chang HC, Doerge DR (1997) Anti-thyroid isoflavaones from soybeans. *Biochemical Pharmacology*, **54**, 1087–96.

Dlugosz L, Belanger K, Hellenbrand K *et al.* (1996) Maternal caffeine consumption and spontaneous abortion: a prospective cohort study. *Epidemiology*, **7**, 250–5.

Doell BH, Ebden CJ, Smith CA (1981) Trypsin inhibitor activity of conventional foods which are part of the British diet and some soya products. *Plant Foods Human Nutrition*, **31**, 139–50.

Donovan JL, Bell JR, Kasim-Karakas S *et al.* (1999) Catechin is present as metabolites in human plasma after consumption of red wine. *Journal of Nutrition*, **129**, 1662–8.

Dragsted LO, Strube M, Leth T (1997) Dietary levels of plant phenols and other non-nutritive components; could they prevent cancer? *European Journal of Cancer Prevention*, **6**, 522–8.

Dreher ML, Maher CV, Kearney P (1996) The traditional and emerging role of nuts in healthful diet. *Nutrition Reviews*, **54**, 241–5.

Drewnowski A, Gomez-Carneros C (2000) Bitter taste, phytonutrients and the consumer: a review. *American Journal of Clinical Nutrition*, **72**, 1424–35.

Drumm TD, Gray JI, Hosfield GI, Uebersax MA (1990) Lipid, saccharide, protein, phenolic acid and saponin contents of four market classes of edible dry beans as influenced by soaking and canning. *Journal of the Science of Food and Agriculture*, **51**, 425.

Duan RD (1996) Distribution of alkaline sphingomyelinase activity in human beings and animals. Tissue and species differences. *Digestive Disease Sciences*, **41**, 1801–6.

Duan RD, Nyberg L, Nilsson A (1995) Alkaline sphingomyelinase in rat gastrointestinal tract; distribution and characteristics. *Biochimica et Biophysica Acta*, **1259**, 49–55.

Dudeja PK, Dahiya R, Brasitus TA (1986) The role of sphingomyelin synthase and sphingomyelinase in 1,2-dimethylhydrazine-induced lipids alterations of rat colonic plasma membranes. *Biochimica et Biophysica Acta*, **863**, 309–12.

DuPont MS, Mondin Z, Williamson G, Price KR (2000) Effect of variety, processing, and storage on the flavonoid glycoside content and composition of lettuce and endive. *Journal of Agricultural and Food Chemistry*, **48**, 3957–3964.

Durgam VR, Fernandes G (1997) The growth inhibitory effect of conjugated linoleic acid on MCF-7 cells is related to estrogen response system. *Cancer Letters*, **116**, 121–30.

Duthie GG, Pedersen MW, Gardner PT *et al.* (1998) The effect of whisky and wine consumption on total phenol content and antioxidant capacity of plasma from healthy volunteers. *European Journal of Clinical Nutrition*, **52**, 733–6.

Duthie GG, Duthie SJ, Kyle JAM (2000) Plant polyphenols in cancer and heart disease: implications as nutritional antioxidants. *Nutrition Research Reviews*, **13**, 79–106.

Dutta PC, Appelqvist L-A (1996) Saturated sterols (stanols) in unhydrogenated and hydrogenated edible vegetable oils and cereal lipids. *Journal of the Science of Food and Agriculture*, **71**, 383–91.

Dwyer JT, Goldin BR, Saul N *et al.* (1994) Tofu and soy drinks contain phytoestrogens. *Journal of the American Dietetic Association*, **94**, 739–43.

Dybing E, Doe J, Groten J *et al.* (2002) Hazard characterisation of chemicals in food and diet: dose repsonse, mechanisms and extrapolation issues. *Food and Chemical Toxicology*, **40**, 237–82.

Edenhardener R, Keller G, Platt KL, Unger KK (2001) Isolation and characterisation of structurally novel antimutagenic flavonoids from spinach (*Spinacia oleracea*). *Journal of Agricultural and Food Chemistry,* **49**, 2767–73.

Edwards MC, Hall MN, Murphy MC, Pitcher R (1990) *A Comparison of the Composition of Fresh, Canned and Frozen Carrots at the Point of Consumption.* Technical Memorandum No. 571. Chipping Campden, Gloucs: Campden & Chorleywood Food Research Association Group.

Elattar TM, Virji AS (1999) The effect of red wine and its components on growth and proliferation of human oral squamous carcinoma cells. *Anticancer Research*, **19**, 5407–14.

Eldridge AL, Smith-Warner SA, Lytle LA, Murray DM (1999) Comparison of 3 methods for counting fruits and vegetables for fourth-grade students in the Minnesota 5 A Day Power Plus Program. *Journal of the American Dietetic Association*, **98**, 777–82.

Elfoul L, Rabot S, Khelifa N *et al.* (2001) Formation of allyl isothiocyanate from sinigrin in the digestive tract of rats monoassociated with a human colonic strain of *Bacteroides thetaiotaomicron*. *FEMS Microbiolical Letters*, **197**, 99–103.

Ellegård L, Bosaeus I (1991) Sterol and nutrient excretion in ileostomists on prudent diets. *European Journal of Clinical Nutrition*, **45**, 451–7.

EPIC (2002) Food consumption, anthropometrics and physical activity in the EPIC cohorts from 10 European countries. Food consumption data derived from the calibration study (special issue coordinator N Slinani; guest eds. DAT Southgate, WA Van Staveren; EPIC Coordinator E Riboli). *Public Health Nutrition* 5, 6(B), 1111–345.

Erdman JW (1999) Variable bioavailability of carotenoids from vegetables. *American Journal of Clinical Nutrition*, **70**, 179–80.

Ernst E, Resch KL (1993) Fibrinogen as a cardiovascular risk factor: a meta-analysis and review of the literature. *Annals of Internal Medicine*, **118**, 956–63.

Esterbauer H, Gebicki J, Puhl H, Jurgens G (1992) The role of lipid peroxidation and antioxidants in oxidative modification of LDL. *Free Radical Biology and Medicine*, **13**, 341–90.

European Commission (2000) *FAIR: Co-operative Research for SMEs.* Brussels: European Commission.

Ewald C, Fjelkner-Modig S, Johansson K, Sjoholm I, Akesson B (1999) Effect of processing on major flavonoids in processed onions, green beans, and peas. *Food Chemistry*, **64**, 231–5.

Fahey JW, Zhang Y, Talalay P (1997) Broccoli sprouts: an exceptionally rich source of inducers of enzymes that protect against chemical carcinogens. *Proceedings of the National Academy of Science*, **94**, 10367–72.

Fantozzi P, Montanari L, Mancini F *et al.* (1998) *In vitro* antioxidant capacity of wort to beer. *Lebensmittel-Wissenschaft & Technologie*, **31**, 221–7.

Farnham MW, Simon PW, Stommel JR (1999) Improved phytonutrient content through plant genetic improvement. *Nutrition Reviews*, **57**, S19–S26.

Favell DJ (1998) A comparison of the vitamin C content of fresh and frozen vegetables. *Food Chemistry*, **62**, 59–64.

Fehily AM, Johns AP (2002) Designing questionnaires for nutrition research. http://www.tinuviel.u-net.com/kbase/khome.htm, Article 22, Tinuviel Software (accessed February 2003).

Fenster L, Eskenazi B, Windham GC, Swan SH (1991) Caffeine consumption during pregnancy and fetal growth. *American Journal of Public Health*, **81**, 458–61.

Fenwick GR, Hanley AB (1985) The genus *Allium* – Part 1. *Critical Reviews in Food Science and Nutrition*, **22**, 199–271.

Fenwick GR, Griffiths NM, Heaney RK (1982) Bitterness in Brussels sprouts (*Brassica oleracea* L. var *gemmifera*): the role of glucosinolates and their breakdown products. *Journal of the Science of Food and Agriculture*, **34**, 73–80.

Fenwick GR, Heaney RK, Mullin WJ (1983) Glucosinolates and their breakdown products in food and food plants. *CRC Critical Reviews in Food Science and Nutrition*, **18**, 123–201.

Ferns GAA, Lamb DJ (2001) Coronary heart disease: pathophysiological events and risk factors. *Nutrition Bulletin*, **26**, 213–8.

Ferreres F, Gil MI, Castañer M, Tomás-Barberán FA (1997) Phenolic metabolites in red pigmented lettuce (*Lactuca sativa*). Changes with minimal processing and cold storage. *Journal of Agricultural and Food Chemistry*, **45**, 4249–54.

Finch S, Doyle W, Lowe C *et al.* (1998) *National Diet and Nutrition Survey: People Aged 65 Years and Over.* London: HMSO.

Fisher C (2002) Spices of life. *Chemistry in Britain*, January, 40–2.

Fitzpatrick DF, Hirschfield SL, Coffey RG (1993) Endothelium-dependent vasorelaxing activity of wine and other grape products. *American Journal of Physiology*, **265**, H774–H778.

Fleischauer AT, Poole C, Arab L (2000) Garlic consumption and cancer prevention: a meta-analysis of colorectal and stomach cancers. *American Journal of Clinical Nutrition*, **72**, 1047–52.

Floyd RA, West MS, Eneff KL *et al.* (1990) Conditions influencing yield and analysis of 8-hydroxy-2′-deoxyguanosine in oxidatively damaged DNA. *Analytical Biochemistry*, **188**, 155–8.

Folsom AR, Rosamond WD, Shahar E *et al.* (1999) Prospective study of markers of hemostatic function with risk of ischaemic stroke. *Circulation*, **100**, 736–42.

Food Standards Agency and Department of Health (2001) *Catering for Health*. London: The Stationery Office.

Food Standards Australia New Zealand (2002) Joint communiqué: Food ministers agree to a range of policy initiatives and approve a number of food standards. *Food Standards News* **37**, 3–4.

Food Standards Agency Wales (2003) *Food and Wellbeing: Reducing Inequalities Through a Nutrition Strategy for Wales*. Cardiff: FSA Wales.

Ford ES, Mokdad AH (2001) Fruit and vegetable consumption and diabetes mellitus incidence among U.S. adults. *Preventive Medicine*, **32**, 33–9.

Forester SB, Gregson J, Beall D *et al.* (1998) The California Children's 5-a-Day – Power Play! Campaign: evaluation of a large scale marketing initiative. *Family and Community Health*, **21**, 46–64.

Fortier I, Marcoux S, Beaulac-Baillargeon L (1993) Relation of caffeine intake during pregnancy to intrauterine growth retardation and preterm birth. *American Journal of Epidemiology*, **137**, 931–40.

Foth D, Cline JM (1998) Effects of mammalian and plant oestrogens on mammary glands and uteri of macaques. *American Journal of Clinical Nutrition*, **68**, 1413S–1417S.

Frankel EN, Kanner J, German JB, Parks E, Kinsella JE (1993) Inhibition of oxidation of human low-density lipoprotein by phenolic substances in red wine. *Lancet*, **341**, 454–7.

Fraser GE (1999) Association between diet and cancer, ischaemic heart disease, and all-cause mortality in non-Hispanic white Californian Seventh-day Adventists. *American Journal of Clinical Nutrition*, **70**, 532S–538S.

Friedrich JE, Lee CY (1998) Phenolic compounds in sweet and sour cherries. *Polyphenol Communications* **527**.

Fritsche J, Steinhart H (1998) Amounts of conjugated linoleic acid (CLA) in German foods and evaluation of daily intake. *Zeitschrift für Lebensmittel-Untersuchung und -Forschung A*, **206**, 77–82.

Fuchs CS, Giovannucci EL, Colditz GA *et al.* (1999) Dietary fiber and the risk of colorectal cancer and adenoma in women. *New England Journal of Medicine*, **340**, 169–76.

Gamet L, Daviaud D, Denis-Pouxviel C, Remesy C, Murat JC (1992) Effects of short-chain fatty acids on growth and differentiation of the human colon-cancer cell line HT29. *International Journal of Cancer*, **52**, 286–9.

Gardner PT, McPhail DB, Crozier A, Duthie GG (1999) Electron spin resonance (ESR) spectroscopic assessment of the contribution of quercetin and other flavonols to the antioxidant capacity of red wines. *Journal of the Science of Food and Agriculture*, **79**, 1011–14.

Gardner PT, McPhail DB, Duthie GG (1997) Electron spin resonance spectroscopic assessment of the antioxidant potential of teas in aqueous and organic media. *Journal of the Science of Food and Agriculture*, **76**, 257–62.

Gaziano JM, Manson JE, Branch LG *et al.* (1995) A prospective study of consumption of carotenoids in fruits and vegetables and decreased cardiovascular mortality in the elderly. *Annals of Epidemiology*, **5**, 255–60.

Gee JM, Faulks RM, Johnson IT (1991) Physiological effects of retrograded, alpha-amylase-resistant cornstarch in rats. *Journal of Nutrition*, **121**, 44–9.

Gee JM, DuPont MS, Day AJ *et al.* (2000a) Intestinal transport of quercetin glycosides in rats involves both deglycosylation and interaction with the hexose transport pathway. *Journal of Nutrition*, **130**, 2765–71.

Gee JM, Noteborn HPJM, Polley ACJ, Johnson IT (2000b) Increased induction of aberrant crypt foci by DMH in rats fed diets containing purified genistein or genistein-rich soya protein. *Carcinogenesis*, **21**, 2255–9.

Geleijnse JM, Launer LJ, Hofman A, Pols HAP, Witteman JCM (1999) Tea flavonoids may protect against atherosclerosis – The Rotterdam study. *Archives of Internal Medicine*, **159**, 2170–4.

Getahun SM, Chung F-L (1999) Conversion of glucosinolates to isothiocyanates in humans after ingestion of cooked watercress. *Cancer Epidemiology Biomarkers and Prevention*, **8**, 447–51.

Gey KF, Brubacher GB, Stahelin HB (1987) Plasma levels of antioxidant vitamins in relation to ischaemic heart disease and cancer. *American Journal of Clinical Nutrition*, **45**, 1368–77.

Gey KF, Moser UK, Jordan P *et al.* (1993a) Increased risk of cardiovascular disease at suboptimal plasma concentrations of essential antioxidants: an epidemiological update with special attention to carotene and vitamin C. *American Journal of Clinical Nutrition*, **57** (Suppl 5), 787S–797S.

Gey KF, Stahelin HB, Eichholzer M (1993b) Poor plasma status of carotene and vitamin C is associated with higher mortality from ischaemic heart disease and stroke: Basel Prospective Study. *Clinical Investigation*, **71**, 3–6.

Geypens B, Claus D, Evenepoel P *et al.* (1997) Influence of dietary protein supplements on the formation of bacterial metabolites in the colon. *Gut*, **41**, 70–6.

Ghiselli A, Natella F, Guidi A *et al.* (2000) Beer increases plasma antioxidant capacity in humans. *Journal of Nutritional Biochemistry*, **11**, 76–80.

Gibson GR, Beatty ER, Wang X, Cummings JH (1995) Selective stimulation of bifidobacteria in the human colon by oligofructose and inulin. *Gastroenterology*, **108**, 975–82.

Gibson GR, Fuller R (2000) Aspects of *in vitro* and *in vivo* research approaches directed toward identifying probiotics and prebiotics for human use. *Journal of Nutrition*, **130**, 391S–395S.

Gibson S (on behalf of the Food Standards Agency) (2002) Report from the Folic Acid Public Stakeholder Meeting. *Nutrition Bulletin*, **27**, 107–15.

Gil MI, Ferreres F, Tomas-Barberan FA (1998) Effect of modified atmosphere packaging on the flavonoids and vitamin C content of minimally processed Swiss chard. *Journal of Agricultural and Food Chemistry*, **46**, 2007–12.

Gil MI, Ferreres F, Tomas-Barberan FA (1999) Effect of postharvest storage and processing on the antioxidant constituents (flavonoids and vitamin C) of fresh cut spinach. *Journal of Agricultural and Food Chemistry*, **47**, 2213–17.

Giovannucci E, Stampfer MJ, Colditz GA *et al.* (1998) Multivitamin use, folate, and colon cancer in women in the Nurses' Health Study. *Annals of Internal Medicine*, **129**, 517–24.

Giovannucci E, Rimm EB, Liu Y, Stampfer MJ, Willett WC (2002) A prospective study of tomato products, lycopene, and prostate cancer risk. *Journal of the National Cancer Institute*, **94**, 391–8.

Glanz K, Basil M, Maibach E, Goldberg J, Snyder D (1998) Why Americans eat what they do: taste, nutrition, cost, convenience and weight control concerns as influences on food consumption. *Journal of the American Dietetic Association*, **98**, 1118–26.

Glinghammar B, Venturi M, Rowland I, Rafter J (1997) Shift from a dairy product-rich to a dairy product-free diet: influence on cytotoxicity and genotoxicity of fecal water-potential risk factors for colon cancer. *American Journal of Clinical Nutrition*, **66**, 1277–82.

Goldberg J, Flowerdew G, Smith E, Brody JA, Tso MOM (1998) Factors associated with age-related macular degeneration: an analysis of data from the first National Health and Nutrition Examination Survey. *American Journal of Epidemiology*, **128**, 700–10.

Goldin BR, Adlercreutz HA, Gorbach SL *et al.* (1986) The relationship between estrogen levels and diets of caucasian American and Oriental immigrant women. *American Journal of Clinical Nutrition*, **44**, 945–53.

Gonther MP, Cheynier V, Donovan JL *et al.* (2003) Microbial aromatic acid metabolites formed in the gut account for a fraction of the polyphenols excreted in urine of rats fed red wine polyphenols. *J Nutrition*, **133**, 461–7.

Goodlad RA (2001) Dietary fibre and the risk of colorectal cancer. *Gut*, **48**, 587–9.

Goodman MT, Wilkens LR, Hankin JH *et al.* (1997) Association of soy and fiber consumption with the risk of endometrial cancer. *American Journal of Epidemiology*, **146**, 294–306.

Goodrich RM, Anderson JL, Stoewsand GS (1989) Glucosinolate changes in blanched broccoli and Brussel sprouts. *Journal of Food Processing and Preservation*, **13**, 275–80.

Greenway HT, Pratt SG (2001) Fruit and vegetable micronutrients in diseases of the eye. In: *Fruits, Vegetables and Herbs in Health Promotion* (ed. R Watson). Boca Raton, FL: CRC Press.

Gregory J, Foster K, Tyler H, Wiseman M (1990) *The Dietary and Nutritional Survey of British Adults*. London: HMSO.

Gregory J, Collins D, Davies P, Hughes J, Clarke P (1995) *National Diet and Nutrition Survey. Children Aged 1½ to 4½ Years*. London: HMSO.

Gregory J, Lowe S, Bates CJ *et al.* (2000) *National Diet and Nutrition Survey, Young People Aged 4 to 18 Years. Volume 1: Report of the Diet and Nutrition Survey*. London: The Stationery Office.

Grey-Wilson C (1987) *Collins Gem. Herbs for Cooking and Health*. Glasgow: HarperCollins.

Grobbee DE, Rimm EB, Keil U, Renaud S (1999) Alcohol and the cardiovascular system. In: *Health Issues Related to Alcohol Consumption*, 2nd edn (ed. I Macdonald), pp. 125–79. Oxford: Blackwell Science.

Grolier P, Bartholin G, Broers L, Caris-Veyrat C, Dadomo M, Di Lucca G, Dumas Y, Meddens F, Sandei L, Scuch W (2001) Composition of tomatoes and tomato products in antioxidants. In: *The White Book on Antioxidants in Tomatoes and Tomato Products and Their Health Benefits* (eds Bilton R, Gerber M, Grolier P, Leoni C), pp 1–104. *Tomato news*, CMITI Avignon Edition.

Gronbaek M, Becker U, Johansen D *et al.* (1998) Population based cohort study of the association between alcohol intake and cancer of the upper digestive tract. *British Medical Journal*, **317**, 844–7.

Groot PH, Stiphout WA van, Krauss XH *et al.* (1991) Postprandial lipoprotein metabolism in normolipidemic men with and without coronary artery disease. *Arteriosclerosis Thrombosis and Vascular Biology*, **11**, 653–62.

Gross GG (1992) Enzymes in the biosynthesis of hydrolysable tannins. In: *Plant Polyphenols* (eds. R Heminway, P Laks, S Branham), pp. 43–60. New York: Plenum Press.

Grubben MJ, Boers GH, Blom HJ *et al.* (2000) Unfiltered coffee increases plasma homocysteine concentrations in healthy volunteers: a randomized trial. *American Journal of Clinical Nutrition*, **71**, 480–4.

Grundy SM, Mok HYI (1977) Determination of cholesterol absorption in man by intestinal perfusion. *Journal of Lipid Research*, **18**, 263–71.

Grusak MA, DellaPenna D, Welch RM (1999) Physiologic processes affecting the content and distribution of phytonutrients in plants. *Nutrition Reviews*, **57**, S27–S33.

Gryglewski RJ, Korbut R, Robak J, Swies J (1987) On the mechanism of antithrombotic action of flavonoids. *Biochemical Pharmacology*, **36**, 317–22.

Gurr MI, Harwood JL (1991) *Lipid Biochemistry. An Introduction*, 4th edn. London: Chapman and Hall.

Guyton KZ, Kensler KW (1993) Oxidative mechanisms in carcinogenesis. *British Medical Bulletin*, **49**, 523–44.

Gylling H, Miettinen TA (1992) Serum cholesterol lowering by sitostanol ester is associated with reduced absorption and enhanced synthesis of cholesterol with subsequently altered LDL apoB kinetics in type II diabetic men. *Circulation*, **86**, 1404.

Gylling H, Miettinen TA (1997) New biologically active lipids in food, health food and pharmaceuticals. In: *Proceedings of the 19th Nordic Lipid Forum* (ed. O Lambertsen), pp. 81–6. Bergen: Lipidforum.

Gylling H, Miettinen TA (1999a) Cholesterol reduction by different plant stanol mixtures and with variable fat intake. *Metabolism*, **48**, 575–80.

Gylling H, Miettinen TA (1999b) Phytosterols, analytical and nutritional aspects. In: *Functional Foods – A New Challenge for the Food Chemist. Proceedings of the Euro Food Chem X*, Vol. 1 (eds. R Lasztity, W Pfannhauser, L Simon-Sarkadi, S Tömösközi), p. 109. Budapest: Publishing Company of TUB.

Ha YL, Storkson J, Pariza MW (1990) Inhibition of benzo(*a*)pyrene-induced mouse forestomach neoplasia by conjugated dienoic derivatives of linoleic acid. *Cancer Research*, **50**, 1097–101.

Hague A, Manning AM, Hanlon KA *et al.* (1993) Sodium butyrate induces apoptosis in human colonic tumour cell lines in a p53-independent pathway: implications for the possible role of dietary fibre in the prevention of large bowel cancer. *International Journal of Cancer*, **55**, 498–505.

Hague A, Butt AJ, Paraskeva C (1996) The role of butyrate in human colonic epithelial cells: an energy source or inducer of differentiation and apoptosis. *Proceedings of the Nutrition Society*, **55**, 937–43.

Hallberg L, Hulthen L (2000) Prediction of dietary iron absorption: an algorithm for calculating absorption and bioavailability of dietary iron. *American Journal of Clinical Nutrition*, **71**, 1147–60.

Halliday J, Johnson H (1992) *The Art and Science of Wine*. London: Mitchell Beazley.

Hallikainen MH, Uutsitupa MIJ (1999) Effects of a 2 low-fat stanol-ester containing margarine on serum cholesterol concentrations as part of a low-fat diet in hypercholesterolemic subjects. *American Journal of Clinical Nutrition*, **69**, 403–10.

Hallikainen SH, Karenlampi SO, Heinonen IM, Mykkanen HM, Torronen AR (1999) Content of the flavonols quercetin, myricetin and kaempherol in 25 edible berries. *Journal of Agricultural and Food Chemistry*, **47**, 2274–9.

Hallikainen MA, Sarkkinen ES, Uusitupa MIJ (2000) Plant stanol esters affect serum cholesterol concentrations of hypercholesterolaemic men and women in a dose-dependent manner. *Journal of Nutrition*, **130**, 767–76.

Hamilton IM, Gilmore WS, Benzie IF, Mulholland CW, Strain JJ (2000) Interactions between vitamins C and E in human subjects. *British Journal of Nutrition*, **84**, 261–7.

Hammerstone JF, Lazarus SA, Mitchell AE, Rucker R, Schmitz HH (1999) Identification of procyanidins in cocoa (*Theobroma cacao*) and chocolate using high performance liquid chromatography/mass spectrometry. *Journal of Agricultural and Food Chemistry*, **47**, 490–6.

Hammerstone JF, Lazarus SA, Schmitz HH (2000) Procyanidin content and variation in some commonly consumed foods. *Journal of Nutrition*, **130**, 2086S–2092S.

Hammond BR, Johnson EJ, Russell RM *et al.* (1997) Dietary modification of human macular pigment density. *Investigative Ophthalmology and Visual Science*, **38**, 1795–801.

Hanada K, Nishijima M, Kiso M *et al.* (1992) Sphingolipids are essential for the growth of Chinese hamster ovary cells. Restoration of the growth of a mutant defective in sphingoid base biosynthesis by exogenous sphingolipids. *Journal of Biological Chemistry*, **267**, 23527–33.

Hankinson SE, Stampfer MJ, Seddon JM *et al.* (1992) Nutrient intake and cataract extraction in women: a prospective study. *British Medical Journal*, **305**, 335–9.

Harborne JB (1993) *The Flavonoids: Advances in Research Since 1986*. London: Chapman and Hall.

Hasegawa S, Lam LKT, Miller E.G. (2000) Citrus limonoids: biochemistry and possible importance to human nutrition. In: *Phytochemicals and Phytopharmaceuticals* (eds. F Shahidi, C-T Ho). Champaign, IL: AOCS Press.

Haslam E (1998) *Practical Polyphenols – From Structure to Molecular Recognition and Physiological Action*. Cambridge: Cambridge University Press

Hasler CM, Blumberg JB (1999) Phytochemicals: biochemistry and physiology. Introduction. *Journal of Nutrition*, **129**, 756S–757S.

Havas S, Heimendinger J, Damron D *et al.* (1995) 5 A Day for better health – nine community research projects to increase fruit and vegetable consumption. *Public Health Report*, **110**, 68–79.

Havas S, Anliker J, Damron D *et al.* (1998a) Final results of the Maryland WIC 5-A-Day Promotion Program. *American Journal of Public Health*, **88**, 1161–7.

Havas S, Treiman K, Langenberg P *et al.* (1998b) Factors associated with fruit and vegetable consumption among women participating in WIC. *Journal of the American Dietetic Association*, **98**, 1141–8.

Hayatsu H, Hayatsu T (1993) Suppressing effect of *Lactobacillus casei* administration on the urinary mutagenicity arising from ingestion of fried ground beef in the human. *Cancer Letters*, **73**, 173–9.

Health Canada (2001) *Product-Specific Authorization of Health Claims for Foods*. Ottawa: Health Canada.

Hecht SS (1999) Chemoprevention of cancer by isothiocyanates, modifiers of carcinogen metabolism. *Journal of Nutrition*, **129**, 768S–774S.

Heinecke JW, Baker L, Rosen H, Chait A (1986) Superoxide-mediated modification of low density lipoprotein by arterial smooth muscle cells. *Journal of Clinical Investigation*, **77**, 757–61.

Heinemann T, Leiss O, von Bergmann K (1986) Effect of low-dose sitostanol on serum cholesterol in patients with hypercholesterolemia. *Atherosclerosis*, **61**, 219–23.

Heinemann T, Kullak-Ublinck GA, Pietruk B, von Bergmann KL (1991) Mechanism of action of plant sterols on inhibition of cholesterol absorption: comparison of sitosterol and sitostanol. *European Journal of Clinical Pharmacology*, **40** (Suppl), S59–S63.

Heinemann T, Axtmann G, von Bergmann KL (1993) Comparison of intestinal absorption of cholesterol with different plant sterols in man. *European Journal of Clinical Investigation*, **23**, 827–31.

Heitmann BL, Lissner L, Osler M (2000) Do we eat less fat, or just report so? *International Journal of Obesity*, **24**, 435–42.

Henderson L, Gregory J, Swan G (2002) *The National Diet and Nutrition Survey; Adults Aged 19 to 64 Years. Volume 1: Types and Quantities of Foods Consumed.* London: The Stationery Office.

Hendriks HFJ, Weststrate JA, van Vlet T, Meijer OW (1999) Spreads enriched with three different levels of vegetable oil sterols and the degree of cholesterol lowering in normocholesterolemic and mildly hypercholesterolemic subjects. *European Journal of Clinical Nutrition*, **53**, 319–27.

Hennekens CH, Buring JE, Manson JE *et al.* (1996) Lack of effect of long-term supplementation with beta carotene on the incidence of malignant neoplasms and cardiovascular disease. *New England Journal of Medicine*, **334**, 1145–9.

Hernandez C, Howard LR (1996) Modified atmosphere packaging affects antioxidant content and market quality of jalapeno pepper rings. In: *IFT Annual Meeting: Book of Abstracts*, 101.

Herrmann K (1976) Flavonols and flavones in food plants: a review. *Journal of Food Technology*, **11**, 433–48.

Hertog MG, Hollman PC (1996) Potential health effects of the dietary flavonol quercetin. European *Journal of Clinical Nutrition*, **50**, 63–71.

Hertog MGL, Hollman PCH, Katan MB (1992) Content of potentially anticarcinogenic flavonoids of 28 vegetables and 9 fruits commonly consumed in The Netherlands. *Journal of Agricultural and Food Chemistry*, **40**, 2379–83.

Hertog MGL, Freskens EJM, Hollman PCH, Katan MB, Kromhout D (1993a) Dietary antioxidant flavonoids and risk of coronary heart disease: the Zutphen Elderly Study. *Lancet*, **342**, 1007–11.

Hertog MGL, Hollman PCH, Katan MB, Kromhout D (1993b) Intake of potentially anticarcinogenic flavonoids and their determinants in adults in The Netherlands. *Nutrition and Cancer*, **20**, 21–9.

Hertog MGL, Hollman PCH, van de Putte B (1993c) Content of potentially anticarcinogenic flavonoids of tea, infusions, wines, and fruit juices. *Journal of Agricultural and Food Chemistry*, **41**, 1242–6.

Hertog MGL, Feskens EJM, Hollman PCH, Katan MB, Kromhout D (1994) Dietary antioxidant flavonoids and cancer risk in the Zutphen Elderly Study. *Nutrition and Cancer*, **22**, 175–84.

Hertog MG, Kromhout D, Aravanis C *et al.* (1995) Flavonoid intake and long-term risk of coronary heart disease and cancer in the Seven Countries Study. *Archives of Internal Medicine*, **155**, 381–6.

Hertog MG, Sweetnam PM, Fehily AM, Elwood PC, Kromhout D (1997) Antioxidant flavonols and ischaemic heart disease in a Welsh population of men: the Caerphilly Study. *American Journal of Clinical Nutrition*, **65**, 1489–94.

Hill MJ, BC Morsen, Bussey HJR (1978) Etiology of adenoma–carcinoma sequence in the large bowel. *Lancet*, **i**, 245–7.

Hirose M, Hoshiya T, Akagi K, Futakuchi M, Ito N (1994) Inhibition of mammary gland carcinogenesis by green tea catechins and other naturally occurring antioxidants in female Sprague–Dawley rats pre-treated with 7,12-dimethylbenz-*a*-anthracene. *Cancer Letters*, **83**, 149–56.

Hodgson JM, Puddey IB, Beilin LJ *et al.* (1999) Effects of isoflavonoids on blood pressure in subjects with high-normal ambulatory blood pressure levels: a randomized control trial. *American Journal of Hypertension*, **12**, 47–53.

Hodgson JM, Puddey IB, Burke V *et al.* (2002) Acute effects of ingestion on black tea on postprandial platelet aggregation in human subjects. *British Journal of Nutrition*, **87**, 141–5.

Hokanson JE, Austin MA (1996) Plasma triglyceride level is a risk factor for cardiovascular disease independent of high-density lipoprotein cholesterol level: a meta-analysis of population-based prospective studies. *Journal of Cardiovascular Risk*, **3**, 213–19.

Hollman PCH (1997) Bioavailability of flavonoids. *European Journal of Clinical Nutrition*, **51** (Suppl. 1), S66–S69.

Hollman PCH (2000) Bioavailability of flavonoids. In: *Wake Up to Flavonoids: Proceedings of a Conference. International Congress and Symposium Series 226* (ed. CR Evans), pp. 45–52. London: Royal Society of Medicine Press.

Hollman PCH, Arts ICW (2000) Flavonols, flavones, and flavanols – nature, occurrence and dietary burden. *Journal of the Science of Food and Agriculture*, **80**, 1081–93.

Hollman PC, Katan MB (1999) Health effects and bioavailability of dietary flavonols. *Free Radical Research*, Suppl, S75–S80.

Hollman PCH, de Vries JHM, van Leeuwen SD, Mengelers MJB, Katan MB (1995) Absorption of dietary quercetin glycosides and quercetin in healthy ileostomy volunteers. *American Journal of Clinical Medicine*, **62**, 1276–82.

Hollman PCH, van der Gaag M, Mengelers MJ *et al.* (1996) Absorption and disposition kinetics of the dietary antioxidant quercetin in man. *Free Radical Biology and Medicine*, **21**, 703–7.

Hollman PC, Tijburg LB, Yang CS (1997a) Bioavailability of flavonoids from tea. *Critical Reviews in Food Science and Nutrition*, **37**, 719–38.

Hollman PCH, Trijp JMP van, Buysman MNCP *et al.* (1997b) Relative bioavailability of the dietary antioxidant flavonol quercetin in man. *FEBS Letters*, **418**, 152–6.

Hollman PCH, van Trijp JMP, Mengelers MJB, de Vries JHM, Katan MB (1997c) Bioavailability of the dietary antioxidant flavonol quercetin in man. *Cancer Letters*, **114**, 139–40.

Holt PR, Atillasoy EO, Gilman J *et al.* (1998) Modulation of aberrant colonic epithelial cell proliferation and differentiation by low-fat dairy foods. *Journal of the American Medical Association*, **280**, 2074–9.

Hopkins CY (1972) Fatty acids with conjugated unsaturation. In: *Topics in Lipid Chemistry* (ed. Gunstone FD), Vol. 3, pp. 37–87. London: Elek Science.

Hoppner K, Lampi B (1993) Folate retention in dried legumes after different methods of meal preparation. *Food Research International*, **26**, 45–8.

Horne PJ, Lowe CF, Fleming PF, Dowey AJ (1995) An effective procedure for changing food preferences in 5–7-year-old children. *Proceedings of the Nutrition Society*, **54**, 441–52.

Hornstra G, Rand ML (1986) Influence of dietary lipids on platelet–vessel wall interaction: possible role of eicosanoids and platelet membrane fluidity. *Haemostasis*, **16**, 41–2.

Horwath CC (1999) Applying the transtheoretical model to eating behaviour change: challenges and opportunities. *Nutrition Research Reviews*, **12**, 281–317.

Howard L, Dewi T (1996) Minimal processing and edible coating effects on consumption and sensory quality of mini-peeled carrots. *Journal of Food Science*, **61**, 643–5.

Howard LR, Smith RT, Wagner AB, Villalon B, Burns EE (1994) Provitamin A and ascorbic acid content of fresh pepper cultivars (*Capsicum annuum*) and processed jalopenos. *Journal of Food Science*, **59**, 362–5.

Hu FB, Stampfer MJ (1999) Nut consumption and risk of coronary heart disease: a review of epidemiologic evidence. *Current Atherosclerosis Reports*, **1**, 204–9.

Hu FB, Rimm EB, Stampfer MJ *et al.* (2000) Prospective study of major dietary patterns and risk of coronary heart disease in men. *American Journal of Clinical Nutrition*, **72**, 912–21.

Huei JW (1995) Thesis. Quantification of potentially anticarcinogenic isoflavones in soy foods and soybeans and the effect of processing on the composition of isoflavones. *Dissertation Abstracts International B*, **55**, 2462–3.

Huei JW, Murphy PA (1996) Mass balance study of isoflavones during soybean processing. *Journal of Agricultural and Food Chemistry*, **44**, 2377–83.

Hughes J (2001) Assisting dietary change: current research. *Nutrition Bulletin*, **26**, 91–4.

Hughes J, Buttriss J (2000) An update on folates and folic acid: contribution of MAFF funded research. *Nutrition Bulletin*, **25**, 113–24.

Huhle G, Abletshauser C, Mayer N *et al.* (1999) Reduction of platelet activity markers in type II hypercholesterolemic patients by a HMG-CoA-reductase inhibitor. *Thrombosis Research*, **95**, 229–34.

Hussein O, Rosenblat M, Schlezinger S, Keidar S, Aviram M (1997) Reduced platelet aggregation after fluvastatin therapy is associated with altered platelet lipid composition and drug binding to the platelets. *British Journal of Clinical Pharmacology*, **44**, 77–84.

Ibern-Gomez M, Roig-Perez S, Lamuela-Raventos RM, de la Torre-Boronat MC (2000) Resveratrol and piceid levels in natural and blended peanut butters. *Journal of Agricultural and Food Chemistry*, **48**, 6352–4.

Ilow R, Regulska-Ilow B, Szymczak J (1995) Assessment of vitamin C losses in conventionally cooked and microwave processed vegetable. *Bromatologia i Chemia Toksykologiczna*, **28**, 317–21.

Innis SM, Sprecher H, Hachey D, Edmond J, Anderson RE (1999) Neonatal polyunsaturated fatty acid metabolism. *Lipids*, **34**, 139–49.

International Life Sciences Institute, Europe (2002) Process for the Assessment of Scientific Support for Claims on Foods (PASSCLAIM). A European Commission Concerted Action Programme. ILSI Europe, 83, avenue E. Mounier, B-1200 Brussels.

International Olive Oil Council (2002). Six monthly report accessed February 2003. www.internationaloliveoil.org

Ip C, Scimeca JA (1997) Conjugated linoleic acid and linoleic acid are distinctive modulators of mammary carcinogenesis. *Nutrition and Cancer*, **27**, 131–5.

Ip C, Chin SF, Scimeca JA, Pariza MW (1991) Mammary cancer prevention by conjugated dienoic derivative of linoleic acid. *Cancer Research*, **51**, 6118–24.

Ip C, Singh M, Thompson HJ, Scimeca JA (1994) Conjugated linoleic acid suppresses mammary carcinogenesis and proliferative activity of the mammary gland in the rat. *Cancer Research*, **54**, 1212–5.

Ip C, Scimeca JA, Thompson H (1995) Effect of timing and duration of dietary conjugated linoleic acid on mammary cancer prevention. *Nutrition and Cancer*, **24**, 241–7.

Irzyniec Z, Klimczak J, Michalowski S (1993) Effect of storage temperature on vitamin C and total anthocyanins of freeze-dried strawberry juices. In: *Bioavailability '93 – Nutritional, Chemical and Food Processing Implications of Nutrient Availability*. Nutrient Bioavailability Symposium Part 2. Federation of European Chemical Societies, pp. 398–403.

Izumi T, Piskula MK, Osawa S *et al.* (2000) Soy isoflavone aglycones are absorbed faster and in higher amounts than their glucosides in humans. *Journal of Nutrition*, **130**, 1695–9.

Jackson K (1999) In: *Industrial Chocolate Manufacture and Use*, 3rd edn (ed. S Beckett). Oxford: Blackwell Science.

Jacobs DR, Meyer KA, Kushi LH, Folsom AR (1999) Is whole grain intake associated with reduced total and cause-specific death rates in older women? The Iowa Women's Health Study. *American Journal of Public Health*, **89**, 322–9.

Jacobs DR, Murtaugh MA (2000) It's more than an apple a day: an appropriately processed plant-centered dietary pattern may be good for your health. *American Journal of Clinical Nutrition*, **72**, 899–900.

Jacques PF, Tucker KL (2001) Are dietary patterns useful for understanding the role of diet in chronic disease? *American Journal of Clinical Nutrition*, **73**, 1–2.

Jacques PF, Taylor A, Hankinson SE *et al.* (1997) Long-term vitamin C supplement use and prevalence of early age-related lens opacities. *American Journal of Clinical Nutrition*, **66**, 911–16.

Janssen PL, Hollman PC, Venema DP, van Staveren WA, Katan MB (1996a) Salicylates in foods. *Nutrition Reviews*, **54**, 357–9.

Janssen PL, Hollman PC, Venema DP, van Staveren WA, Katan MB (1996b) Urinary salicylate excretion in subjects eating a variety of diets shows that amounts of bioavailable salicylates in foods are low. *American Journal of Clinical Nutrition*, **64**, 743–7.

Janssen PLTMK, Mensink RP, Cox FJJ *et al.* (1998) Effects of the flavonoids quercetin and apigenin on hemostasis in healthy volunteers: results from man *in vitro* and a dietary supplement study. *American Journal of Clinical Nutrition*, **67**, 255–62.

Jardine NJ (1999) Phytochemicals and phenolics. In: *Chocolate and Cocoa: Health and Nutrition* (ed. I Knight), pp. 119–42. Oxford: Blackwell Science.

Jayo MJ, Anthon, Register TC *et al.* (1996) Dietary soy isoflavones and bone loss: a study in ovariectomized monkeys. *Journal of Bone Mineral Research*, **11**, S228.

Jenkins DJ, Kendall CW, Vuksan V *et al.* (2000) Effect of cocoa bran on low-density lipoprotein oxidation and fecal bulking. *Archives of Internal Medicine*, **160**, 2374–9.

Jensen RO (1989) *The Lipids of Human Milk.* Boca Raton, FL: CRC Press.

Jiang J, Wolk A, Vessby B (1999) Relation between the intake of milk fat and the occurrence of conjugated linoleic acid in human adipose tissue. *American Journal of Clinical Nutrition*, **70**, 21–7.

Joffe M, Robertson A (2001) The potential contribution of increased vegetable and fruit consumption to health gain in the European Union. *Public Health Nutrition*, **4**, 893–901.

Johnson EJ, Hammond BR, Yeum KJ *et al.* (2000) Relation among serum and tissue concentrations of lutein and zeaxanthin and macular pigment density. *American Journal of Clinical Nutrition*, **71**, 1555–62.

Johnson IT (2001) Mechanisms and anticarcinogenic effects of diet-related apoptosis in the intestinal mucosa. *Nutrition Research Reviews*, **14**, 229–56.

Johnson JD, Viale HE, Wait DM (1978) Method for extracting carotenoid pigments from citrus oils. US Patent 4 126 709.

Jones F (1995) *The Save Your Heart Wine Guide.* London: Headline Press.

Jones PJ, Raeini-Sarjaz M (2001) Plant sterols and their derivatives: the current spread of results. *Nutrition Reviews*, **59**, 21–4.

Jones PJ, Ntanios FT, Raeini M *et al.* (1999) Similar modulation of plasma lipids by phytosterol and phytostanol esters through reduced cholesterol absorption. *Circulation*, **100** (Suppl), 1–115.

Jood S, Chanhan BM, Kapoor AC (1986) Saponin content of chickpea and black gram: varietal differences and effects of processing and cooking methods. *Journal of the Science of Food and Agriculture*, **37**, 1121.

Joshi MR, Srirangarajan AN, Thomas P (1990) Effects of gamma irradiation and temperature on sugar and vitamin C changes in five Indian potato cultivars during storage. *Food Chemistry*, **35**, 209–16.

Joshipura KJ, Ascherio A, Manson JE *et al.* (1999) Fruit and vegetable intake in relation to risk of ischaemic stroke. *Journal of the American Medical Association*, **282**, 1233–9.

Juan ME, Lamuela-Raventós RM, de la Torre-Boronat MC, Planas JM (1999) Determination of *trans*-resveratrol in plasma by HPLC. *Analytical Chemistry*, **71**, 747–50.

Kala-Yadav S, Sehgal S (1995) Effect of home processing on ascorbic acid and beta-carotene content of spinach and amaranth leaves. *Plant Foods for Human Nutrition*, **47**, 125–31.

Kanazawa K, Sakakibara H (2000) High content of dopamine, a strong antioxidant, in Cavendish banana. *Journal of Agricultural and Food Chemistry*, **48**, 844–8.

Kanematsu H, Ushigusa T, Maruyama T *et al.* (1983) Studies on the improvement of antioxidant effect of tocopherols. I. Addition levels of tocopherols and oxidative stability of edible fats. *Journal of the Japanese Chemical Society*, **32**, 475–9.

Karim M, McCormick K, Kappagoda CT (2000) Effects of cocoa extracts on endothelium-dependent relaxation. *Journal of Nutrition*, **130**, 2105S–2108S.

Kato M, Mizuno K, Crozier A, Fujimura T, Ashihara H (2000) Caffeine synthase gene from tea leaves. *Nature*, **406**, 956–7.

Kaufmann WK (1998) Human topoisomerase II function, tyrosine phosphorylation and cell cycle checkpoints. *Proceedings of the Society for Experimental Biology and Medicine*, **217**, 327–34.

Keil U, Chambless LE, Doring A, Filipiak B, Stieber J (1997) The relation of alcohol intake to coronary heart disease and all-cause mortality in beer-drinking population. *Epidemiology*, **8**, 150–6.

Keli SO, Hertog MG, Feskens EJ, Kromhout D (1996) Dietary flavonoids, antioxidant vitamins, and incidence of stroke: the Zutphen study. *Archives of Internal Medicine*, **156**, 637–42.

Kelly CNM, Smith RD, Williams CM (2001) Dietary monounsaturated fatty acids and haemostasis. *Proceedings of the Nutrition Society*, **60**, 161–70.

Kelly GE, Nelson C, Waring MA, Joannou GE, Reeder AY (1993) Metabolites of dietary (soya) isoflavones in human urine. *Clinica Chimica Acta*, **31**, 9–22.

Kerry N, Rice-Evans C (1998) Peroxynitrite oxidises catechols to *o*-quinones. *FEBS Letters*, **437**, 167–71.

Key TJA, Pike MC (1988) The role of oestrogens and progestagens in the epidemiology and prevention of breast cancer. *European Journal of Cancer, Clinical Oncology*, **24**, 29–34.

Key TJA, Chen J, Wang D, Pike MC, Boroeham JJ (1990) Sex hormones in women in rural china and in Britain. *British Journal of Cancer*, **62**, 631–6.

Key TJ, Thorogood M, Appelby PN, Burr ML (1996) Dietary habits and mortality in 11,000 vegetarians and health conscious people: results of a 17 year follow up. *British Medical Journal*, **313**, 775–9.

Key TJ, Fraser GE, Thorogood M *et al.* (1998) Mortality in vegetarians and non-vegetarians: a collaborative analysis of 8300 deaths among 76,000 men and women in five prospective studies. *Public Health Nutrition*, **1**, 33–41.

Keys A (1980) Wine, garlic and CHD in seven countries. *Lancet*, **i**, 145–6.

Khaw KT, Bingham S, Welch A *et al.* (2001) Relation between plasma ascorbic acid and mortality in men and women in EPIC-Norfolk prospective study. European Prospective Investigation into Cancer and Nutrition. *Lancet*, **357**, 657–63.

Khaza Ai H (1997) Modulation of polyunsaturated fatty acid metabolism in human umbilical vein endothelial cell cultures by antioxidants. PhD Thesis, University of Aberdeen.

Kidmose U, Knuthsen P, Edelenbos M, Justesen U, Hegelund E (2001) Carotenoids and flavonoids in organically grown spinach (*Spinacia oleracea* L) genotypes after deep frozen storage. *Journal of the Science of Food and Agriculture*, **81**, 918–23.

Kim H, Keeney PG (1984) (–)-Epicatechin content in fermented and unfermented cocoa beans. *Journal of Food Science*, **49**, 1090–2.

Kinzler KW, Vogelstein B (1996) Lessons from hereditary colorectal cancer. *Cell*, **87**, 159–70.

Klatsky AL, Armstrong MA, Friedman GD, Hiatt RA (1989) The relations of alcoholic beverage use to colon and rectal cancer. *American Journal of Epidemiology*, **126**, 1007–13.

Klatsky AL, Friedman GD, Armstrong MA (1990) Coffee use prior to myocardial infarction restudied: heavier intake may increase the risk. *American Journal of Epidemiology*, **132**, 479–88.

Kleijnen J, Knipschild P, ter Riet G (1989) Garlic, onions and cardiovascular risk factors. A review of the evidence from human experiments with emphasis on commercially available preparations. *British Journal of Clinical Pharmacology*, **28**, 535–44.

Klus K, Barz W (1998) Formation of polyhydroxylated isoflavones from the isoflavones genistein and biochanin A by bacteria isolated from tempeh. *Phytochemistry*, **47**, 1045–8.

Knekt P, Jarvinen R (1999) Intake of dairy products and breast cancer risk. In: *Advances in Conjugated Linoleic Acid Research*, Vol. 1 (eds. M Yurawecz, M Mossoba, J Kramer, M Pariza, G Nelson), pp. 444–70. Champaign, IL: American Oil Chemists Society.

Knekt P, Jarvinen R, Reunanen A, Maatela J (1996) Flavonoid intake and coronary mortality in Finland: a cohort study. *British Medical Journal*, **312**, 478–81.

Kobayashi T, Shimizugawa T, Osakabe T, Watanabe S, Okuyama H (1997) A long-term feeding of sphingolipids affected the level of plasma cholesterol and hepatic triacylglycerol but not tissue phospholipids and sphingolipids. *Nutrition Research*, **17**, 111–14.

Kochhar SP (1983) Influence of processing on sterols of edible vegetable oils. *Progress in Lipid Research*, **22**, 161–8.

Kochian LV, Garvin DF (1999) Agricultural approaches to improving phytonutrient content in plants. *Nutrition Reviews*, **57**, S13–S18.

Koes RE, Quattrocchio F, Mol JNM (1994) The flavonoid biosynthetic pathway in plants: function and evolution. *BioEssays*, **16**, 123–32.

Koletzko B, Agostoni C, Carlson SE *et al.* (2001) Long chain polyunsaturated fatty acids (LC-PUFA) and perinatal development. *Acta Paediatrica*, **90**, 460–4.

Komatsu Y, Suematsu S, Hisanobu Y *et al.* (1993) Effects of pH and temperature on reaction kinetics of catchins in green tea infusion. *Bioscience, Biotechnology and Biochemistry*, **57**, 907–10.

Kondo K, Hirano R, Matsumoto A, Igarashi O, Itakura H (1998) Inhibition of LDL oxidation by cocoa. *Lancet*, **348**, 1514.

Kopas-Lane LM, Warthesen JJ (1995) Carotenoid photostability in raw spinach and carrots during cold storage. *Journal of Food Science*, **60**, 773–6.

Kris-Etherton PM, Yu S (1997) Individual fatty acid effects on plasma lipids and lipoproteins: human studies. *American Journal of Clinical Nutrition*, **65** (5 Suppl), 1628S–1644S.

Kris-Etherton PM, Derr J, Mitchell DC *et al.* (1993) The role of fatty acid saturation on plasma lipids, lipoproteins, and apolipoproteins: I. Effects of whole food diets high in cocoa butter, olive oil, soybean oil, dairy butter, and milk chocolate on the plasma lipids of young men. *Metabolism*, **42**, 121–9.

Kris-Etherton PM, Zhao G, Binkoski AE, Coval SM, Etherton TD (2001) The effects of nuts on coronary heart disease risk. *Nutrition Reviews*, **59**, 103–11.

Kritchevsky D (2000) Antimutagenic and some other effects of conjugated linoleic acid. *British Journal of Nutrition*, **83**, 459–65.

Kritchevsky D, Tepper SA, Wright S, Tso P, Czarnecki SK (2000) Influence of conjugated linoleic acid (CLA) on establishment and progression of atherosclerosis in rabbits. *Journal of the American College of Nutrition*, **19**, 472S–477S.

Kroon PA, Williamson G (1999) Hydroxycinnamates in plants and food: current and future perspectives. *Journal of the Science of Food and Agriculture*, **79**, 355–61.

Kudou S, Fleury Y, Welti D *et al.* (1991) Malonyl isoflavone glycosides in soybean seeds. *Agricultural and Biological Chemistry*, **55**, 2227–34.

Kühnau J (1976) The flavonoids: a class of semi-essential food components: their role in human nutrition. *World Review of Nutrition and Dietetics*, **24**, 117–91.

Lamartiniere CA, Moore JB, Brown NM *et al.* (1995) Genistein suppppresses mammary cancer in rats. *Carcinogenesis*, **16**, 2833–40.

Lamartinere CA, Zhang J-X, Cotroneo MS (1998) Genistein studies in rats: potential for breast cancer prevention and reproductive and development toxicity. *American Journal of Clinical Nutrition*, **68**, 1400S–1405S.

Lampe JW (1999) Health effects of vegetables and fruit: assessing mechanisms of action in human experimental studies. *American Journal of Clinical Nutrition*, **70** (suppl), 475S–490S.

Lampe JW, Karr SC, Hutchins AM, Slavin JL (1998) Urinary equol excretion with a soy challenge: influence of habitual diet. *Proceedings of the Society for Experimental Biology and Medicine*, **217**, 335–9.

Landman J, Butriss J, Margetts B (1998) Curriculum design for professional development in public health nutrition, in Britain. *Public Health Nutrition*, **1**, 69–74.

Langham S, Thorogood M, Normand C *et al.* (1996) Costs and cost effectiveness of health checks conducted by nurses in primary care: the Oxcheck study. *British Medical Journal*, **312**, 1265–8.

Lass RA (1999) Cacao growing and harvesting practices. In: *Chocolate and Cocoa, Health and Nutrition* (ed. I Knight), pp. 11–42. Oxford: Blackwell Science.

Law M (2000) Plant sterol and stanol margarines and health. *British Medical Journal*, **320**, 861–4.

Law MR, Morris JK (1998) By how much does fruit and vegetable consumption reduce the risk of ischaemic heart disease? *European Journal of Clinical Nutrition*, **52**, 549–56.

Leaf A, Webber PC (1987) A new era for science in nutrition. *American Journal of Clinical Nutrition*, **45**, 1048–53.

Lean ME, Noroozi M, Kelly I *et al.* (1999) Dietary flavonols protect diabetic human lymphocytes against oxidative damage to DNA. *Diabetes*, **48**, 176–81.

Lechner L, Brug J (1997) Consumption of fruit and vegetables: how to motivate the population to change their behaviour. *Cancer Letters*, **114**, 335–6.

Lees C-J, Ginn T-A (1998) Soy isolate diet does not prevent increased cortical bone turnover in ovariectomized macaques. *Calcified Tissue International*, **62**, 557–8.

Leger AS St, Cochrane AL, Moore F (1979) Factors associated with cardiac mortality in developed countries with particular reference to the consumption of wine. *Lancet*, **1**, 1017–20.

Leichter J, Switzer BP, Landymore AF (1978) Effect of cooking on folate content of vegetables. *Nutrition Reports International*, **18**, 475–9.

Leppala JM, Virtamo J, Fogelholm R *et al.* (2000) Controlled trial of alpha-tocopherol and beta-carotene supplements on stroke incidence and mortality in male smokers. *Arteriosclerosis, Thrombosis, and Vascular Biology*, **20**, 230–5.

Leung AY, Foster S (1996) *Encyclopedia of Common Natural Ingredients Used in Food, Drugs and Cosmetics*, 2nd edn. New York: Wiley.

Lewis CE, Walker JRL, Lancaster E (1996) Effect on cooking treatments on pigment loss coloured potato tubers. *Food Technologist*, **26**, 63–5.

Lidbeck A, Nord CE, Gustafsson JA, Rafter J (1992) Lactobacilli, anticarcinogenic activities and human intestinal microflora. *European Journal of Cancer Prevention*, **1**, 341–53.

Liew C, Schut HA, Chin SF, Pariza MW, Dashwood RH (1995) Protection of conjugated linoleic acids against 2-amino-3-methylimidazo[4,5-*f*]quinoline-induced colon carcinogenesis in the F344 rat: a study of inhibitory mechanisms. *Carcinogenesis*, **12**, 3037–43.

Lin DS, Connor WE, Phillipson E (1983) Sterol composition of normal human bile. Effects of feeding shellfish (marine) sterols. *Gastroenterology*, **86**, 611–7.

Ling WE, Jones PJH (1995) Enhanced efficacy of sitostanol-containing versus sitostanol-free phytosterol mixtures in altering of lipoprotein cholesterol levels and synthesis in rats. *Atherosclerosis*, **118**, 319–31.

Lishaut ST-v, Rechkemmer G, Rowland I *et al.* (1999) The carbohydrate crystalean and colonic microflora modulate expression of glutathione S-transferase subunits in colon of rats. *European Journal of Nutrition*, **38**, 76–83.

Lisiewska Z, Kmiecik W (1996) Effects of level of nitrogen fertiliser, processing conditions and period of storage of frozen broccoli and cauliflower on vitamin C retention. *Food Chemistry*, **57**, 267–70.

Lissner L, Heitmann BL, Bengtsson C (2000) Population studies of diet and obesity. *British Journal of Nutrition*, **83**, Suppl 1, S21–S24.

Lister CE, Podivinsky EP (1998) Antioxidants in New Zealand grown fruit and vegetables. *Polyphenol Communications*, **98**, 273.

Liu S, Stampfer MJ, Hu FB et al. (1999) Whole-grain consumption and risk of coronary heart disease; results from the Nurses' Health Study. *American Journal of Clinical Nutrition*, **70**, 412–19.

Liu S, Manson JE, Lee IM et al. (2000) Fruit and vegetable intake and risk of cardiovascular disease: the Women's Health Study. *American Journal of Clinical Nutrition*, **72**, 922–8.

London SJ, Yuan J-M, Chung F-L et al. (2000) Isothiocyanates, glutathione S-transferase M1 and T1 polymorphisms, and lung cancer risk: a prospective study of men in Shanghai, China. *Lancet*, **356**, 724–9.

Lorenz KJ, Kulp K (1991) *Handbook of Cereal Science and Technology*. New York: Marcel Dekker.

Lu LJW, Anderson KE, Grady JJ, Kohen F, Nagamani M (2000) Decreased ovarian hormones during a soya diet: implications for breast cancer prevention. *Cancer Research*, **60**, 4112–21.

Lutjohann D, Björkhem I, Beil UF, von Bergmann KL (1995) Sterol absorption and sterol balance in phytosterolaemia evaluated by deuterium-labeled sterols: effect of sitostanol treatment. *Journal of Lipid Research*, **36**, 1763–73.

Lyle BJ, Mares-Perlman JA, Klein BE et al. (1999) Serum carotenoids and tocopherols and incidence of age-related nuclear cataract. *American Journal of Clinical Nutrition*, **69**, 272–7.

Määttä K, Lampi A-M, Petterson J et al. (1999) Phytosterol content in seven oat cultivars grown at three locations in Sweden. *Journal of the Science of Food and Agriculture*, **79**, 1021–7.

MacCallum PK, Meade TW (1999) Haemostatic function, arterial disease and the prevention of arterial thrombosis. *Baillière's Best Practice and Research. Clinical Haematology*, **12**, 577–99.

Macdonald I (ed.) (1999) *Health Issues Related to Alcohol Consumption*, 2nd edn. Oxford: Blackwell Science.

MacLeod AJ, MacLeod G (1968) Volatiles of cooked cabbage. *Journal of the Science of Food and Agriculture*, **19**, 273–7.

MAFF (1975) *National Food Survey 1974*. London: HMSO.

MAFF (1980) *National Food Survey 1979*. London: HMSO.

MAFF (1985) *National Food Survey 1984*. London: HMSO.

MAFF (1990) *National Food Survey 1989*. London: HMSO.

MAFF (1995) *National Food Survey 1994*. London: The Stationery Office.

MAFF (1997) *Food Information. Surveillance Sheet 127. Dietary Intake of Iodine and Fatty Acids*. London: MAFF.

MAFF (1998) *Fatty Acids. Seventh Supplement to the Fifth Edition of McCance and Widdowson's The Composition of Foods*. Cambridge: Royal Society of Chemisty and London: MAFF.

MAFF (1999) 1997 *Total Diet Study – Aluminium, Arsenic, Cadmium, Chromium, Copper, Lead, Mercury, Nickel, Selenium, Tin and Zinc. Food Surveillance Information Sheet 191*. London: MAFF.

MAFF (2000a) *Multi-element Survey of Wild Edible Fungi and Blackberries. Surveillance Information Sheet 1999*. www.food.gov.uk/science/surveillance.

MAFF (2000b) *National Food Survey 1999*. London: The Stationery Office.

MAFF (2000c) *Duplicate Diet Study of Vegetarians – Dietary Exposure to 12 Metals and Other Elements. Food Surveillance Information Sheet 193*. London: MAFF.

Mahungu SM, Diaz-Mercado S, Li J et al. (1999) Stability of isoflavones during extrusion processing of corn/soy mixture. *Journal of Agricultural and Food Chemistry*, **47**, 279–84.

Majima T, Tsutsumi M, Nishino H, Tsunoda T, Konishi Y (1998) Inhibitory effects of β-carotene, palm carotene and green tea polyphenols on pancreatic carcinogenesis initiated by N-nitrosobis(2-oxopropyl)amine in Syrian golden hamsters. *Pancreas*, **16**, 13–18.

Majumder B, Wahle KWJ, Moir S et al. (2002) Conjugated linoleic acids (CLAs) regulate the expression of key apoptotic genes in human breast cancer cells. *FASEB Journal*, **16**, 1447–9.

Maki KC, Davidson MH, Umporowicz DM et al. (2001) Lipid responses to plant-sterol-enriched reduced-fat spreads incorporated into a National Cholesterol Education Program Step 1 diet. *American Journal of Clinical Nutrition*, **74**, 33–43.

Malin JD (1977) Total folate activity in Brussels sprouts: the effects of storage, processing, cooking and ascorbic acid content. *Journal of Food Technology*, **12**, 623–32.

Manzi P, Panfili G, Esti M, Pizzaferrato L (1998) Natural antioxidants in the unsaponifiable fraction of virgin oil oils from different cultivars. *Journal of Food Science and Agriculture*, **77**, 115–20.

Mao TK, Powell JJ, van de Water J *et al.* (1999) The influence of cocoa procyanidins on the transcription of interleukin-2 in peripheral blood mononuclear cells. *International Journal of Immunotherapy*, **15**, 23–9.

Mao TK, Powell JJ, van der Water J *et al.* (2000a) Effect of cocoa procyanidins on the secretion of interleukin-4 in peripheral blood mononuclear cells. *Journal of Medicinal Food*, **3**, 107–14.

Mao TK, Powell JJ, van der Water J *et al.* (2000b) The effect of cocoa procyanidins on the transcription and secretion of interleukin-1 beta in peripheral blood mononuclear cells. *Life Sciences*, **66**, 1377–86.

Margetts BM, Jackson AA (1996) The determinants of plasma β-carotene: interactions between smoking and other lifestyle factors. *European Journal of Clinical Nutrition*, **50**, 236–8.

Margetts BM, Thompson RL, Key T *et al.* (1995) Development of a scoring system to judge the scientific quality of information from case-control and cohort studies of nutrition and disease. *Nutrition and Cancer*, **24**, 231–9.

Marsman KE, McBurney MI (1996) Dietary fiber and short-chain fatty acids affect cell proliferation and protein synthesis in isolated rat colonocytes. *Journal of Nutrition*, **126**, 1429–37.

Mason L, Brown C (1999) *Traditional Foods of Britain: an Inventory*. Devon: Prospect Books.

Matsui T, Y Matsukawa, Saka T *et al.* (1995) Effect of ammonia on cell-cycle progression of human gastric cancer cells. *European Journal of Gastroenterology and Hepatology*, **7** (Suppl 1), S79–S81.

Mattson FH, Volpenheim RA, Erickson BA (1977) Effect of plant sterol esters on the absorption of dietary cholesterol. *Journal of Nutrition*, **107**, 1139–46.

McBain AJ, Macfarlane GT (1997) Investigations of bifidobacterial ecology and oligosaccharide metabolism in a three-stage compound continuous culture system. *Scandinavian Journal of Gastroenterology*, **222** (Suppl), 32–40.

McCance RA, Widdowson EM (1991) *The Composition of Foods*, 5th edn. Cambridge: Royal Society of Chemistry and London: MAFF.

McClelland JW, Demark-Wahnefried W, Mustian RD, Cowan AT, Campbell MK (1998) Fruit and vegetable consumption of rural African Americans: baseline survey results of the Black Churches United for Better Health 5 A Day Project. *Nutrition and Cancer*, **30**, 148–57.

McCullough ML, Robertson AS, Jacobs EJ *et al.* (2001) A prospective study of diet and stomach cancer mortality in United States men and women. *Cancer Epidemiology, Biomarkers and Prevention*, **10**, 1201–5.

McDonnell WM, Hitom E, Askari FK (1996) Identification of bilirubin UDP-GTs in the human alimentary tract in accordance with the gut as a putative metabolic organ. *Biochemical Pharmacology*, **51**, 483–8.

McMichael-Philips DE (1998) Effects of soy protein supplementation on epithelial proliferation in the histologically normal human breast. *American Journal of Clinical Nutrition*, **68**, 1431S–1436S.

McPhail DB, Gardner PT, Duthie GG, Steele M, Reid K (1999) Assessment of the antioxidant potential of Scotch whiskies by electron spin resonance (ESR) spectroscopy: relationship to hydroxyl-containing aromatic components. *Journal of Agricultural and Food Chemistry*, **47**, 1937–41.

Meade TW, Vickers MV, Thompson SG, Seghatchian MJ (1985a) The physiological effects of fibrinogen on platelet aggregation. *Thrombosis Research*, **38**, 527–34.

Meade TW, Vickers MV, Thompson SG *et al.* (1985b) Epidemiological characteristics of platelet aggregability. *British Medical Journal*, **290**, 428–32.

Meade TW, Cooper JA, Stirling Y *et al.* (1994) Factor VIII, ABO blood group and the incidence of ischaemic heart disease. *British Journal of Haematology*, **88**, 601–7.

Mellies MJ, Ishikawa TT, Glueck CJ, Bove K, Morrison J (1976) Phytosterols in aortic tissue in adults and infants. *Journal of Clinical, Laboratory Medicine*, **88**, 914–21.

Mensink RP, Katan MB (1992) Effect of dietary fatty acids on serum lipids and lipoproteins. A meta-analysis of 27 trials. *Arteriosclerosis and Thrombosis*, **12**, 911–19.

Merrill AH, Schmelz EM, Wang E *et al.* (1995) Role of dietary sphingolipids and inhibitors of sphingolipid metabolism in cancer and other diseases. *Journal of Nutrition*, **125** (Suppl), 1677S–1682S.

Merrill AH, Schmelz EM, Dillehay DL *et al.* (1997) Sphingolipids – the enigmatic lipid class: biochemistry, physiology, and pathophysiology. *Toxicology and Applied Pharmacology*, **142**, 208–25.

Mesquita HB, Maisonneuve P, Moerman CJ, Runia S, Boyle P (1992) Lifetime consumption of alcoholic beverages, tea and coffee and exocrine carcinoma of the pancreas: a population based case-control study in the Netherlands. *International Journal of Cancer*, **50**, 514–22.

Meursing EH (1994) Cocoa mass, cocoa butter, cocoa powder. In: *Industrial Chocolate Manufacturing and Use* (ed. S Beckett). Glasgow: Blackie Academic and Professional.

Michaelsen S, Otte J, Simonsen L-O, Sorensen H (1994) Absorption and degradation of individual intact glucosinolates in the digestive tract of rodents. *Acta Agriculturae Scandinavica, Section A. Animal Science*, **44**, 25–37.

Miettinen TA (1999) Stanol esters in the treatment of hypercholesterolemia. *European Heart Journal*, Suppl. 1, 550–7.

Miettinen TA, Gylling H (1998) Regulation of cholesterol metabolism by dietary plant sterols. *Current Opinion in Lipidology*, **10**, 9–14.

Miettinen TA, Ahrens EH Jr, Grundy SM (1964) Quantitative isolation and gas–liquid chromatographic analysis of total dietary and fecal neutral steroids. *Journal of Lipid Research*, **6**, 411–24.

Miettinen TA, Puska P, Gylling H, Vanhanen H, Vartiainen E (1995) Reduction of serum cholesterol with sitostanol-ester margarine in a mildly hypercholesterolemic population. *New England Journal of Medicine*, **333**, 1308–12.

Miettinen TA, Vuoristo M, Nissinen M, Jarvinen HJ, Gylling H (2000) Serum, biliary, and fecal cholesterol and plant sterols in colectomized patients before and during consumption of stanol ester margarine. *American Journal of Clinical Nutrition*, **71**, 1095–102.

Miller EC, Giovannucci E, Erdman JW et al. (2002) Tomato products, lycopene, and prostate cancer risk. *Urology Clinics of North America*, **29**, 83–93.

Miller TL, Wolin MJ (1986) Methanogens in human and animal digestive tracts. *Systematic and Applied Microbiology*, **7**, 223–9.

Miller TL, Weaver GA, Wolin MJ (1984) Methanogens and anaerobes in a colon segment isolated from the normal fecal stream. *Applied and Environmental Microbiology*, **48**, 449–50.

Minguez-Mosquera MI, Jaren-Galan M, Garrido-Fernandez J (1993) Effect of processing of paprika on the main carotenes and esterified xanthophylls present in fresh fruit. *Journal of Agricultural and Food Chemistry*, **41**, 2120–4.

Mithen RF, Dekker M, Verkerk R, Rabot S, Johnson IT (2000) The nutritional significance, biosynthesis and bioavailability of glucosinolates in human foods. *Journal of the Science of Food and Agriculture*, **80**, 967–84.

Miyazama T, Nakagawa K, Kudo M, Muraishi K, Someya K (1999) Direct intestinal absorption of red fruit anthocyanins, cyanidin-3-glucoside and cyanidin-3,5-diglucoside, into rats and humans. *Journal of Agricultural and Food Chemistry*, **47**, 1083–91.

Mohede I, Albers R, van der Wielen R, Brink L, Dorovska-Taran V (2001) Immuno-modulation: CLA stimulates antigen specific antibody production in humans. 1st International Conference on CLA, Aleslund, Norway, 12.

Moisyadi S, Neupane KR, Stiles JL (1999) Cloning and characterization of xanthosine-N7-methyltransferase, the first enzyme in the caffeine biosynthesis pathway. In: *18th ASIC Proceedings*, 1999, Helsinki. Paris: ASIC.

Mondy NI, Munshi CB (1993) Effect of maturity and storage on ascorbic acid and tyrosine concentrations and enzymatic discoloration of potatoes. *Journal of Agricultural and Food Chemistry*, **41**, 1868–71.

Montedoro M, Servili M, Baldoli M et al. (1993) Simple and hydrolysable compounds in virgin olive oil. 3. Spectroscopic characterizations of the secoiridoid derivatives. *Journal of Agricultural and Food Chemistry*, **41**, 2228–34.

Moore L, Paisley CM, Dennehy A (2000) Are fruit tuck shops in primary schools effective in increasing pupils' fruit consumption? A randomised controlled trial. *Nutrition and Food Science*, **30**, 35–9.

Moore WEC, Holdeman LV (1974) Human faecal flora: the normal flora of 20 Japanese-Hawaiians. *Applied Microbiology*, **27**, 961–79.

Morishita Y, Yoshimi N, Kawabata K et al. (1997) Regressive effects of various chemopreventive agents on azoxymethane-induced aberrant crypt foci in the rat colon. *Japanese Journal of Cancer Research*, **88**, 815–20.

Morton GM, Lee SM, Buss DH, Lawrence P (1995) Intakes and major dietary sources of cholesterol and phytosterols in the British diet. *Journal of Human Nutrition and Dietetics*, **8**, 429–40.

Morton MS, Matos-Ferreira A, Abranches-Monteiro L et al. (1997) Measurement and metabolism of isoflavanoids and lignans in human make. *Cancer Letters*, **114**, 145–51.

Moynihan PJ, Anderson AS, Stacy R et al. (2001) The effect of an after-school 'Food Club' on food preparation skills and nutritional knowledge. *Proceedings of the Nutrition Society*, **60 OCB**, 181A.

Mueller H, Diehl JF (1996) Effects of ionizing radiation on folates in food. *Lebensmittel-Wissenschaft & Technologie*, **29**, 187–90.

Muir AD, Westcott ND (2000) Quantitation of the lignan secoisolariciresinol diglucoside in baked goods containing flax seed or flax meal. *Journal of Agricultural and Food Chemistry*, **48**, 4048–52.

Mullen W, McGinn J, Lean MEJ et al. (2002) Ellagitannins, flavonoids, and other phenolics in red raspberries and their contribution to antioxidant capacity and vasorelaxation properties. *Journal of Agricultural and Food Chemistry*, **50**, 6902–9.

Mulvihill B (2001) Ruminant meat as a source of conjugated linoleic acid (CLA). *Nutrition Bulletin*, **26**, 295–9.

Munday JS, Thompson KG, James KA (1999) Dietary conjugated linoleic acids promote fatty streak formation in the C57BL/6 mouse atherosclerosis model. *British Journal of Nutrition*, **81**, 251–5.

Nadathur SR, Carney JR, Gould SJ, Bakalinsky AT (1996) Palmitic acid is the major fatty acid responsible for significant anti-*N*-methyl-*N'*-nitro-*N*-nitroguanidine (MNNG) activity in yogurt. *Mutation Research*, **359**, 179–89.

Nagata C, Kabuto M, Kuriso Y, Shimizu H (1997) Decreased serum estradiol concentration associated with high dietary intake of soy products in premenopausal Japanese women. *Nutrition and Cancer*, **29**, 228–33.

Nagel CW, Baranowski JD, Wulf LW, Powers JR (1979) The hydroxycinnamic acid tartaric acid ester content of musts and grape varieties grown in the Pacific Northwest. *American Journal of Enology and Viticulture*, **30**, 198–201.

Nagiec MM, Lester RL, Dickson RC (1996) Sphingolipid synthesis: identification and characterisation of mammalian cDNA encoding the Lcb2 subunit of serine palmitoyltransferase. *Gene*, **177**, 237–41.

Nanji AA, French SW (1985) Hepatocellular carcinoma. Relationship to wine and pork consumption. *Cancer*, **56**, 2711–12.

Naska A, Vasdekis VG, Trichopoulou A *et al.* (2000) Fruit and vegetable availability among ten European countries: how does it compare with the 'five a day' recommendation? DAFNE I and II projects of the European Commission. *British Journal of Nutrition*, **84**, 549–56.

National Academy of Sciences Food and Nutrition Board (2000) *Dietary Reference Intakes for Vitamin C, Vitamin E, Selenium and Carotenoids*. Washington, DC: National Academy Press.

National Audit Office (2001) *Tackling Obesity in England*. London: The Stationery Office.

Nelson M (2001) *Tea Drinking and Iron Status; a Review*. London: King's College London.

Nesbitt PD, Lam Y, Thompson LU (1999) Human metabolism of mammalian lignan precursors in raw and processed flaxseed. *American Journal of Clinical Nutrition*, **69**, 549–55.

Ness AR, Powles JW (1997) Fruit and vegetables, and cardiovascular disease: a review. *International Journal of Epidemiology*, **26**, 1–13.

Ness AR, Powles JW (1999) The role of diet, fruit and vegetables and antioxidants in the aetiology of stroke. *Journal of Cardiovascular Risk*, **4**, 229–34.

Ness A, Egger M, Powles J (1999) Fruit and vegetables and ischaemic heart disease: systematic review or misleading meta-analysis? *European Journal of Clinical Nutrition*, **53**, 900–4.

New SA (2001) Fruit and vegetable consumption and skeletal health: is there a positive link? *Nutrition Bulletin*, **26**, 121–5.

Nguyen TT (1999) Recent clinical trial evidence for the cholesterol-lowering efficacy of plant stanol ester spread in a USA population. *European Heart Journal*, Suppl. 1, 573–9.

Nicklas TA, Johnson CC, Myers L, Farris RP, Cunningham A (1998) Outcomes of a high school program to increase fruit and vegetable consumption: Gimme 5 – a fresh nutrition concept for students. *Journal of School Health*, **68**, 248–53.

Nicolosi RJ, Rogers EJ, Kritchevsky D, Scimeca JA, Huth PJ (1997) Dietary conjugated linoleic acid reduces plasma lipoproteins and early aortic atherosclerosis in hypercholesterolemic hamsters. *Artery*, **22**, 266–77.

Nigdikar SV, Williams NR, Griffin BA, Howard AN (1998) Consumption of red wine polyphenols reduces the susceptibility of low-density lipoproteins to oxidation *in vivo*. *American Journal of Clinical Nutrition*, **68**, 258–65.

Niinikoski H, Vukari J, Palmu T (1997) Cholesterol-lowering effect and sensory properties of sitostanol ester margarine in normocholesterolemic adults. *Scandinavian Journal of Nutrition*, **41**, 9–12.

Nijhoff WA, Grubben MJ, Nagengast FM *et al.* (1995) Effects of consumption of Brussels sprouts on intestinal and lymphocytic glutathione S-transferases in humans. *Carcinogenesis*, **16**, 2125–8.

Nilsson A (1969a) Metabolism of cerebroside in the intestinal tract of the rat. *Biochimica et Biophysica Acta*, **187**, 113–21.

Nilsson A (1969b) The presence of spingomyelin- and ceramide-cleaving enzymes in the small intestinal tract. *Biochimica et Biophysica Acta*, **176**, 339–47.

Normén L, Johnson M, Andersson H, van Gameren Y, Dutta P (1999) Plant sterols in vegetables and fruits commonly consumed in Sweden. *European Journal of Clinical Nutrition*, **38**, 84–9.

Novak WK, Haslberger AG (2000) Substantial equivalence of antinutrients and inherent plant toxins in genetically modified foods. *Food, Chemical Toxicology*, **38**, 473–83.

NúñezSellés AJ, Vélez Castro HT, Agüero JA. *et al.* (2002) Isolation and quantitative analysis of phenolic antioxidants, free sugars, and polyols from mango (*Mangifera indica* L.) stem bark aqueous decoction used in Cuba as a nutritional supplement. *Journal of Agricultural and Food Chemistry*, **50**, 762–6.

Nurminen M-L, Niittynen L, Korpela R, Vapaatalo H (1999) Coffee, caffeine and blood pressure. *European Journal of Clinical Nutrition*, **53**, 831–9.

Nyberg L, Nilsson A, Lundgren P, Duan RD (1997) Localization and capacity of sphingomyelin digestion in the rat intestinal tract. *Journal of Nutritional Biochemistry*, **8**, 112–18.

Ochoa J, Majumder B, Hey S *et al.* (2002) ISSFAL, Montreal, Abstract E6.

Oldreive S (2003) Safe intakes of vitamins and minerals: recommendations from the Expert Group on Vitamins and Minerals. *Nutrition Bulletin*, **28**, 199–203.

Olsen SF, Sorensen JD, Secher NJ *et al.* (1992) Randomised controlled trial of effect of fish-oil supplementation on pregnancy duration. *Lancet*, **339**, 1003–7.

Olthof MR, Hollman PCH, Katan MB (2001) Chlorogenic acid and caffeic acid are absorbed in humans. *Journal of Nutrition*, **131**, 66–71.

Omenn GS, Goodman GE, Thornquist MD *et al.* (1996) Effects of a combination of beta carotene and vitamin A on lung cancer and cardiovascular disease. *New England Journal of Medicine*, **334**, 1150–5.

O'Neill ME, Carroll Y, Corridan B *et al.* (2001) A European carotenoid database to assess carotenoid intakes and its use in a five-country comparative study. *British Journal of Nutrition*, **85**, 499–507.

Ooghe WC, Ooghe SJ, Detaverier CM, Huyghebaert A (1994) Characterization of orange juice (*Citrus sinensis*) by polymethoxylated flavones. *Journal of Agricultural and Food Chemistry*, **42**, 2191–5.

Oufedjikh H, Mahrouz M, Amiot MJ, Lacroix M (2000) Effect of gamma-irradiation on phenolic compounds and phenylalanine ammonia-lyase activity during storage in relation to peel injury from peel of *Citrus clementina* Hort. Ex. Tanaka. *Journal of Agricultural and Food Chemistry*, **48**, 559–65.

Pace-Asciak CR, Hahn S, Diamandis EP, Soleas G, Goldberg DM (1995) The red wine phenolics *trans*-resveratrol and quercetin block human platelet aggregation and eicosanoid synthesis: implications for protection against coronary heart disease. *Clinica Chimica Acta*, **235**, 207–19.

Paganga G, Rice-Evans CA (1997) The identification of flaronoids as glycosides in human plasma. *FEBS Letters*, **401**, 78–82.

Paganga G, Miller NJ, Rice-Evans CA (1999) The polyphenolic content of fruit and vegetables and their antioxidant activities. What does a serving constitute? *Free Radical Research*, **30**, 153–62.

Painter J, Rah J-H, Lee Y-K (2002) Comparison of international food guide pictorial representations. *Journal of the American Dietetic Association*, **102**, 483–9.

Pan GG, Kilmartin PA, Smith BG, Melton LD (2002) Detection of orange juice adulteration by tangelo juice using multivariate analysis of polymethoxylated flavones and carotenoids. *Journal of the Science of Food and Agriculture*, **82**, 421–7.

Pandjaitan N, Hettiarachchy N, Ju ZY (2000a) Enrichment of genistein in soy protein concentrate with beta-glucosidase. *Journal of Food Science*, **65**, 403–7.

Pandjaitan N, Hettiarachchy N, Ju ZY *et al.* (2000b) Evaluation of genistin and genistein contents in soybean varieties and soy protein concentrate prepared with 3 basic methods. *Journal of Food Science*, **65**, 399–402.

Pannala AS, Razaq R, Halliwell B, Singh S, Rice-Evans CA (1998) Inhibition of peroxynitrite dependent tyrosine nitration by hydroxycinnamates: nitration or electron donation. *Free Radical Biology and Medicine*, **24**, 594–606.

Pannelli F, Rosa F La, Saltamacchia G *et al.* (1989) Tobacco smoking, coffee, cocoa and tea consumption in relation to urinary bladder cancer in Italy. *European Journal of Epidemiology*, **5**, 392–7.

Pariza MW (1999) The biological activities of conjugated linoleic acid. In: *Advances in Conjugated Linoleic Acid Reseach*, Vol. 1 (eds. M Yurawecz, M Mossoba, J Kramer, M Pariza, G Nelson), pp. 12–20. Champaign, IL: American Oil Chemists Society.

Pariza MW, Hargraves WA (1985) A beef-derived mutagenesis modulator inhibits initiation of mouse epidermal tumors by 7,12-dimethylbenz[*a*]anthracene. *Carcinogenesis*, **6**, 591–3.

Pariza MW, Ashoor SH, Chu FS, Lund DB (1979) Effects of temperature and time on mutagen formation in pan-fried hamburger. *Cancer Letters*, **7**, 63–9.

Park Y (1999) Changes in body composition in mice during feeding and withdrawal of conjugated linoleic acid. *Lipids*, **34**, 243–8.

Parker RS, Swanson JE, You CS, Edwards AJ, Huang T (1999) Bioavailability of carotenoids in human subjects. *Proceedings of the Nutrition Society*, **58**, 155–62.

Parodi PW (1997) The French paradox unmasked: the role of folate. *Medical Hypotheses*, **49**, 313–18.

Parodi PW (1999) Conjugated linoleic acid: the early years. *In Advances in Linoleic Acid Research*, Vol. 1 (eds. M Yurawecz, M Mossoba, J Kramer, M Pariza, G Nelson), pp. 1–11. Champaign, IL: American Oil Chemists Society.

Passmore R and Eastwood MA (eds) (1980) *Davidson and Passmore's Human Nutrition and Dietetics*, 8th edn. Edinburgh: Churchill Livingstone.

Patel SB, Salen G, Hideka H *et al.* (1998) Mapping a gene involved in regulation of dietary cholesterol absorption. The sitosterolemia locus is found at chromosome 2p2 1. *Journal of Clinical Investigation*, **102**, 1041–4.

Paterson JR, Lawrence JR (2001) Salicylic acid: a link between aspirin, diet and the prevention of colorectal cancer. *Quarterly Journal of Medicine*, **94**, 445–8.

Patsch JR, Miesenbock G, Hopferwieser T *et al.* (1992) Relation of triglyceride metabolism and coronary artery disease. Studies in the postprandial state. *Arteriosclerosis Thrombosis and Vascular Biology*, **12**, 1336–45.

Pavoro A (1999) *The New Kitchen Garden*. London: Dorling Kindersley.

Pelletier X, Belbraouet S, Mirabel D *et al.* (1995) A diet moderately enriched in phytosterols lowers plasma cholesterol concentrations in normocholesterolemic humans. *Annals of Nutrition and Metabolism*, **39**, 291–5.

Perry CL, Bishop DB, Taylor G *et al.* (1998) Changing fruit and vegetable consumption among children: 5-a-Day Power Plus program in St. Paul, Minnesota. *American Journal of Public Health*, **88**, 603–9.

Perry IJ, Refsum H, Morris RW *et al.* (1995) Prospective study of serum total homocysteine concentration and risk of stroke in middle-aged British men. *Lancet*, **346**, 1395–8.

Peter KV (2001) Introduction. In: *Handbook of Herbs and Spices* (ed. KV Peter), pp. 1–12. Cambridge: Woodhead Publishing.

Peters U, Poole C, Arab L (2001) Does tea affect cardiovascular disease? A meta-analysis. *American Journal of Epidemiology*, **154**, 495–503.

Peters WH, Boon CE, Roelofs HM *et al.* (1992) Expression of drug-metabolizing enzymes and P-170 glycoprotein in colorectal carcinoma and normal mucosa. *Gastroenterology*, **103**, 448–55.

Petersen MA, Berends H (1993) Ascorbic acid and dehydroascorbic acid content of blanched sweet green pepper during chilled storage in modified atmospheres. *Zeitschrift für Lebensmittel-Untersuchung und -Forschung*, **197**, 546–9.

Peterson J, Dwyer J (1998a) Flavonoids: dietary occurrence and biochemical activity. *Nutrition Research*, **18**, 1995–2018.

Peterson J, Dwyer J (1998b) Taxonomic classification helps identify flavonoid-containing foods on a semi-quantitative food frequency questionnaire. *Journal of the American Dietetic Association*, **98**, 677–82.

Petrakis NL, Barnes S, King EB *et al.* (1996) Stimulatory influence of soy protein isolate on breast secretion in pre- and postmenopausal women. *Cancer Epidemiology Biomarkers and Prevention*, **10**, 785–94.

Petroni A, Blasevich M, Salami M *et al.* (1994) A phenolic antioxidant extracted from olive oil inhibits platelet aggregation and arachidonic acid metabolism *in vitro*. *World Review of Nutrition and Dietetics*, **75**, 169–71.

Phillips KM, Toivo JI, Swank MA, Whiton RS, Ruggio DM (1999a) Free and esterified sterol content of food oils and fats. Presented at the 90th AOCS Annual Meeting and Expo, Orlando, FL. *A Special Supplement to INFORM*, **10**, (5), S101. Champaign, IL: AOCS.

Phillips KM, Tarragó-Trani MT, Stewart KK (1999b) Phytosterol content of experimental diets differing in fatty acid composition. *Food Chemistry*, **64**, 415–22.

Pierpoint WS (2000) Why do plants make medicines. *The Biochemist*, **22**, 37–40.

Pietinen P, Rimm EB, Korhonen P *et al.* (1996) Intake of dietary fibre and risk of coronary heart disease in a cohort of Finnish men. The Alpha-Tocopherol, Beta-carotene Cancer Prevention Study. *Circulation*, **94**, 2720–7.

Piggott JR, Conner JM, Paterson A, Clyne J (1993) Effects on Scotch whisky composition and flavour of maturation in oak casks with varying histories. *International Journal of Food Science and Technology*, **28**, 303–18.

Piironen V, Lindsay DG, Miettinen TA, Toivo J, Lampi A-M (2000) Plant sterols: biosynthesis, biological function and their importance in human nutrition. *Journal of the Science of Food and Agriculture*, **80**, 939–66.

Pither RJ, Edwards MC (1995) *The Effects of Domestic Cooking and Preparation Techniques on the Nutritional Composition of Vegetables*. Chipping Campden, Gloucs: Campden & Chorleywood Food Research Association Group.

Plat J, Mensink RP (1998) Safety aspects of dietary plant sterols and stanols. A special report. *Postgraduate Medicine*.

Plat J, Mensink RP (2000) Vegetable oil based versus wood based stanol ester mixtures: effects on serum lipids and hemostatic factors in non-hypercholesterolemic subjects. *Atherosclerosis*, **148**, 101–12.

Plat J, van Onselen ENM, Mensink RP (1999) Dietary plant stanol ester mixtures. Effects on safety parameters and erytrocyte membrane fatty acid composition in non-hypercholesterolaemic subjects. *European Heart Journal*, Suppl. 1, S58–S63.

Plumb GW, Price KR, Rhodes MJC, Williamson G (1997) Antioxidant properties of the major phenolic compounds in broccoli. *Free Radical Research*, **27**, 429–35.

Podsedek A, Wilskajeszka J, Anders B (1998) Characterization of proanthocyanidins of apple, quince and strawberry fruits. *Polyphenol Communications*, 319–20.

Pollak OJ, Kritchevsky D (1981) Sitosterol. In: *Monographs on Atherosclerosis*, Vol. 10 (eds. T Clarkson, D Kritchevsky, O Pollak), pp. 1–219. Basel: Karger.

Pomeranz Y (1992) Biochemical, functional, and nutritive changes during storage. In: *Storage of Cereals Grains and Their Products* (ed. D Sauer), pp. 65–141. St. Paul, MN: American Association of Cereal Chemists.

Pool-Zobel BL, Neudecker C, Domizlaff I *et al.* (1996) Lactobacillus- and bifidobacterium-mediated antigenotoxicity in the colon of rats. *Nutrition and Cancer,* **26**, 365–80.

Poppitt SD, Swann D, Black AE, Prentice AM (1998) Assessment of selective under-reporting of food intake by both obese and non-obese women in a metabolic facility. *International Journal of Obesity,* **22**, 303–11.

Potter JD, Finnegan JR, Guinard J-X *et al.* (2000) *5-A-Day Better Health Program Evaluation Report. NIH Publication No. 01-4904.* Bethesda, MD: National Institutes of Health and National Cancer Institute.

Poulter J (1998) Antioxidants in tea. *Nutrition Bulletin,* **23**, 203–10.

Powell SM, Zilz N, Beazer-Barclay Y *et al.* (1992) APC mutations occur early during colorectal tumorigenesis. *Nature,* **359**, 235–7.

Prescott E, Gronbaek M, Becker U, Sorensen TI (1999) Alcohol intake and risk of lung cancer. Influence of alcoholic beverage. *American Journal of Epidemiology,* **149**, 463–70.

Price KR, Fenwick GR (1985) Naturally occurring oestrogens in food – a review. *Food Additives and Contaminants,* **2**, 73–106.

Price KR, Johnson IT, Fenwick GR (1987) The chemistry and biological significance of saponins in foods and feedingstuffs. *CRC Critical Reviews in Food Science and Nutrition,* **26**, 1.

Price KR, Casuscelli F, Colquhoun IJ, Rhodes MJC (1998a) Composition and content of flavonol glycosides in broccoli florets (*Brassica olearacea*) and their fate during cooking. *Journal of the Science of Food and Agriculture,* **77**, 468–72.

Price KR, Colquhoun IJ, Barnes KA, Rhodes MJC (1998b) Composition and content of flavonol glycosides in green beans and their fate during processing. *Journal of Agricultural and Food Chemistry,* **46**, 4898–903.

Prochaska JO, DiClemente CC (1983) Stages and processes of self-change of smoking: toward an integrative model of change. *Journal of Consulting, Clinical Psychology,* **51**, 390–5.

Puska P, Isokääntä M, Korpelainen V, Vartialnen E (1999) Village competition as an innovative method for lowering population cholesterol. *European Heart Journal,* Suppl. 1, S64–S72.

Putnam SD, Cerhan JR, Parker AS *et al.* (2000) Lifestyle and anthropometric risk factors for prostate cancer in a cohort of Iowa men. *Annals of Epidemiology,* **10**, 361–9.

Quinsac A, Charrier A, Ribaillier D (1994) Glucosinolates in etiolated sprouts of sea kale. *Journal of the Science of Food and Agriculture,* **65**, 201–7.

Rabot S, Nugon-Baudon L, Raibaud P, Szylit O (1993) Rapeseed meal toxicity in gnotobiotic rats; influence of a whole human faecal flora or single human strains of *Escherichia coli* and *Bacteroides vulgatus. British Journal of Nutrition,* **70**, 323–31.

Rabot S, Guerin C, Nugon-Baudon L, Szylit O (1995) Glucosinolate degradation by bacterial strains isolated from a human intestinal microflora. In: *Proceedings of the 9th International Rapeseed Congress,* Vol. 1, pp. 212–4.

Radtke J, Linseisen J, Wolfram G (1998) Phenolic acid intake of adults in a Bavarian subgroup of the national food consumption survey. *Zeitschrift für Ernährungswissenschaft,* **37**, 190–7.

Rankin SM, Parthasarathy S, Steinberg D (1991) Evidence for a dominant role of lipoxygenase(s) in the oxidation of LDL by mouse peritoneal macrophages. *Journal of Lipid Research,* **32**, 449–56.

Rayman MP (1997) Dietary selenium: time to act. *British Medical Journal,* **314**, 387–8.

Rayman MP (2000) The importance of selenium to human health. *Lancet,* **356**, 233–41.

Readers Digest Association Ltd. (2000) *The Readers Digest Guide to Vitamins, Minerals and Supplements.* London: Readers Digest Association Ltd.

Reaven P, Parthasarathy S, Grasse BJ *et al.* (1991) Feasibility of using an oleate-rich diet to reduce the susceptibility of low-density lipoprotein to oxidative modification in humans. *American Journal of Clinical Nutrition,* **54**, 701–6.

Rechner AR, Pannala AS, Rice-Evans CA (2001) Caffeic acid derivatives in artichoke extract are metabolised to phenolic acids *in vivo. Free Radical Research,* **35**, 195–202.

Rein D, Lotito S, Holt RR *et al.* (2000a) Epicatechin in human plasma: *in vivo* determination and effect of chocolate consumption on plasma oxidation status. *Journal of Nutrition,* **130**, 2109S–2114S.

Rein D, Paglieroni TG, Wun T *et al.* (2000b) Cocoa inhibits platelet activation and function. *American Journal of Clinical Nutrition,* **72**, 30–5.

Reinli K, Block G (1996) Phytoestrogen content of foods – a compendium of literature values. *Nutrition and Cancer,* **26**, 123–48.

Renaud SC, Gueguen R, Schenker J, d'Houtaud A (1998) Alcohol and mortality in middle-aged men from Eastern France. *Epidemiology*, **9**, 184–8.

Revill SA, Adamson AJ, Stacy R, Hooper J, Moynihan PJ (2001) The effect of an after-school 'Food Club' on intake of foods and nutrients by children from deprived social backgrounds. *Proceedings of the Nutrition Society*, **60 OCB**, 189A.

Reynolds KD, Franklin FA, Binkley D et al. (2000a) Increasing the fruit and vegetable consumption of fourth-graders: results from the high 5 project. *Preventative Medicine*, **30**, 309–19.

Reynolds KD, Franklin FA, Leviton LC, et al. (2000b) Methods, results, and lessons learned from process evaluation of the high 5 school-based nutrition intervention. *Health Education and Behaviour*, **27**, 177–86.

Rhodes MJ (1996) Physiologically-active compounds in plant foods: an overview. *Proceedings of the Nutrition Society*, **55** (1B), 371–84.

Rhodes, Price (1998) Phytochemicals; classification and occurrence. In: *Encyclopaedia of Human Nutrition*. (eds. MJ Sadler, JJ Strain, B Caballero), Vol. 3, pp. 1539–49. New York: Academic Press.

Riboli E, Cornee J, Macquart-Moulin G et al. (1991) Cancer and polyps of the colorectum and lifetime consumption of beer and other alcoholic beverages. *American Journal of Epidemiology*, **134**, 157–66.

Rice-Evans C, (1995) Free radicals and antioxidants in atherosclerosis. In: *Immunopharmacology of Free Radical Species* (eds DR Blake, PG Winyard). New York: Academic Press.

Richelle M, Tavazzi I, Enslen M, Offord EA (1999) Plasma kinetics in man of epicatechin from black chocolate. *European Journal of Clinical Nutrition*, **53**, 22–6.

Rimm EB, Ascherio A, Giovannucci E et al. (1996a) Vegetable, fruit, and cereal fiber intake and risk of coronary heart disease among men. *Journal of the American Medical Association*, **275**, 447–51.

Rimm EB, Katan MB, Ascherio A, Stampfer MJ, Willett WC (1996b) Relation between intake of flavonoids and risk for coronary heart disease in male health professionals. *Annals of Internal Medicine*, **125**, 384–9.

Rimm EB, Klatsky A, Grobbee D, Stampfer MJ (1996c) Review of moderate alcohol consumption and reduced risk of coronary heart disease: is the effect due to wine, beer or spirits? *British Medical Journal*, **312**, 713–36.

Ring SG, Gee JM, Whittam M, Orford P, Johnson IT (1988) Resistant starch: its chemical form in foodstuffs and effect upon digestibility *in vitro*. *Food Chemistry*, **28**, 97–109.

Riserus U, Bergland L, Vessby B (2001) Conjugated linoleic acid (CLA) reduced abdominal adipose tissue in obese middle-aged men with signs of the metabolic syndrome: a randomised controlled trial. *International Journal of Obesity*, **25**, 1129–35.

Roche HM, Gibney MJ (1999) Long chain n-3 polyunsaturated fatty acids and triglycerol metabolism in the postprandial state. *Lipids*, **34**, S259–S265.

Roche HM, Zampelas A, Knapper JME et al. (1998) Effect of long-term olive oil dietary intervention on postprandial triacylglycerol and factor VII metabolism. *American Journal of Clinical Nutrition*, **68**, 552–60.

Rock CL, Lovalvo JL, Emenhiser C et al. (1998) Bioavailability of beta-carotene is lower in raw than in processed carrots and spinach in women. *Journal of Nutrition*, **128**, 913–16.

Roediger WE (1980a) Anaerobic bacteria, the colon and colitis. *Australian and New Zealand Journal of Surgery*, **50**, 73–5.

Roediger WE (1980b) The colonic epithelium in ulcerative colitis: an energy-deficiency disease? *Lancet*, **8197**, 712–15.

Rolfe RD (2000) The role of probiotic cultures in the control of gastrointestinal health. *Journal of Nutrition*, **130**, 396S–402S.

Rommel A, Heatherbell DA, Wrolstad RE (1990) Red raspberry juice and wine: effect of processing and storage on anthocyanin pigment composition, colour and appearance. *Journal of Food Science*, **55**, 1011–17.

Rosenberg DW (1991) Tissue-specific induction of the carcinogen inducible cytochrome P450 isoform, P450IAI, in colonic epithelium. *Archives of Biochemistry and Biophysics*, **284**, 223–6.

Rotondo D (1995) Fatty acid modulation of cell responsiveness. *Biochemical Society Transactions*, **23**, 291–6.

Rous C, Aldersen B (1983) Phenolic extraction curves for white wine aged in French and American oak barrels. *American Journal of Enology and Viticulture*, **34**, 211–15.

Rubnov S, Kashman Y, Rabinowitz R, Schlesinger M, Mechoulam R (2001) Suppressers of cancer cell proliferation from fig (*Ficus caria*) resin: isolation and structure elucidation. *Journal of Natural Products*, **64**, 993–6.

Ryan D, Robards K (1998) Phenolic compounds in olives. *Analyst*, **123**, 31–44.

Sacks FM, Svetkey LP, Vollmer WM et al. (2001) Effects on blood pressure of reduced dietary sodium and the Dietary Approaches to Stop Hypertension (DASH) diet. DASH–Sodium Collaborative Research Group. *New England Journal of Medicine*, **344**, 3–10.

Sahay TB, Rootman I, Ashbury FD (2000). *Review of Nutrition Interventions for Cancer Prevention*. Ontario Cancer Care, Canada.

Saltmarsh M (2001) Thirst: or, why do people drink? *Nutrition Bulletin*, **26**, 53–8.

Sanbongi C, Suzuki N, Sakane T (1997) Polyphenols in chocolate, which have antioxidant activity, modulate immune functions in humans *in vitro*. *Cellular Immunology*, **177**, 129–36.

Sanbongi C, Osakabe N, Natsume M *et al.* (1998) Antioxidant polyphenols isolated from *Theobroma cacao*. *Journal of Agricultural and Food Chemistry*, **46**, 454–7.

Sanders ME (2000) Considerations for use of probiotic bacteria to modulate human health. *Journal of Nutrition*, **130**, 384S–390S.

Sanderson P, Finnegan YE, Williams CM *et al.* (2002a) UK Food Standards Agency alpha-linolenic acid workshop report. *British Journal of Nutrition*, **88**, 573–9.

Sanders TH, McMichael RW, Hendrix KW (2000b) Occurrence of resveratrol in edible peanuts. *Journal of Agricultural and Food Chemistry*, **48**, 1243–6.

Sanderson P, Gill JM, Packard CJ, Sanders TA, Vessby B, Williams CM (2002b) UK Food Standards Agency cis-monounsaturated fatty acid workshop report. *British Journal of Nutrition*, **88**, 99–104.

SanGiovanni JP, Berkey CS, Dwyer JT, Colditz GA (2000) Dietary essential fatty acids, long-chain polyunsaturated fatty acids, and visual resolution acuity in healthy fullterm infants: a systematic review. *Early Human Development*, **57**, 165–88.

Sanoner P, Guyot S, Drilleau JF (1998) Characterisation of the phenolic compound classes in four cider apples cultivars by thiolysis and HPLC. *Polyphenol Communications*, 401–3.

Santos-Buelga C, Scalbert A (2000) Proanthocyanidins and tannin-like compounds – nature, occurrence, dietary intake and effects on nutrition and health. *Journal of the Science of Food and Agriculture*, **80**, 1094–117.

Sargent JR (1997) Fish oils and human diet. *British Journal of Nutrition*, **78** (Suppl 1), S5–S13.

Scalbert A, Williamson G (2000) Dietary intake and bioavailability of polyphenols. *Journal of Nutrition*, Suppl, 2073S–2085S.

Schatzkin A, Lanza E, Corle D *et al.* (2000) Lack of effect of a low-fat, high-fiber diet on the recurrence of colorectal adenomas. Polyp Prevention Trial Study Group. *New England Journal of Medicine*, **342**, 1149–55.

Scheline RR (1973) Metabolism of foreign compounds by gastrointestinal microorganisms. *Pharmacological Reviews*, **25**, 451–523.

Schenker S (2000) The nutritional and physiological properties of chocolate. *Nutrition Bulletin*, **25**, 303–13.

Schenker S (2001) Cranberries. *Nutrition Bulletin*, **26**, 115–16.

Scheppach W, Bartram P, Richter A *et al.* (1992a) Effect of short-chain fatty acids on the human colonic mucosa *in vitro*. *Journal of Parenteral and Enteral Nutrition*, **16**, 43–8.

Scheppach W, Sommer H, Kirchner T *et al.* (1992b) Effect of butyrate enemas on the colonic mucosa in distal ulcerative colitis. *Gastroenterology*, **103**, 51–6.

Schmelz EM (2000) Dietary sphingomyelin and other sphingolipids in health and disease. *Nutrition Bulletin*, **25**, 135–9.

Schmelz EM, Merrill AH (1998) Ceramides and ceramide metabolites in cell regulation: evidence for dietary sphingolipids as inhibitors of colon carcinogenesis. *Nutrition and Cancer*, **14**, 717–19.

Schmelz EM, Crall KL, LaRocque R, Dillehay DL, Merrill AH (1994) Uptake and metabolism of sphingolipids in isolated loops of mice? *Journal of Nutrition*, **124**, 702–12.

Schmelz EM, Dillehay DL, Webb SK *et al.* (1996) Sphingomyelin consumption suppresses aberrant crypt foci and increases the proportion of ademomas versus adenocarcinomsa in CF1 mice treated with 1,2-dimethylhydrazine; implications for dietary sphingolipids and colon carcinogenesis. *Cancer Research*, **56**, 4936–41.

Schmelz EM, Bushnev AS, Dillehay DL *et al.* (1999) Ceremide B-glucuronide: synthesis, digestion and suppression of early markers of colon carcinogenesis. *Cancer Research*, **59**, 7568–72.

Schothorst RC, Jekel AA (1999) Oral sterol intake in the Netherlands: evaluation of the results obtained by GC analysis of duplicate 24-h diet samples collected in 1994. *Food Chemistry*, **64**, 561–6.

Schulz T, Chew B, Seaman W (1992) Differential stimulatory and inhibitory responses of human MCF-7 breast cancer cells to linoleic acid and conjugated linoleic acid in culture. *Anticancer Research*, **12**, 21–43.

Schunemann HJ, Grant BJ, Freudenheim JL *et al.* (2001) The relation of serum levels of antioxidant vitamins C and E, retinol and carotenoids with pulmonary function in the general population. *American Journal of Respiratory and Critical Care Medicine*, **163**, 1246–55.

Schuurman AG, Goldbohm RA, van den Brandt PA (1999) A prospective cohort study on consumption of alcoholic beverages in relation to prostate cancer incidence (The Netherlands). *Cancer Causes Control*, **10**, 597–605.

Scottish Executive. *Scottish Diabetes Framework*. Edinburgh: NHS Scotland.

Seddon JM, Ajaani UA, Sperduto RD *et al.* (1994) Dietary carotenoids, vitamin A, C and E and advanced age-related macular degeneration. *Journal of the American Medical Association*, **272**, 1413–20.

Seitz LM (1989) Stanol and sterol esters of ferulic and *p*-coumaric acids in wheat, corn, rye, and triticale. *Journal of Agricultural and Food Chemistry*, **37**, 662–7.

Sellers TA, Kushi LH, Cerhan JR *et al.* (2001) Dietary folate intake, alcohol, and risk of breast cancer in a prospective study of postmenopausal women. *Epidemiology*, **12**, 420–8.

Serafini M, Bugianesi R, Salucci M, Azzini E, Raguzzini A, Maiani G (2002) Effect of acute ingestion of fresh and stored lettuce (Laktuscasative) on plasma total antioxidant capacity and antioxidant levels in human subjects. *British Journal of Nutrition*, **88**, 615–23.

Sesso HD, Gaziano JM, Buring JE, Hennekens CH (1999) Coffee and tea intake and the risk of myocardial infarction. *American Journal of Epidemiology*, **149**, 162–7.

Setchell KDR, Cassidy A (1999) Dietary isoflavones – biological effects and relevance to human health. *Journal of Nutrition*, **129**, 758S–767S.

Setchell KDR, Lawson AM, Borriello SP *et al.* (1981) Lignan formation in man–microbial involvement and possible roles in relation to cancer. *Lancet*, **8236**, 4–7.

Setchell KDR, Borriello SP, Hulme P, Kirk DN, Axelson M (1984) Non-steroidal oestrogens of dietary origin: possible roles in hormone dependent disease. *American Journal of Clinical Nutrition*, **40**, 569–78.

Setchell KDR, Nechemias-Zimmer L, Cai J, Heubi JE (1997) Exposure of infants to phytoestrogens from soy infant formulas. *Lancet*, **350**, 23–7.

Setchell KDR, Brown NM, Desai P *et al.* (2001) Bioavailability of pure isoflavones in healthy humans and analysis of commercial soy isoflavone supplements. *Journal of Nutrition*, **131**, 1362S–1375S.

Shaheen SO, Sterne JA, Thompson RL *et al.* (2001) Dietary antioxidants and asthma in adults: population-based case-control study. *American Journal of Respiratory Critical Care Medicine*, **164**, 1823–8.

Shapiro TA, Fahey JW, Wade KL, Stephenson KK, Talalay P (1998) Human metabolism and excretion of cancer chemoprotective glucosinolates and isothiocyanates of cruciferous vegetables. *Cancer Epidemiology Biomarkers and Prevention*, **7**, 1091–100.

Sharma A, Sehgal A (1992) Effect of domestic processing, cooking and germination on the trypsin inhibitor activity and tannin content of faba bean. *Plant Foods in Human Nutrition*, **42**, 127–33.

Shaw PE, Wilson CW (1983) Debittering citrus juices with beta cyclodextrin polymer. *Journal of the Science of Food and Agriculture*, **48**, 646.

Shepherd R (1999) Social determinants of food choice. *Proceedings of the Nutrition Society*, **58**, 807–12.

Shepherd R (2001) Eating, Food and Health LINK Programme: progress on funded projects. *Nutrition Bulletin*, **26**, 147–51.

Shewfelt RL (1990) Sources of variation in the nutrient content of agricultural commodities from the farm to the consumer. *Journal of Food Quality*, **13**, 37–54.

Shi J, Le Maguer M (2000) Lycopene in tomatoes: chemical and physical properties affected by food processing. *Critical Reviews in Food Science and Nutrition*, **40**, 1–42.

Shibutani S, Takeshita M, Grollman AP (1991) Insertion of specific bases during DNA synthesis past the oxidation-damaged base 8-oxodG. *Nature*, **349**, 431–4.

Shirsat SG, Thomas P (1998) Effect of irradiation and cooking methods on ascorbic acid levels of four potato cultivars. *Journal of Food Science and Technology – India*, **35**, 509–14.

Silva KDRR, Jones AE, Smith RD *et al.* (2001) Lower postprandial apolipoprotein B48 and increased chylomicron particle size in subjects on a high monounsaturated fat diet. *Proceedings of the Nutrition Society*, **60 OCA**, 106A.

Simmer K (2001a) Long chain polyunsaturated fatty acid supplementation in preterm infants (Cochrane Review). In: *The Cochrane Library. Issue 3: Update Software*. Oxford.

Simmer K (2001b) Long chain polyunsaturated fatty acid supplementation in infants born at term (Cochrane Review). In: *The Cochrane Library. Issue 3: Update Software*. Oxford.

Simon JA, Hudes ES (1999) Serum ascorbic acid and other correlates of self-reported cataract among older Americans. *Journal of Clinical Epidemiology*, **52**, 1207–11.

Simopoulos AP (1999) Essential fatty acids in health and chronic disease. *American Journal of Clinical Nutrition*, **70** (3 Suppl), 560S–569S.

Simopoulos AP, Leaf A, Salem N (2000) Workshop statement on the essentiality of and recommended dietary intakes for omega-6 and omega-3 fatty acids. *Prostaglandins, Leukotrienes and Essential Fatty Acids*, **63**, 119–21.

Simpson BB, Conner-Ogorzaly M (1986) *Economic Botany Plants in Our World*. New York: McGraw-Hill International.

Singleton VL (1982) Grape and wine phenolics: background and prospects. In: *Proceedings of the University of California, Davis, Grape and Wine Centennial Symposium* (ed. A Webb), pp. 215–27. Davis, CA: University of California Press.

Singleton VL (1995) Maturation of wines and spirits – comparisons, facts, and hypotheses. *American Journal of Enology and Viticulture*, **46**, 98–115.

Sinha R, Chow WH, Kulldorff M *et al.* (1999) Well-done, grilled red meat increases the risk of colorectal adenomas. *Cancer Research*, **59**, 4320–4.

Sivaraman L, Leatham MP, Yee J *et al.* (1994) CYP1A1 genetic polymorphisms and *in situ* colorectal cancer. *Cancer Research*, **54**, 3692–5.

Smith FB, Lee AJ, Fowkes FG *et al.* (1997) Hemostatic factors as predictors of ischaemic heart disease and stroke in the Edinbury Artery Study. *Arteriosclerosis Thrombosis and Vascular Biology*, **17**, 3321–5.

Smith TK, Lund EK, Johnson IT (1998) Inhibition of dimethylhydrazine-induced aberrant crypt foci and induction of apoptosis in rat colon following oral administration of the glucosinolate sinigrin. *Carcinogenesis*, **19**, 267–73.

Smith WL (1992) Prostanoid biosynthesis and mechanisms of action. *American Journal of Physiology*, **263**, F181–F191.

Smith-Warner SA, Spiegelman D, Yaun SS *et al.* (2001) Intake of fruits and vegetables and risk of breast cancer, a pooled analysis of cohort studies. *Journal of the American Medical Association*, **285**, 769–76.

Sobel A (1999) *Galileo's Daughter. A Drama of Science, Fate and Love*. London: Fourth Estate.

Soleas GJ, Diamandis EO, Goldberg DM (1997a) Wine as a biological fluid: history, production, and role in disease prevention. *Journal of Clinical Laboratory Analysis*, **11**, 287–313.

Soleas GJ, Diamandis EP, Goldberg DM (1997b) Resveratrol: a molecule whose time has come and gone? *Clinical Chemistry*, **30**, 91–113.

Sommerburg O, Keunen JEE, Bird AC, van Kuijjk FJGM (1994) Fruits and vegetables that are sources for lutein and zeaxanthin: the macular pigment in human eyes. *British Journal of Ophthalmology*, **82**, 907–10.

Sorensen G, Hunt MK, Cohen N *et al.* (1998) Worksite and family education for dietary change: the Treatwell 5-a-day program. *Health Education Resources*, **13**, 577–91.

Southgate DAT (2000) Beverages. In: *Human Nutrition and Dietetics*, 10th edn (eds. J Garrow, W James, A Ralph), pp. 385–395. London: Churchill Livingstone.

Spencer AP, Carson DS, Crouch MA (1999) Vitamin E and coronary artery disease. *Archives of Internal Medicine*, **159**, 1313–20.

Sprecher H (2000) Metabolism of highly unsaturated *n*-3 and *n*-6 fatty acids. *Biochimica et Biophysica Acta*, **1486**, 219–31.

Stagg GV, Millin DJ (1975) The nutritional and therapeutic value of tea. *Journal of the Science of Food and Agriculture*, **26**, 1439–59.

Stampfer MJ, Malinow MR (1995) Can lowering homocysteine levels reduce cardiovascular risk? *New England Journal of Medicine*, **332**, 328–9.

Stampfer MJ, Malinow MR, Willett WC *et al.* (1992) A prospective study of plasma homocyst(e)ine and risk of myocardial infarction in US physicians. *Journal of the American Medical Association*, **268**, 877–81.

Stanner S (2001) Highlights of the European conference on nutrition and cancer. *Nutrition Bulletin*, **26**, 337–9.

Stanner S (2002) Food, nutrition and the prevention of cancer: getting the message across. *Nutrition Bulletin*, **27**, 199–202.

Steinberg D, Parthasarathy S, Carew TE, Khoo JC, Witztum JL (1989) Beyond cholesterol. Modifications of low-density lipoprotein that increase its atherogenicity. *New England Journal of Medicine*, **320**, 915–24.

Steiner M, Khan AH, Holbert D, Lin RIS (1996) A double-blind crossover study in moderately hypercholesterolemic men that compared the effect of aged garlic extract and placebo administration on blood lipids. *American Journal of Clinical Nutrition*, **64**, 866–70.

Steinmetz KA, Kushi LH, Bostick RM, Folsom AR, Potter JD (1994) Vegetables, fruit and colon cancer in the Iowa Women's Health Study. *American Journal of Epidemiology*, **139**, 1–8.

Stensvold I, Tverdal A, Solvoll K, Foss OP (1992) Tea consumption: relationship to cholesterol, blood pressure, and coronary and total mortality. *Preventative Medicine*, **21**, 546–53.

Stephen AM, Cummings JH (1980) The microbial contribution to human faecal mass. *Journal of Medical Microbiology*, **13**, 45–56.

Stephen AM, Wiggins HS, Cummings JH (1987) Effect of changing transit time on colonic microbial metabolism in man. *Gut*, **28**, 601–9.

Stephens NG, Parsons A, Schofield PM *et al.* (1996) Randomised controlled trial of vitamin E in patients with coronary disease: Cambridge Heart Antioxidant Study (CHAOS). *Lancet*, **347**, 781–6.

Stewart AJ, Bozonnet S, Mullen W *et al.* (2000) Occurrence of flavonols in tomato fruits and tomato-based products. *Journal of Agricultural and Food Chemistry*, **48**, 2663–9.

Strack D (1997) Phenolic metabolism. In: *Plant Biochemistry* (eds. P Dey, J. Harborne), pp. 387–416. London: Academic Press.

Strack D, Wray V (1994) Anthocyanins. In: *The Flavonoids: Advances in Research Since 1986* (ed. J Harborne), pp. 1–22. London: Chapman and Hall.

Strandhagen E, Hansson PO, Bosaeus I, Isaksson B, Eriksson H (2000) High fruit intake may reduce mortality among middle-aged and elderly men. The Study of Men Born in 1913. *European Journal of Clinical Nutrition*, **54**, 337–41.

Subar AF, Heimendinger J, Patterson BH *et al.* (1995) Fruit and vegetable intake in the United States: the baseline survey of the Five A Day for Better Health Program. *American Journal of Health Promotion*, **9**, 352–60.

Suganuma M, Okabe S, Oniyama M *et al.* (1998) Wide distribution of [^{3}H]-epigallocatechin gallate, a cancer preventative tea polyphenol, in mouse tissue. *Carcinogenesis*, **19**, 1771–6.

Suter PM (1999) The effects of potassium, magnesium, calcium, and fiber on risk of stroke. *Nutrition Reviews*, **57**, 84–8.

Swain AR, Dutton SP, Truswell AS (1985) Salicylates in foods. *Journal of the American Dietetic Association*, **85**, 950–60.

Takahama U (1985) O$_2$-dependent and -independent photooxidation of quercetin in the presence and absence of riboflavin and effects of ascorbate on the photooxidation. *Photochemistry and Photobiology*, **42**, 89–91.

Talcott ST, Howard L, Brenes (2000) Antioxidant changes and sensory properties of carrot puree processed with and without periderm tissue. *Journal of Agricultural and Food Chemistry*, **48**, 1315–21.

Tannahill R (1988) *Food in History*. London: Penguin.

Tapadia SB, Arya AB, Rohini-Devi P (1995) Vitamin C content of processed vegetables. *Journal of Food Science and Technology – India*, **32**, 513–15.

Tavani A, La Vecchia C (1999) Beta-carotene and risk of coronary heart disease. A review of observational and intervention studies. *Biomedical Pharmacotherapy*, **53**, 409–16.

Tawfiq N, Heaney RK, Plumb JA *et al.* (1995) Dietary glucosinolates as blocking agents against carcinogenesis: glucosinolate breakdown products assessed by induction of quinone reductase activity in murine hepa1c1c7 cells. *Carcinogenesis*, **16**, 1191–4.

Taylor A, Takahama U (2000) Nutritional influences on risk for cataract. *International Ophthalmology Clinics*, **40**, 17–49.

The Scottish Office Department of Health (1996) *Eating for Health; a Diet Action Plan for Scotland*. Edinburgh: The Scottish Office.

Thom E, Wadstein J, Gudmundsen O (2001) Conjugated linoleic acid reduces body fat in healthy exercising humans. *Journal of International Medical Research*, **29**, 392–6.

Thomas DB, Uhk CN, Hartge P (1983) Bladder cancer and alcoholic beverage consumption. *American Journal of Epidemiology*, **720**, 720–7.

Thompson LU, Robb P, Serrano M, Cheung F (1991) Mammalian lignan production from various foods. *Nutrition and Cancer*, **16**, 43–52.

Thorn J, Robertson J, Buss DH, Bunton NG (1978) Trace nutrients. Selenium in British food. *British Journal of Nutrition*, **39**, 391–6.

Tijburg LBM, Wiseman SA, Meijer GW, Weststrate JA (1997) Effect of green tea, black tea and dietary lipophilic antioxidants on LDL oxidizability and atherosclerosis in hypercholesterolaemic rabbits. *Atherosclerosis*, **135**, 37–47.

Toivonen PMA, Zebarth BJ, Bowen PA (1994) Effect of nitrogen fertilization on head size, vitamin C content and storage life of broccoli. *Canadian Journal of Plant Science*, **74**, 607–10.

Tomás-Barberán FA, Clifford MN (2000a) Flavanones, chalcones and dihydrochalcones – nature, occurrence and dietary burden. *Journal of the Science of Food and Agriculture*, **80**, 1073–80.

Tomás-Barberán FA, Clifford MN (2000b) Dietary hydroxybenzoic acid derivatives – nature, occurrence and dietary burden. *Journal of the Science of Food and Agriculture*, **80**, 1024–32.

Tomás-Barberán FA, Gil MI, Cremin P *et al.* (2001) HPLC–DAD–ESIMS analysis of phenolic compounds in nectarines, peaches, and plums. *Journal of Agricultural and Food Chemistry*, **49**, 4748–60.

Tomlinson IP, Bodmer WF (1995) Failure of programmed cell death and differentiation as causes of tumors: some simple mathematical models. *Proceedings of the National Academy of Science, USA*, **92**: 11130–4.

Toniolo P, Kappel AL Van, Akhmedkhanov A *et al.* (2001) Serum carotenoids and breast cancer. *American Journal of Epidemiology*, **153**, 1142–7.

Trenga CA, Koenig JQ, Williams PV (2001) Dietary antioxidants and ozone-induced bronchial hyper-responsiveness in adults with asthma. *Archives of Environmental Health*, **56**, 242–9.

Treptow van Lishaut S, Rechkemmer G, Rowland I, Dolara P, Pool-Zobel BL (1999) The carbohydrate crystalean and colonic microflora modulate expression of glutathione S-transferase subunits in colon of rats. *European Journal of Nutrition*, **38**, 76–83.

Trichopoulou A, Katsouyanni K, Stuver S *et al.* (1995) Consumption of olive oil and specific foods in relation to breast cancer in Greece. *Journal of the National Cancer Institute*, **87**, 110–16.

Trudeau E, Kristal AR, Li S, Patterson RE (1998) Semographic and psychosocial predictors of fruit and vegetable intakes differ; implications for dietary interventions. *Journal of the American Dietetic Association*, **98**, 1412–17.

Truswell AS (2002) Cereal grains and coronary heart disease. *European Journal of Clinical Nutrition*, **56**, 1–14.

Tsimidou M (1998) Polyphenols and quality of olive oil in retrospect. *Italian Journal of Food Science*, **10**, 99–116.

Tsuda T, Horio F, Osawa T (1999) Absorption and metabolism of cyanidin 3-*O*-β-D-glucoside in rats. *FEBS Letters*, **449**, 179–82.

Tsushida T, Suzuki M (1995) Isolation of flavonoid-glycosides in onion and identification by chemical synthesis of the glycoside (Flavonoids in fruits and vegetables Part 1). *Nippon Shokuhin Kagaku Kaishi*, **42**, 100–8.

Uauy-Dagach R, Birch EE, Birch DG, Hoffman DR (1994) Significance of ω-3 fatty acids for retinal and brain development of preterm and term infants. *World Review of Nutrition and Dietetics*, **75**, 52–62.

USDA (1999) *USDA Nutrient Database, Release 12.* Issued February 1999. Washington, DC: US Department of Agriculture, Agricultural Research Service.

van Dam RM , Rimm EB, Willett WC, Stampfer MJ, Hu FB (2002) Dietary patterns and risk for type 2 diabetes mellitus in U.S. men. *Annals of Internal Medicine*, **136**, 201–9.

van den Berg H , Faulks R, Fernando Granado H *et al.* (2000) The potential for the improvement of carotenoid levels in foods and the likely systemic effects. *Journal of the Science of Food and Agriculture*, **80**, 880–912.

van der Meer R, Lapre JA, Govers MJ, Kleibeuker JH (1997) Mechanisms of the intestinal effects of dietary fats and milk products on colon carcinogenesis. *Cancer Letters*, **114**, 75–83.

van Echten G, Birk R, Brenner-Weiss G, Schmidt RR, Sandhoff K (1990) Modulation of sphingolipid biosynthesis in primary cultured neurons by long chain bases. *Journal of Biological Chemistry*, **265**, 9333–9.

van het Hof KH, Wiseman SA, Yang CS, Tijburg LB (1999) Plasma and lipoprotein levels of tea catechins following repeated tea consumption. *Proceedings of the Society of Experimental Biology and Medicine*, **220**, 203–9.

van Vliet T, Schreurs WHP, van den Berg H (1995) Intestinal β-carotene absorption and cleavage in men: response of β-carotene and retinyl esters in the triglyceride-rich lipoprotein fraction after a single oral dose of β-carotene. *American Journal of Clinical Nutrition*, **62**, 110–16.

Vanhanen H, Miettinen TA (1991) Effects of sitostanol esters, dissolved in dietary oil, on serum cholesterol, plant sterols and cholesterol precursors. *Circulation*, **84**, II-601.

Vanhanen HT, Miettinen TA (1992) Effects of unsaturated and saturated dietary plant sterols on their serum contents. *Clinica Chimica Acta*, **205**, 97–107.

Vanhanen HT, Miettinen TA (1995) Cholesterol absorption and synthesis during pravastatin, gemfibrozil and their combination. *Atherosclerosis*, **115**, 135–46.

Vanhanen HT, Blomqvist S, Ehnholm C *et al.* (1993) Serum cholesterol, cholesterol precursors, and plant sterols in hypercholesterolemic subjects with different apoE phenotypes during dietary sitostanol ester treatment. *Journal of Lipid Research*, **34**, 1535–44.

van't Veer P, Jansen MC, Klerk M, Kok FJ (2000) Fruits and vegetables in the prevention of cancer and cardiovascular disease. *Public Health Nutrition*, **3**, 103–7.

Venema DP, Hollman PCH, Janssen KPLTM, Katan MB (1996) Determination of acetylsalicylic acid and salicylic acid in foods using HPLC with fluorescence detection. *Journal of Agriculture and Food Chemistry*, **44**, 1762–7.

Verhoeven DT, Verhagen H, Goldbohm RA, Brand PA van den, Poppel GA van (1997) Review of mechanisms underlying anticarcinogenicity by brassica vegetables. *Chemical Biological Interactions*, **103**, 79–129.

Verkerk R (2002) PhD Thesis. Evaluation of glucosinolate levels throughout the production chain of Brassica vegetables, University of Wageningen.

Verkerk R, Dekker M, Jongen WMF (2001) Postharvest increase of indolyl glucosinolates in response to chopping and storage of Brassica vegetables. *Journal of the Science of Food and Agriculture*, **81**, 953–8.

Verkerk R, van der Gaag MS, Dekker M, Jongen WMF (1997) Effects of processing conditions on glucosinolates in cruciferous vegetables. *Cancer Letters*, **114**, 193–4.

Vesper H, Schmelz EM, Nikolova-Karakashian MN *et al.* (1999) Sphingolipids in food and the emerging importance of sphingolipids to nutrition. *Journal of Nutrition*, **129**, 1239–50.

References

Vidal-Valverde C, Frias J, Estrella I *et al.* (1994) Effect of processing on some antinutritional factors of lentils. *Journal of Agricultural and Food Chemistry*, **42**, 2291–5.

Vinson JA (1998) Flavonoids in foods as *in vitro* and *in vivo* antioxidants. *Advances in Experimental Medicine and Biology*, **439**, 151–64.

Vinson JA, Proch J, Zubik L (1999) Phenol antioxidant quantity and quality in foods: cocoa, dark chocolate, and milk chocolate. *Journal of Agricultural and Food Chemistry*, **47**, 4822–4.

Visioli F, Galli C (2001) Antiatherogenic components of olive oil. *Current Atherosclerosis Reports*, **3**, 64–7.

Visioli F, Bellomo G, Montedoro GF, Gallio C (1995) Low density lipoprotein oxidation is inhibited *in vitro* by olive oil constituents. *Atherosclerosis*, **117**, 25–32.

Visioli F, Bellosta S, Galli C (1998a) Oleuropein, the bitter principle of olives, enhances nitric oxide production by mouse macrophages. *Life Sciences*, **62**, 541–6.

Visioli F, Galli C (1998b) The effect of minor constituents of olive oil on cardiovascular disease: New findings. *Nutrition Reviews*, **56**, 142–7.

Visioli F, Galli C (1998c) Olive oil phenols and their potential effects on human health. *Journal of Agricultural and Food Chemistry*, **46**, 4292–6.

Visioli F, Galli C, Bornet F *et al.* (2000) Olive oil phenolics are dose-dependently absorbed in humans. *FEBS Letters*, **468**, 159–60.

Visonneau S, Cesano A, Tepper SA *et al.* (1997) Conjugated linoleic acid suppresses the growth of human breast adenocarcinoma cells in SCID mice. *Anticancer Research*, **2A**, 969–73.

Vogelstein B, Fearon ER, Hamilton SR *et al.* (1988) Genetic alterations during colorectal-tumour development. *New England Journal of Medicine*, **319**, 525–33.

Vogt TM, Mayne ST, Graubard BI *et al.* (2002) Serum lycopene, other serum carotenoids, and risk of prostate cancer in US Blacks and Whites. *American Journal of Epidemiology*, **155**, 1023–32.

Wahle KWJ, Heys SD (2002) Cell signal mechanisms, conjugated linoleic acids (CLAs) and anti-tumorigenesis. *Prostaglandins, Leukotrienes and Essential Fatty Acids*, **67**, 183–6.

Wahle KWJ, Rotondo D (1999) Fatty acids and endothelial cell function: regulation of adhesion molecule and redox enzyme expression. *Current Opinion in Clinical Nutrition and Metabolic Care*, **2**, 109–15.

Wahle KWJ, Heys SD, Majumder B *et al.* (2001) Conjugated linoleic acids modulate apoptotic and anti-signal mechanisms in breast and prostate cells.

1st International Conference on CLA, Aleslund, Norway, 11.

Wald NJ (1987) Retinol, beta-carotene and cancer. *Cancer Surveys*, **4**, 635–51.

Wald NJ, Thompson SG, Ensem JW, Boreham J, Bailey A (1988) Serum beta-carotene and subsequent risk of cancer: results from the BUPA study. *British Journal of Cancer*, **57**, 428–33.

Walker R (2002) Risk assessment of ochratoxin: current views of the European Scientific Committee on Food, the JEFCA and the Codex Committee on Food Additives and Contaminants. *Advances in Experimental Medicine and Biology*, **504**, 249–55.

Wanasundara PKJPD, Shahidi F, Shukla VKS (1997) Endogenous antioxidants from oilseeds and edible oils. *Food Reviews International*, **13**, 225–92.

Wang C, Ma Q, Pagadala S, Sherrard MS, Krishnan PG (1998) Changes of isoflavones during processing of soy protein isolates. *Journal of the American Oil Chemists' Society*, **75**, 337–42.

Wang H, Nair MG, AF Lezzoni *et al.* (1997) Quantification and characterisation of anthocyanins in Balaton tart cherries. *Journal of Agricultural and Food Chemistry*, **45**, 2556–60.

Wang JF, Schramm DD, Holt RR *et al.* (2000) Dose response effect from chocolate consumption on plasma epicatechin and oxidative damage. *Journal of Nutrition*, **130**, 2115S–2119S.

Warm D *et al.* (2002) Food deserts. Proceedings of the Nutrition Society.

Wasan HS, Goodlad RA (1996) Fibre-supplemented foods may damage your health. *Lancet*, **348**, 319–20.

Waterhouse A, Teissedre P-L (1997) Levels of phenolics in California varietal wines. In: *Wine: Nutritional and Therapeutic Benefits, ACS Symposium Series 661* (ed. T Watkins), pp. 12–23. Washington, DC: American Chemical Society.

Watkins TR (ed.) (1997) *Wine: Nutritional and Therapeutic Benefits. ACS Symposium Series 661*. Washington, DC: American Chemical Society.

Watson DG, Oliveira EJ (1999) Solid-phase extraction and gas chromatography mass spectrometry determination of kaempferol and quercetin in human urine after consumption of *Ginkgo biloba* tablets. *Journal of Chromatography B*, **723**, 203–10.

Wearne S (2000) Estimating dietary intake of flavonoids. In: *Wake up to Flavonoids* (ed. C Rice-Evans). International Congress Series. London: Royal Society of Medicine.

Weihrauch JL, Gardner JM (1978) Sterol content of foods of plant origin. *Journal of the American Dietetic Association*, **73**, 39–47.

Weisburger JH (1997) Tea and health: a historical perspective. *Cancer Letters*, **114**, 315–17.

Welsh Assembly (2001a) *National Service Framework for Diabetes (Wales)*. Cardiff: Welsh Assembly.

Welsh Assembly (2001b) *Tackling Coronary Heart Disease in Wales: Implementing Through Evidence*. Cardiff: Welsh Assembly.

Wenham JE (ed.) (1995) *Post-harvest Deterioration of Cassava: A Biotechnology Perspective*. FAO Plant Production and Protection Paper 130. Rome: Food and Agriculture Organization of the United Nations.

Wensing AG, Mensink RP, Hornstra G (1999) Effects of dietary *n*-3 polyunsaturated fatty acids from plant and marine origin on platelet aggregation in healthy elderly subjects. *British Journal of Nutrition*, **82**, 183–91.

Weststrate JA, Meijer GW (1998) Plant sterol-enriched margarines and reduction of plasma total and LDL-cholesterol concentrations in normocholesterolemic and mildly hypercholesterolemic subjects. *European Journal of Clinical Nutrition*, **52**, 334–43.

Whiteman K (1999) *The Definitive Guide to the Fruits of the World*. London: Hermes House.

Wilcox JN, Blumenthal BF (1995) Thrombotic mechanisms in atherosclerosis: potential impact of soy proteins. *Journal of Nutrition*, **125**, 631S–638S.

Willett WC (2001a) Diet and breast cancer. *Journal of Internal Medicine*, **249**, 395–411.

Willett WC (2001b) Diet and cancer: one view at the start of the millennium. *Cancer Epidemiology Biomarkers and Prevention*, **10**, 3–8.

Williams C (1995) Healthy eating: clarifying advice about fruit and vegetables. *British Medical Journal*, **310**, 1453–5.

Williams CA, Harborne JB (1992) Flavone and flavonol glycosides. In: *The Flavonoids. Advances in Research Since 1986* (ed. J Harborne), pp. 337–85. London: Chapman and Hall.

Williams CL, Bollella M, Strobino BA, Boccia L, Campanaro L (1999a) Lipid-lowering effects of a plant stanol ester spread in young children. *European Heart Journal*, Suppl. 1, S96–S103.

Williams CM (2000) Dietary fatty acids and human health. *Annals Zoologies*, **49**, 165–80.

Williams CM, Francis-Knapper JA, Webb D *et al.* (1999b) Cholesterol reduction using manufactured foods high in monounsaturated fatty acids; a randomised crossover study. *British Journal of Nutrition*, **81**, 439–46.

Williams DE, Prevost AT, Whichelow MJ *et al.* (2000) A cross-sectional study of dietary patterns with glucose intolerance and other features of the metabolic syndrome. *British Journal of Nutrition*, **83**, 257–66.

Wills RBH, Bone K, Morgan M (2000) Herbal products: active constituents, modes of action and quality control. *Nutrition Research Reviews*, **13**, 47–77.

Withy LM, Heatherbell DA, Fisher BM (1993) Red raspberry wine – effect of processing and storage on colour and stability. *Fruit Processing*, **3**, 303–7.

Witthoft CM, Forssen K, Johannesson L, Jargerstad M (1999) Folates – food sources, analyses, retention and bioavailability. *Scandinavian Journal of Nutrition*, **43**, 138–46.

Witztum JL (1994) The oxidation hypothesis of atherosclerosis. *Lancet*, **344**, 793–5.

Wojciechowski ZA (1991) Biochemistry of phytosterol conjugates. In: *Physiology and Biochemistry of Sterols* (eds. C Patterson, W Nes), pp. 361–95. Champaign, IL: American Oil Chemists Society.

Wollenweber E (1992) Flavones and flavonols. In: *The Flavonoids: Advances in Research Since 1986* (ed. J Harborne), pp. 259–335. London: Chapman and Hall.

Woodward M, Tunstall-Pedoe H (1999) Coffee and tea consumption in the Scottish Heart Health Study conflicting relations with coronary risk factors, coronary disease and all cause mortality. *Journal of Epidemiology and Community Health*, **53**, 481–7.

World Cancer Research Fund (1997) *Food, Nutrition and the Prevention of Cancer: a Global Perspective*. Washington DC: American Institute for Cancer Research.

World Health Organisation (1990) *Diet, Nutrition, and the Prevention of Chronic Diseases. Report of a WHO Study Group. Technical Report Series 797*. Geneva: World Health Organization.

World Health Organisation/FAO (2003). *Diet, Nutrition and the Prevention of Chronic Diseases. Report of a Joint WHO/FAO Expert Consultation. WHO Technical Report Series 916*. Geneva: World Health Organisation.

Wu SY, Leske MC (2000) Antioxidants and cataract formation: a summary review. *International Ophthalmology Clinics*, **40**, 71–81.

Wursch P, Del Vedovo S, Koellreutter B (1986) Cell structure and starch nature as key determinants of the digestion rate of starch in legume. *American Journal of Clinical Nutrition*, **43**, 25–9.

Würsch P, Finot P-A (1999) Carbohydrate and protein. In: *Chocolate and Cocoa: Health and Nutrition* (ed. I Knight), pp. 105–15. Oxford: Blackwell Sciences.

Wyate CJ, Carballido S, Mendez RO (1998) Alpha and gamma tocopherol content of selected foods in the Mexican diet: effects of cooking. *Journal of Agricultural and Food Chemistry*, **46**, 4657–61.

Yang CS, Yang GY, Landau JM, Kim S, Liao J (1998) Tea and tea polyphenols inhibit cell hyperproliferation, lung tumorigensis and tumour progression. *Experimental Lung Research*, **24**, 629–39.

Yatomi Y, Ruan F, Hakomori S, Igarashi Y (1995) Sphingosine-1-phosphate: a platelet-activating sphingolipid released from agonist-stimulated human platelets. *Blood*, **86**, 193–202.

Yochum L, Kushi LH, Meyer K, Folsom AR (1999) Dietary flavonoid intake and risk of cardiovascular disease in postmenopausal women. *American Journal of Epidemiology*, **149**, 943–9.

Yoshie Y, Suzuki T (2000) Antioxidant activity of polyphenolic compounds from seaweed and tea in oil emulsion model. *Polyphenol Communications*, 381–3.

Young AM (1994) *The Chocolate Tree*. Washington, DC: Smithsonian Institution Press.

Yusuf S, Dagenais G, Pogue J, Bosch J, Sleight P (2000) Vitamin E supplementation and cardiovascular events in high-risk patients. The Heart Outcomes Prevention Evaluation Study Investigators. *New England Journal of Medicine*, **342**, 154–60.

Zampelas A, Roche H, Knapper JME *et al.* (1998) Differences in postprandial lipaemic response between Northern and Southern Europeans. *Atherosclerosis*, **139**, 83–93.

Zane E, Wender SH (1961) Flavonols in spinach leaves. *Journal of Organic Chemistry*, **26**, 4718–19.

Zhang Y, Talalay P (1994) Anticarcinogenic activities of organic isothiocyanates: chemistry and mechanisms. *Cancer Research*, **54** (7 Suppl), 1976s–1981s.

Zhang Y, Talalay P, Cho C-G, Posner GH (1992) A major inducer of anticarcinogenic protective enzymes from broccoli: solation and elucidation of structure. *Proceedings of the National Academy of Sciences, USA*, **89**, 2399–403.

Zijp IM, Korver O, Tijburg LBM (2000) Effect of tea and other dietary factors on iron absorption. *Critical Reviews in Food Science and Nutrition*, **40**, 371–98.

Index

Note: readers are directed to the Key Points at the end of each chapter, the Task Force recommendations on pages 282–5, Answers to the Commonly Asked Questions (pages 286–97) and the Glossary on page 300.